CURRENT CLINICAL NEUROLOGY

Daniel Tarsy, MD, SERIES EDITOR

More information about this series at http://www.springer.com/series/7630

Hrayr P. Attarian
Editor

Clinical Handbook of Insomnia

Third Edition

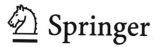 Springer

Editor
Hrayr P. Attarian
Sleep Disorders Center, Department of Neurology
Northwestern University Feinberg School of Medicine
Chicago, IL, USA

Current Clinical Neurology
ISBN 978-3-319-82345-4   ISBN 978-3-319-41400-3   (eBook)
DOI 10.1007/978-3-319-41400-3

Printed on acid-free paper

This Springer imprint is published by Springer Nature
The registered company is Springer International Publishing AG Switzerland

Preface

Insomnia is the second most common complaint, after pain, in the primary care setting. Chronic insomnia, as defined by the 2015 edition International Classification of Sleep Disorders (ICSD 3), affects 9–12 % of the population, is a risk factor for significant psychiatric morbidity, and is associated with higher mortality in men. Insomnia also leads to overutilization of health care services, decreased productivity in the workplace, more accidents, and more absenteeism from work. All this costs about $100 billion annually. Hence, persistent insomnia is both a public health and an economic problem. Chronic insomnia is a complex illness with many comorbidities each, naturally, requiring a different method of evaluation and treatment. Patients with insomnia frequently self-treat with alcohol or over-the-counter medications. There is very little scientific evidence for the efficacy of these medications in insomnia and there is growing evidence of significant long-term adverse effects with their use. Additionally, those taking these medications may suffer impaired daytime functioning caused by lingering feelings of sedation. Newer data also points to increased mortality and morbidity risks even with prescription sleep aids of proven efficacy. Most medical school curricula suffer a dearth of material on sleep medicine as well as insomnia. Primary care text and reference books often do not include chapters that address the evaluation and treatment of insomnia. When we published the *Clinical Handbook of Insomnia* 12 years ago it represented the first clinically oriented, easily readable textbook dedicated to the evaluation and treatment of insomnia in the primary care setting. Our goal was to provide practitioners in general and primary care providers specifically with an easily accessible handbook to serve as a reference for the evaluation and treatment of this important yet poorly recognized medical problem. The volume was very well received by the medical community, so we decided to update and expand it for the second edition. Now, 6 years hence, the diagnostic criteria of insomnia have completely changed with the advent of ICSD3. The third edition of the *Clinical Handbook of Insomnia* is divided into two parts. The first includes chapters on nomenclature, epidemiology, pathophysiology, diagnosis and differential diagnosis, complications and prognosis, and both pharmacological and behavioral treatments. The second includes chapters on insomnia in special populations including ones on children and adolescents, cancer sufferers and survivors, in pregnancy, in menopausal women, and in patients with neurological disorders and those with psychiatric illnesses.

We hope the third edition of the *Clinical Handbook of Insomnia* will continue to fill an important niche in the medical literature by providing a comprehensive publication that addresses insomnia in its multiple forms, summarizes the findings published in different medical journals, and presents these to the practicing health care provider in an easily accessible format.

Chicago, IL, USA   Hrayr P. Attarian, M.D.

Series Editor Introduction

This is the third edition of Dr. Attarian's *Clinical Handbook of Insomnia,* which is being published 6 years after the second edition and 11 years after the first edition when the field of insomnia was in its infancy as a scientific discipline. The need to regularly update this field is a testament to the rapid growth of interest in the insomnias. At one time this subset of sleep disorders was relatively neglected in contrast with disorders causing excessive daytime sleepiness. Thanks to the efforts of Dr. Attarian and the investigators and authors he has recruited to contribute scholarly chapters to all three volumes, this is no longer the case. The impact of disturbances in sleep on daytime mood, energy, and cognitive function is now much more widely recognized than it has been in the past. A new chapter on the complications of insomnia points out the significant burden of insomnia as a public health issue affecting work productivity, disability, accidents, and the costs of health care. As a result, there has been a major growth in efforts to understand and properly deal with insomnia.

As explained in the opening chapter concerning the definition of insomnia, the classification of insomnia has undergone revision and simplification with *chronic insomnia* now encompassing what previously had been considered a variety of insomnias occurring with other medical conditions. The new chapter on the clinical features, diagnosis, and differential diagnosis of insomnia provides a very useful overview of the subject. As detailed in the series of chapters on insomnia in special populations, impaired sleep accompanies a broad spectrum of medical, neurological, and psychiatric conditions, which increasingly demand the attention of specialists who practice in these areas. The chapter on insomnia associated with comorbid medical problems importantly emphasizes that insomnia appears as a result of many of these conditions but also contributes to the morbidity they produce. Insomnia as a special problem in normal childhood, pregnancy, and menopause also receives special attention in this volume. Updates in the diagnostic workup of insomnia and methods of sleep testing are also provided. The chapter on the pathophysiology of insomnia emphasizes new information concerning the role of brain arousal areas on awake-sleep physiology. The chapter on the pharmacological treatment of insomnia has been considerably updated to reflect the explosion of new pharmacological treatments and the mechanisms of action of these agents while also appropriately emphasizing the art of using medications to treat insomnia.

This volume continues to be a very useful resource for both the general and specialty physician who wishes to properly address the difficult area of insomnia in a responsible and informed manner.

Beth Israel Deaconess Medical Center   Daniel Tarsy, M.D.
Harvard Medical School
Boston, MA, USA

Contents

Part I Chronic Insomnia Disorder

1 **Defining Insomnia** 3
   Annise Wilson and Hrayr P. Attarian

2 **Epidemiology of Insomnia** 13
   Ritu G. Grewal and Karl Doghramji

3 **Clinical Features, Diagnosis, and Differential Diagnosis** 27
   Mary B. O'Malley and Edward B. O'Malley

4 **Pathophysiology of Insomnia** 41
   Michael H. Bonnet and Donna L. Arand

5 **Prognosis and Complications** 59
   Ramadevi Gourineni

6 **Cognitive Behavioral Therapy for Insomnia** 75
   Kelly Glazer Baron, Michael L. Perlis, Sara Nowakowski,
   Michael T. Smith Jr., Carla R. Jungquist, and Henry J. Orff

7 **Pharmacological Treatment of Insomnia** 97
   Paula K. Schweitzer and Stephen D. Feren

Part II Insomnia in Special Populations

8 **Insomnias of Childhood: Assessment and Treatment** 135
   Daniel S. Lewin and Edward Huntley

9 **Pregnancy-Related Sleep Disturbances and Sleep Disorders** 159
   Beth Ann Ward

10 **Insomnia and Menopause** 181
   Helena Hachul, Andréia Gomes Bezerra, and Monica Levy Andersen

11   Insomnia in Patients with Comorbid Medical Problems 199
      Rachel Paul and Ron C. Anafi

12   Sleep Disturbance in Cancer Survivors 221
      Heather L. McGinty, Allison J. Carroll, and Stacy D. Sanford

13   Insomnia in Comorbid Neurological Problems 243
      Federica Provini and Carolina Lombardi

14   Insomnia in Psychiatric Disorders 267
      Zachary L. Cohen and Katherine M. Sharkey

Index 283

List of Editor and Contributors

Editor

Hrayr P. Attarian, M.D. Sleep Disorders Center, Department of Neurology, Northwestern University Feinberg School of Medicine, Chicago, IL, USA

Contributors

Ron C. Anafi, M.D., Ph.D. Division of Sleep Medicine and Center for Sleep and Circadian Neurobiology, University of Pennsylvania, Philadelphia, PA, USA

Monica Levy Andersen, Ph.D. Department of Psychobiology, Universidade Federal de São Paulo, São Paulo, SP, Brazil

Donna L. Arand, Ph.D. Department of Neurology, Wright State Boonshoft School of Medicine, Dayton, OH, USA

Kelly Glazer Baron, Ph.D., M.P.H., C.B.S.M. Department of Neurology, Feinberg School of Medicine, Rush University, Chicago, IL, USA

Andréia Gomes Bezerra, M.Sc. Department of Psychobiology, Universidade Federal de São Paulo, São Paulo, SP, Brazil

Michael H. Bonnet, Ph.D. Department of Neurology, Wright State Boonshoft School of Medicine, Dayton, OH, USA

Sycamore Kettering Sleep Disorders Center, Miamisburg, OH, USA

Allison J. Carroll, M.S. Department of Preventive Medicine, Northwestern University Feinberg School of Medicine, Chicago, IL, USA

Zachary L. Cohen, B.A. The Warren Alpert Medical School of Brown University, Providence, RI, USA

Karl Doghramji, M.D. Jefferson Sleep Disorders Center, Thomas Jefferson University, Philadelphia, PA, USA

Stephen D. Feren, M.D. Department of Neurology and Sleep Medicine, Kaiser Permanente, Atlanta, GA, USA

Ramadevi Gourineni, M.D. Department of Neurology, Northwestern Feinberg Hospital, Northwestern Feinberg School of Medicine, Chicago, IL, USA

Ritu G. Grewal, M.D. Pulmonary Division, Department of Internal Medicine, Jefferson Sleep Disorders Center, Thomas Jefferson University, Philadelphia, PA, USA

Helena Hachul, M.D., Ph.D. Departments of Gynecology and Psychobiology, Head of the Women's Sleep Division, Universidade Federal de São Paulo, São Paulo, SP, Brazil

Edward Huntley, Ph.D. Survey Research Center, Institute for Social Research, University of Michigan, Ann Arbor, MI, USA

Carla R. Jungquist, A.N.P., Ph.D. School of Nursing, University of Buffalo, Buffalo, NY, USA

Daniel S. Lewin, Ph.D. Department of Pulmonary and Sleep Medicine, Children's National Medical Center, George Washington University School of Medicine, Washington, DC, USA

Carolina Lombardi, M.D., Ph.D. Department of Cardiology, Sleep Disorder Center, Instituto Auxologico Italiano IRCCS, Milan, Italy

Heather L. McGinty, Ph.D. Department of Medical Social Sciences, Northwestern University Feinberg School of Medicine, Chicago, IL, USA

Sara Nowakowski, Ph.D. Department of Obstetrics and Gynecology, University of Texas Medical Branch, Galveston, TX, USA

Edward B. O'Malley, Ph.D. Your Optimal Nature, Great Barrington, MA, USA

Mary B. O'Malley, M.D., Ph.D. Berkshire Medical Center, Pittsfield, MA, USA

Henry J. Orff, Ph.D. Department of Psychology, VA San Diego Healthcare System, San Diego, CA, USA

Rachel Paul, M.D. Department of Sleep Medicine, University of Pennsylvania, Philadelphia, PA, USA

Michael L. Perlis, Ph.D. Department of Psychiatry and School of Nursing, UPENN Behavioral Sleep Medicine Program, University of Pennsylvania, Philadelphia, PA, USA

Federica Provini, M.D., Ph.D. Department of Biomedical and Neuromotor Sciences, University of Bologna, Bologna, Italy

IRCCS Institute of Neurological Sciences, Bellaria Hospital, Bologna, Italy

Stacy D. Sanford, Ph.D. Department of Medical Social Sciences, Northwestern University Feinberg School of Medicine, Chicago, IL, USA

Department of Psychiatry and Behavioral Sciences, Northwestern University Feinberg School of Medicine, Chicago, IL, USA

Paula K. Schweitzer, Ph.D. Sleep Medicine and Research Center, St. Luke's Hospital, Chesterfield, MO, USA

Katherine M. Sharkey, M.D., Ph.D. Sleep for Science Research Laboratory, Division of Pulmonary, Critical Care, and Sleep Medicine, Rhode Island Hospital, Brown University, Providence, RI, USA

Michael T. Smith Jr., Ph.D. Department of Psychiatry, Johns Hopkins School of Medicine, Baltimore, MD, USA

Beth Ann Ward, M.D. Department of Sleep Medicine, St. Luke's Sleep Medicine and Research Center, Chesterfield, MO, USA

Annise Wilson, M.D. Sleep Disorders Center, Department of Neurology, Northwestern University Feinberg School of Medicine, Chicago, IL, USA

Part I
Chronic Insomnia Disorder

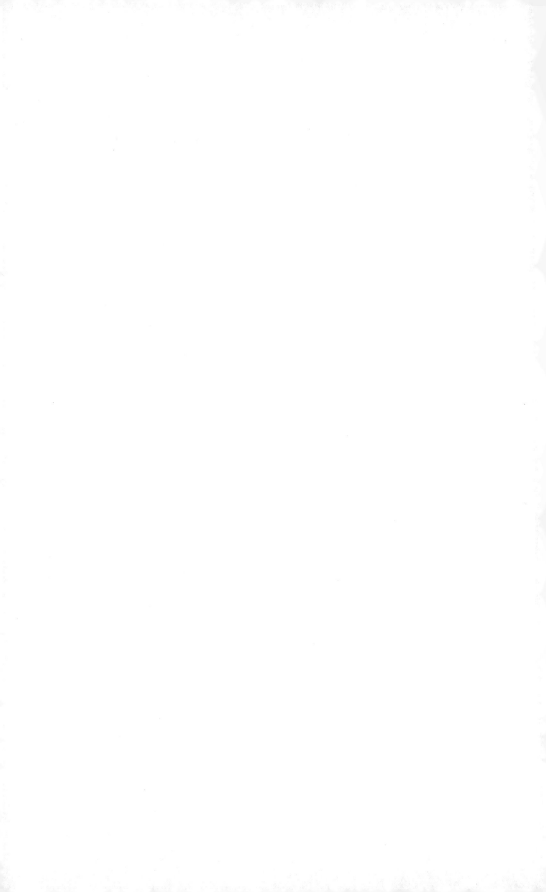

Chapter 1
Defining Insomnia

Annise Wilson and Hrayr P. Attarian

Abstract Insomnia is one of the most common sleep complaints with a prevalence of 3–22 % depending on the classification system.

The classification of insomnia has an ever-changing definition, currently based on the recent International Classification of Sleep Disorders: Diagnostic and Coding Manual-3rd Edition (ICSD-3), International Classification of Diseases (ICD-10), and DSM-V. As of now, it is described as difficulty initiating or maintaining sleep for a specified period of time with adequate time given for sleep but ultimately resulting in daytime disruption. Insomnia is commonly associated with comorbid medical and psychiatric conditions and with exposure to drugs or other substances but should be appropriately treated regardless of whether it is associated with a comorbid condition.

Keywords Insomnia • International Classification of Sleep Disorders: Diagnostic and Coding Manual-3rd Edition (ICSD-3) • Diagnostic and Statistical Manual on Mental Disorders-5th Edition (DSM-V) • Nomenclature • Classification • Nosology

Introduction

In the early 1980s, as the sleep medicine movement was just gathering steam, there was perhaps no rallying cry as popular as "insomnia is a symptom, not a disorder." Presumably, this position was taken in part for medico-political reasons, but also because it was genuinely believed that the polysomnographic study of sleep was

A. Wilson, M.D. • H.P. Attarian, M.D. (✉)
Sleep Disorders Center, Department of Neurology, Northwestern University Feinberg School of Medicine, 710 N Lake Shore Drive, Suite 1111, Chicago, IL 60611, USA
e-mail: h-attarian@northwestern.ed

© Springer International Publishing Switzerland 2017
H.P. Attarian (ed.), *Clinical Handbook of Insomnia*, Current Clinical Neurology,
DOI 10.1007/978-3-319-41400-3_1

destined to reveal all the underlying pathologies that give rise to the "symptoms" of insomnia, fatigue, and sleepiness. After two decades or more of sleep research and sleep medicine, it is interesting to find that "all things old are new again": Insomnia is once again considered a distinct nosological entity. The ICSD-3 has deviated from the prior edition in that primary and secondary insomnias have been eliminated as it was difficult to distinguish the conditions given that patients did not exclusively fit in either category and there was considerable overlap between primary and secondary insomnias. The subtypes of primary insomnia have also been removed in the most recent ICSD-3 as it was increasingly difficult to discriminate among the subtypes. The manual now classifies three categories of insomnia: chronic, short-term, and other insomnia disorder [1]. Prevalence rates for insomnia vary widely, from 3.9 to 22.1 % [2].

Historical Perspectives

The first references in the Western culture to insomnia, the inability to initiate and or maintain sleep, date back to the ancient Greeks. The earliest mention of it is in the pre-Hippocratic Epidaurian tablets that list 70 cases, one of which is a patient with insomnia. The first scientific approach is found in the writings of Aristotle from circa 350 BC, and the first records of treatment of insomnia come from the first-century BC Greek physician, Heraclides of Taras, who lived in Alexandria and recommended opium for the treatment of insomnia. Although there had been significant amount of research and interest in insomnia in the twentieth century it was not until the 1970s that distinct diagnostic criteria were created to describe different forms of insomnia.

Over the years insomnia has featured in the writings of several prominent literary figures including William Shakespeare, who alluded to it in several of his plays, to the pop culture icons the Beatles who referred to it in their song "I am so tired." Prominent historical figures that have suffered from insomnia include Churchill, Charles Dickens, Napoleon Bonaparte, Marcel Proust, Alexander Dumas, and Benjamin Franklin to name a few.

Definitions of Insomnia

Insomnia is the most common sleep-related complaint and the second most common overall complaint (after pain) reported in primary care settings with about 30–50 % of adults reporting sleep trouble in a given year [3]. The general consensus based on many population studies is that one-third of adults have frequent trouble falling sleep, staying asleep, or overall poor sleep quality [2]. NIH State-of-the-Science Conference held in June 2005 concluded that the prevalence of chronic, persistent insomnia that also causes daytime fatigue and impairment is 10 % [4] and is a cause of significant morbidity [1]. It costs the American public about $100 billion annually in medical expenses, ramifications of accidents, and reduced productivity due to absenteeism and decreased work efficiency [5].

Insomnia is not defined by total sleep time but by the inability to obtain sleep of sufficient length or quality to produce refreshment the following morning [6]. For example, a person who needs only 4 h of sleep does not have insomnia if he or she is refreshed in the morning after 4 h of sleep, whereas someone who needs 10 h of sleep may have insomnia if he or she does not feel refreshed after 8 h of fragmented sleep. Previously the underlying psychiatric or psychological condition was thought to be the most common cause of insomnia, but newer studies have refuted this theory. In fact untreated insomnia may adversely affect the course of the associated disorder [6].

Classifications

There are three major classification systems used by sleep medicine professionals: The International Classification of Diseases (ICD-10) by the World Health Organization (WHO), The International Classification of Sleep Disorders-3rd edition (2014) by the American Academy of Sleep Medicine (AASM), and the Diagnostic and Statistical Manual on Mental Disorders-5th edition (DSM-V) (2013) by the American Psychiatric Association (APA) (Table 1.1).

Table 1.1 DSM-V diagnostic criteria for primary insomnia [8]

(A) The primary complaint of poor sleep quality or duration associated with any one of these symptoms:
1. Trouble with sleep onset (in children, this symptom may be trouble falling asleep without the help of a caregiver).
2. Trouble with sleep maintenance (in children, this symptom may be trouble staying asleep without the help of a caregiver).
3. Waking up earlier than desired in the morning.
(B) Troubled sleep causes significant distress or decline in social, occupational, academic, behavioral, or other life areas.
1. Trouble sleeping is happening for at least thrice per week.
2. Trouble sleeping is happening for at least 3 months.
3. The sleep difficulty occurs despite adequate opportunity for sleep.
4. The insomnia is not secondary to another sleep disorder:
(C) The insomnia is not due to the effects of a pharmacological substance.
(D) Comorbid mental and medical disorders are not the cause of the predominant complaint of insomnia.

Table 1.2 ICSD-3 criteria for chronic insomnia disorder [1]

(A) The patient or caregiver report:
1. Sleep onset difficulty.
2. Sleep maintenance difficulty
3. Early morning awakenings.
4. Not going to bed when appropriate.
5. Difficulty sleeping without the intervention of the caregiver.
(B) The patient or caregiver report:
1. Fatigue and/or malaise.
2. Troubles with attention, concentration, or memory.
3. Difficulty with family obligations or social, school, or work performance.
4. Irritability and mood disturbance.
5. Sleepiness during the day.
6. Issues with behavior such as aggression, impulsivity, or hyperactivity.
7. Tendency to make errors or cause accidents.
8. Decreased energy and motivation or lack of initiative.
9. Dissatisfaction and complaints about sleep quality.
(C) The complaints in (A) and (B) are not solely due to inappropriate circumstances or not enough time allotted for sleep.
(D) The symptoms in (A) and (B) occur at least thrice weekly.
(E) The symptoms in (A) and (B) have been ongoing for at least 3 months.
(F) The symptoms above are not due to another sleep disorder.

All the above must be met

WHO-ICD: The World Health Organization defines insomnia as a condition of unsatisfactory quantity and/or quality of sleep, which persists for a considerable period of time, including difficulty falling asleep, difficulty staying asleep, or early final wakening [7].

AASM: The American Academy of Sleep Medicine's nosology (the International Classification of Sleep Disorders-3rd edition [ICSD-3]) classifies insomnia into three categories: chronic, short-term, and other insomnia disorders. Chronic insomnia includes the "primary" and "secondary" insomnia referenced in ICSD-2, comorbid insomnia, behavioral-insomnia of childhood, psychophysiological insomnia, inadequate sleep hygiene, idiopathic insomnia, and paradoxical insomnia [1] (Tables 1.2 and 1.3).

Classification Based on Duration and Severity

Apart from presenting a specific definition of the disorder/disease entity, there is the need to qualify the duration and severity of the defined illness. Typically, duration is framed dichotomously in terms of acute and chronic stages. Severity can be construed in one of the two ways. In one case, standards are set for what constitutes

Table 1.3 ICSD-3 diagnostic criteria for short-term insomnia [1]

(A) The patient or caregiver report:
1. Sleep onset difficulty.
2. Sleep maintenance difficulty.
3. Early morning awakenings.
4. Not going to bed when appropriate.
5. Difficulty sleeping without the intervention of the caregiver.
(B) The patient or caregiver report:
1. Fatigue and or malaise.
2. Troubles with attention, concentration, or memory.
3. Difficulty with family obligations or social, school, or work performance.
4. Irritability and mood disturbance.
5. Sleepiness during the day.
6. Issues with behavior such as aggression, impulsivity, or hyperactivity.
7. Tendency to make errors or cause accidents.
8. Decreased energy and motivation or lack of initiative.
9. Dissatisfaction and complaints about sleep quality.
(C) The complaints in (A) and (B) are not solely due to inappropriate circumstances or not enough time allotted for sleep.
(D) The symptoms in (A) and (B) have been ongoing for less than 3 months.
(E) The symptoms above are not due to another sleep disorder.

All the above must be met

significant deviance from population norms with respect to frequency and intensity of presenting symptoms. In the other case, standards are set by "setting the bar" for "pathologic" at a level which is modal for patients who are help-seeking.

Duration of Illness

Insomnia lasting less than 3 month is generally considered "acute," or by the ICSD-3 criteria short-term insomnia. It is often associated with clearly defined precipitants such as stress, acute pain, or substance abuse. Insomnia is characterized as being chronic when symptoms persist unabated for a duration of at least 3 months with a frequency of at least three times per week. Please note that these cutoffs are relatively arbitrary and correspond to traditional medical definitions of what constitutes short and long periods of time. At this time there are no studies, which use risk models to evaluate the natural course of insomnia. Thus, there is no way of definitively defining "chronicity" in terms which are related to when the disorder becomes severe, persistent, and (for want of a better expression) "self-perpetuating." One clinical cue for differentiating between acute and chronic insomnia resides in the way patients characterize their complaint. When patients stop causally linking their insomnia to its precipitant and instead indicate that their sleep problems seem "to have a life of their own," this change in presentation may (1) serve to define the "cut point" between the acute and chronic phases of the disorder and (2) suggest when CBT should be indicated.

Severity of Illness

Intensity. Although there are no formal diagnostic criteria, most investigators consider 30 or more minutes to fall asleep and/or 30 or more minutes of wakefulness after sleep onset to represent the threshold between normal and abnormal sleep. The criterion should be set at "more than 30 min," as this definition is better related to the occurrence of complaint in population studies [2, 11]. With respect to "how much sleep," many investigators are reluctant to fix a value for this parameter. Of the investigators that are inclined to set minimums, most specify that the amount of sleep obtained on a regular basis be equal to or less than either 6.0 or 6.5 h per night. The reluctance to establish total sleep time parameters is due, in part, to the difficulty in establishing precisely what one considers to be abnormal. Representing what is pathological with a single number is too confounded by factors like age, prior sleep, and the individual's basal level of sleep need. The lack of an established total sleep time cutoff is also related to the possibility that profound sleep initiation or maintenance problems may occur in the absence of sleep loss. This is an important distinction, because it is often assumed that insomnia is synonymous with sleep deprivation. While it is certainly the case that the daytime symptoms associated with insomnia might be explained, in part, by partial chronic sleep loss, daytime symptoms need not be ascribable only to lack of sleep. Studies have also indicated the presence of a 24-h hyperarousal state which includes increased beta activity during NREM, increased cortisol and ACTH secretion during early sleep, and increased metabolic rate during waking and sleep [12–14]. Sleep studies reveal an increased frequency of shifts between NREM and REM and between NREM stages causing microarousals and brief periods of awakening. This correlates well with patient perceptions about their sleep quality and quantity [15].

Frequency. Both DSMV and ICSD-3 require that insomnia-related symptoms be experienced on three or more nights per week for the diagnosis to be made. This may have more to do with increasing the odds of studying the occurrence of the disorder in laboratory than an inherent belief that less than three nights per week is "normal."

Commonalities and Problems with Current Definitions

All of the above definitions show a degree of consistency, both in terms of what "is" and "is not" delineated. Common to all is that (1) insomnia is defined as a subjective complaint, (2) patients must report compromised daytime functioning, (3) there are no specific criteria for how much wakefulness is considered pathologic (prior to desired sleep onset or during the night), and (4) there are no criteria for how little total sleep must be obtained to fall outside the normal range. There are lack of quantitative criteria for sleep-onset latency (SOL), wake after sleep onset (WASO), and total sleep time (TST).

Insomnia as a Subjective Complaint

Defining insomnia as a subjective complaint without requiring objective verification of signs and symptoms has advantages and disadvantages. The advantage of having subjective criteria is that it recognizes the primacy of the patient's experience of distress or disease. That is, ultimately patients seek, comply with, and discontinue treatment based on their perception of wellness. The disadvantage is that such measures, when used alone, do not allow for a complete characterization of either the patient's condition or the disorder in general [10].

Insomnia and Daytime Impairment

The reason that daytime complaints are required for diagnosis is that in the absence of such complaints, it is possible that the phenomena of "short sleep" may be misidentified as insomnia. Frequent complaints associated with insomnia include fatigue, irritability, problems with attention, and concentration and distress directly related to the inability to initiate and/or maintain sleep [9].

The Old Diagnostic Entity of Comorbid or Secondary Insomnia

Secondary insomnia was a term coined to refer to insomnia that was due to another disorder. Since the main diagnostic tool is history and most people present with the insomnia lasting at least 6 months if not more, they are unable to provide a reliable accounting of the course and their relative sequence of the two disorders. Nevertheless incorporating sleep diaries, questionnaires, and other modalities can help rule out various comorbidities in addition to a thorough medical and psychiatric evaluation [16].

Since comorbidity without necessarily implying causality can easily be established and since, from a treatment standpoint, both conditions need to be treated together the tide in 2010 turned in favor of abandoning secondary insomnia and adopting the term comorbid insomnia. Instead of saying insomnia due to a certain disorder they stated that the onset and the temporal course of the insomnia should coincide with the course of the specific disorder for the insomnia to be considered comorbid [1].

The next logical step, however, was to abandon comorbid insomnia as well and just incorporate this into the overarching diagnosis of chronic insomnia, as treatment modalities for insomnia, most of the time, are the same regardless of comorbidities. Also since, regardless of causality, both conditions need to be treated for a successful outcome the terms comorbid or secondary became equally unnecessary.

Summary

We are fortunate to have several nosologies that recognize insomnia as primary disorder. The various classification systems provide us the wherewithal to differentiate types of insomnia both by presenting complaint and by the factors that are thought to precipitate or perpetuate the illness. In the past 2 years there has been more concordance than ever between the two major diagnostic manuals, the ICSD-3 and the DSM-V. Perhaps what remains to still be accomplished, from a definitional point of view, is for scholars and scientists to complete the characterization of this important disorder by providing for the formulation of the ultimate definition based on more objective quantifiable guidelines, one which formally lays out the research diagnostic criteria and does so based on the force of empirical research.

References

1. American Academy of Sleep Medicine. The international classification of sleep disorders: diagnostic and coding manual. 3rd ed. Darien, IL: American Academy of Sleep Medicine; 2014.
2. Roth T, Coulouvrat C, Hajak G, et al. Prevalence and perceived health associated with insomnia based on DSM-IV-TR; International Statistical Classification of Diseases and Related Health Problems, Tenth Revision; and Research Diagnostic Criteria/International Classification of Sleep Disorders, Second Edition criteria, results from the America Insomnia Survey. Biol Psychiatry. 2011;69(6):592–600.
3. Masters PA. In the Clinic. Insomnia. Ann Intern Med. 2014;161(7):ITC1–15.
4. NIH. National Institutes of Health State of the Science Conference statement on manifestations and management of chronic insomnia in adults, June 13–15, 2005. Sleep. 2005;28(9):1049–57.
5. Fullerton DS. The economic impact of insomnia in managed care: a clearer picture emerges. Am J Manag Care. 2006;12(8 Suppl):S246–52.
6. Sateia MJ. International classification of sleep disorders-third edition: highlights and modifications. Chest. 2014;146:1387–94.
7. World Health Organization. The ICD-10 classification of mental and behavioural disorders: clinical descriptions and diagnostic guidelines. Geneva: World Health Organization; 2007.
8. APA. DSM-V. Washington, DC: American Psychiatric Association; 2013.
9. Shekleton JA, Flynn-Evans EE, Miller B, et al. Neurobehavioral performance impairment in insomnia: relationships with self-reported sleep and daytime functioning. Sleep. 2014;37(1):107–16.
10. Bastien CH, Ceklic T, St-Hilaire P, Desmarais F, Pérusse AD, Lefrançois J, Pedneault-Drolet M. Insomnia and sleep misperception. Pathol Biol (Paris). 2014;62(5):241–51.
11. Gross CR, Kreitzer MJ, Reilly-Spong M, et al. Mindfulness-based stress reduction vs. pharmacotherapy for primary chronic insomnia: a pilot randomized controlled clinical trial. Explore (New York, NY). 2011;7(2):76–87.
12. Wu YM, Pietrone R, Cashmere JD, et al. EEG power during waking and NREM sleep in primary insomnia. J Clin Sleep Med. 2013;9(10):1031–7.
13. Covassin N, De ZM, Sarlo M, De Min TG, Sarasso S, Stegagno L. Cognitive performance and cardiovascular markers of hyperarousal in primary insomnia. Int J Psychophysiol. 2011;80:79–86.
14. Riemann D, Spiegelhalder K, Feige B, et al. The hyperarousal model of insomnia: a review of the concept and its evidence. Sleep Med Rev. 2010;14:19–31.

15. Riemann D, Nissen C, Palagini L, Otte A, Perlis ML, Spiegelhalder K. The neurobiology, investigation, and treatment of chronic insomnia. Lancet Neurol. 2015;14(5):547–58.
16. Cunnington D, Junge MF, Fernando AT. Insomnia: prevalence, consequences and effective treatment. Med J Aust. 2013;199(8):36–40.

Chapter 2
Epidemiology of Insomnia

Ritu G. Grewal and Karl Doghramji

Abstract Prevalence of insomnia is variable due to inconsistency in defining the syndrome. It can be seen with or without comorbid illnesses and is now recognized as a distinct clinical syndrome even when associated with an underlying medical or psychiatric disorder. It is more common in women and in people who do shift work. Insomnia is present worldwide but appears to be less common in Asians. Individuals who have an anxiety-prone personality and depression are more prone to develop insomnia. It can have a huge economic impact as insomnia sufferers place a significant economic burden on their employers and health care system. Insomnia may be a risk factor for development of depression, hypertension, diabetes, and coronary artery diseases.

Keywords Prevalence of insomnia • Anxiety • Depression • Fatigue • Shift work • Women and sleep • Difficulty sleeping

Sleep accounts for one-third of human life and insomnia is the most common sleep-related complaint and the second most common overall complaint (after pain) reported in primary care settings [1].

R.G. Grewal, M.D. (✉)
Pulmonary Division, Department of Internal Medicine, Jefferson Sleep Disorders Center, Thomas Jefferson University,
211 South Ninth Street, Suite 500, Philadelphia, PA 19107, USA
e-mail: Ritu.Grewal@jefferson.edu

K. Doghramji, M.D.
Jefferson Sleep Disorders Center, Thomas Jefferson University, Philadelphia, PA, USA

© Springer International Publishing Switzerland 2017
H.P. Attarian (ed.), *Clinical Handbook of Insomnia*, Current Clinical Neurology,
DOI 10.1007/978-3-319-41400-3_2

Estimates of the prevalence of insomnia are variable, owing in part to inconsistencies in definitions and diagnostic criteria for insomnia. These issues also make it difficult to define other dimensions of the condition, such as incidence and remission rates, as a uniform characterization of episode lengths is lacking; a positive finding of insomnia at baseline and at 1-year follow-up may reflect unremitting chronic insomnia or two episodes of transient insomnia [2, 3]. Currently, there are three distinct diagnostic nosologic systems for insomnia; the Diagnostic and Statistical Manual of Mental Disorders (DSM-5) [4], the International Classification of Sleep Disorders (ICSD-3) [5], and the ICD-10 Classification of Mental and Behavioral Disorders [6]. Several changes have been made to the diagnostic criterion of Insomnia in the DSM-5 and ICSD-3. The ICSD-3 classification of insomnia is notably different in terms of elimination of previous subtypes of insomnia as primary vs. secondary insomnia related to an existing psychiatric, medical, or substance-abuse disorder. There are now three distinct categories of insomnia: chronic insomnia, short-term insomnia disorder, and other insomnia disorder. These diagnoses apply to patients with and without comorbidities. Similarly DSM-5 no longer makes a distinction between primary insomnia and insomnia secondary to a psychiatric, medical, or another sleep disorder. DSM-5 criteria for insomnia includes "any sleep dissatisfaction" or early morning awakening. It should last for at least 3 months and be present for more than three nights per week. Importantly insomnia is now regarded as a disorder and DSM-5 states that it can coexist with "comorbid" vs. "secondary" conditions. These changes were made as it was determined that it was difficult to ascertain which disorder was the cause and which is the consequence and the realization that over time insomnia may remain as a clinically significant condition despite the associated condition being resolved.

Mellinger and colleagues presented data from one of the first attempts to quantify the prevalence of the disorder. Their 1979 USA survey, utilizing a nationally representative sample of 3161 people whose ages ranged from 18 to79, found that insomnia affected 35 % of the general adult population in 1 year [7]. About half of these people experienced the problem as severe [7]; yet only 15 % were treated with hypnotic medications [7]. In 1996, another study by Ohayon et al. in Montreal examined the prevalence of insomnia in a representative sample of the population of 5622 subjects, 15 years of age or more. In their cohort 20.1 % of the participants stated that they were unsatisfied with their sleep or were taking medication for sleeping difficulties [8]. A 2000 study by Leger and colleagues, in France, noted that the prevalence of frequent insomnia was 29 % in a representative sample of the population that included 12,778 individuals [9]. A 2001 study by Sutton et al. reported that 24 % of English-speaking Canadians aged 15 and above reported insomnia [10]. In a representative selection of 1997 German citizens older than 13 years of age, 25 % reported occasional difficulties in falling asleep and/or staying asleep not due to external factors and 7 % reported the same symptoms frequently or all the time [11]. A similar survey in Japan, conducted in a group of 6277 new outpatients from 11 hospitals, revealed a prevalence of 20.3 % with 11.7 % of the people suffering from insomnia for over a month. Only 37 % were treated with hypnotics [12]. A second Japanese study, in another representative population sample ($n=3030$), reported almost identical results [13]. A representative adult sample (18 years and above) of the Norwegian population, comprising 2001 subjects, participated in telephone interviews, focusing on the 1-month point prevalence of insomnia and use of prescribed hypnotics. Employment of DSM-IV inclusion criteria of insomnia yielded a prevalence rate of 11.7 % [14]. A prior Norwegian study had queried 14,667 subjects and reported 41.7 % of the women and 29.9 % of the men complaining of occasional insomnia [15].

Another study in Austria in a sample of 1000 revealed a prevalence of 26 % with 21 % of them being severe and chronic with duration of 1 year or more [16]. In a representative sample of the South Korean general population composed of 3719 non-institutionalized individuals aged 15 years or older the prevalence of insomnia symptoms occurring at least three nights per week was reported to be 17.0 % [17]. In Mexico the prevalence of insomnia in a group of a 1000 subjects, aged 18–84, was found to be 36 % with 16 % reporting severe insomnia [18]. In Singapore the prevalence of persistent insomnia for over a year was 15.3 % in subjects between the ages of 15 and 55 [19]. In a group of 1099 subjects representative of the Finnish population, Hyyppa and Kronholm reported a male/female prevalence of 9.6/12.8 % of frequent or nightly insomnia and 57.6–62.7 % of occasional insomnia [20]. The prevalence of severe insomnia was 5–14 %, depending on the age group [20].

There are fewer studies in the pediatric population; yet they reveal, in general, similar prevalence rates. In preadolescent children, one of the earliest studies noted that 14 % of an outpatient US pediatric population between the ages of 6 and 12 had insomnia with a mean duration of 5 years [21]. Archbold et al. at Ann Arbor surveyed parents of 1038 unselected children (554 boys) aged 2.0–13.9 years. Forty-one percent of the children had at least one symptom of insomnia and 18 % had two or more symptoms [22]. The prevalence of frequent insomnia in 1413 Swedish schoolchildren aged 6.2–10.9 years was reported to be 13 % [23].

In adolescent groups, the prevalence of insomnia appears to be similar to that of younger children. In a Chinese study, a total of 1365 adolescents between the ages of 12 and 18 years were surveyed and 16.9 % reported insomnia [24]. A multinational study in Europe, in a representative sample of 1125 adolescents aged 15–18 years, from four countries (France, Great Britain, Germany, and Italy) reported insomnia symptoms in approximately 25 % and DSM-IV insomnia disorder in approximately 4 % [25]. Previous studies had reported prevalence rates of 4–5 % for persistent insomnia in a group of 574 (aged 7–17) [26], 10.8–33.2 % for frequent insomnia (at least twice a week) in a group of 40,202 children aged 11–16 [27], 11–12.6 % for frequent insomnia [28–30], 23–38 % for occasional insomnia, and 1–2 % for persistent insomnia [31]. In summary, studies from different countries suggest that insomnia is a universal complaint, and that it is commonly expressed, making it a major health issue.

In a recent review by Ohayon [32] an attempt was made to determine the prevalence of insomnia based on four categories:

Table 2.1 Prevalence of insomnia by country

Country	No. of subjects	Age (years)	Prevalence (%)	Reference
USA	3161	18–79	35	[7]
Canada-French	5622	>15	20.1	[8]
German	1997	>13	25	[11]
Norway	2001	>18	11.7	[14]
South Korea	3719	>15	17	[17]
Mexico	1000	18–84	36	[18]
China	1365	15–18	25	[25]
Europe (France, UK, Germany, Italy)	1125	15–18	25	[25]

1. Insomnia symptoms of difficulty in initiating and maintaining sleep or non-restorative sleep.
2. Insomnia symptoms accompanied by daytime consequences.
3. Dissatisfaction with sleep quality or quantity.
4. Insomnia diagnosis based on definitions established by DSM-IV, or ICSD.

The first category based on insomnia symptoms alone revealed a prevalence of 30–48%. This dropped to 16–12% when frequency modifiers were added to symptoms such as presence of symptoms to at least three nights a week or "often" or "always." When severity criteria were added to insomnia symptoms the prevalence of insomnia ranged from 10 to 28%. The prevalence of insomnia based on insomnia symptoms with daytime consequences (category 2) was around 10%. The prevalence of insomnia based on dissatisfaction with sleep quality and quantity (category 3) was 8–18% with a higher prevalence being consistently reported in females. The prevalence of insomnia based on DSM-IV classification varied from 4.4 to 6.4%. Primary insomnia was the most frequent diagnosis, its prevalence ranging between 2 and 4% (Table 2.1) [7, 8, 11, 14, 17, 18, 25].

Sociodemographic Determinants

Most epidemiological studies indicate that women, the elderly, and people with coexisting health problems are more likely to suffer from insomnia [33].

Gender

All of the available epidemiological studies that compare the prevalence of insomnia between the genders report a higher prevalence in women [8]. The female-to-male ratio is roughly 1.5/1 [33]. This is especially true when comparing peri- or

Table 2.2 Prevalence of insomnia by gender

Country	Age (years)	Insomnia % female/male	Reference
USA	11–14	30.4/16.8	[36]
Germany	>18	5/3 (severe insomnia)	[39]
Hong Kong	18–65	14/9.3	[38]
South Korea	>15	19.1/14/8	[17]
Singapore	15–55	17.5/12.9	[19]
France	18–65+	12/6.3	[9]

post-menopausal women to age-matched men. One of the most common perimenopausal symptoms in women ranging in age from 35 to 55 is insomnia [34, 35].

There are, however, other studies that report an increased prevalence of insomnia in younger women, and even in adolescent girls, when compared to age-matched male counterparts. When studying a group of children and adolescents between ages of 3 and 14 ($n=452$), Camhi et al. found that the complaints of insomnia were much higher in adolescent girls (ages 11–14) than in the rest of the group (30.4–16.8 %) [36]. This suggests that insomnia, or the processes that produce it, are operant in women as early as adolescence. The increased prevalence of insomnia in adult women of all ages when compared to men seems to be a universal phenomenon. Studies from Hong Kong [37, 38], Germany [39], Canada [8, 13], the USA [2, 40], Norway [15], Scotland [41], and other countries [42, 43] have all reported increased prevalence in adult women when compared to age-matched male counterparts (Table 2.2) [9, 17, 19, 36, 38, 39].

Age

Advancing age is thought to be a risk factor for developing insomnia. The odds ratio was noted to be 1.3 in one study [33]. Despite other reports of increased prevalence of insomnia with aging [13, 14], a few studies that involve elderly populations exclusively have failed to demonstrate this effect [42, 44, 45]. In 2001, Ohayon et al. surveyed 13,057 subjects, whose ages were above 15 years, from three different countries (UK, Germany, and Italy). Insomnia symptoms were reported by more than one-third of the population aged 65 and older. Multivariate models showed that age was not a predictive factor for insomnia symptoms when controlling for activity status and social life satisfaction. The authors concluded that the aging process per se is not responsible for the increase of insomnia often reported in older people. Instead, inactivity, dissatisfaction with social life, and the presence of organic diseases and mental disorders were the best predictors of insomnia, with the contribution of age being insignificant. In this study, the prevalence of insomnia symptoms in healthy seniors was similar to that observed in younger individuals [46].

Ethnocultural Factors

The few studies that have looked at the impact of ethnocultural variables on insomnia have shown that, among the elderly, European-Americans more frequently complained of insomnia than African-Americans [47, 48] and had a greater reliance on sleep medications [48]. In a nationwide sleep survey [49] in the USA of 1007 individuals (aged 25–60) to characterize sleep habits in different ethnic groups, insomnia in adults was diagnosed in 20 % Whites, 18 % Blacks, 14 % Hispanics, and 9 % Asians. Overall, Asians were most likely to report getting a good night sleep [49]. It is possible that people of different ethnicities and cultures experience and perceive their sleep problems differently due to sociocultural influences and what may be experienced as abnormal in one group may be considered as normal in another.

Shift Work

Several studies have demonstrated that rotating daytime shift workers report sleep-onset insomnia more frequently than the fixed daytime-schedule workers (20.1 % vs. 12.0 %) [50], with the complaints of insomnia increasing in proportion to the number of shifts worked. Insomnia and other sleep complaints are significantly more common in three-shift workers than in two-shift workers. By the same token two-shift workers complain more of insomnia than straight-day shift workers [51]. Working the night or third shift may not only acutely cause insomnia but may have persistent deleterious effects on sleep quality, when adhered to for prolonged periods of time, even after reversion to day or evening shifts [52].

Other Factors

Occupation, socioeconomic status, marital status, and mental and physical health also impact the prevalence of insomnia. A few studies have reported a direct relationship between being unemployed [8, 13, 38, 53], lower socioeconomic status [33, 38], lower educational level [38], and increased prevalence of insomnia. Higher prevalence of insomnia complaints has also been reported among single, widowed, or divorced adults as compared to ones who were married or partnered [8, 12, 53]. Noisy environments are associated with increased reports of poor sleep particularly in women [38, 54]. Psychosocial stressors and [24] poor physical health are also associated with higher prevalence of insomnia [12, 24, 33, 37, 43–45] as is poor mental health [12, 42, 44, 45]. Medical problems associated with insomnia include depressive disorders [44, 55], anxiety disorders [55, 56], substance abuse [56], schizophrenia [55], congestive heart failure, sleep-disordered breathing [57], back and hip problems, and prostate problems [58]. In the 2015 Sleep in America poll,

Table 2.3 Factors impacting prevalence of insomnia

Low unemployment	[8, 13, 38, 53]
Lower socioeconomic status	[33, 38]
Lower educational level	[38]
Single/divorced/widowed status	[8, 12, 53]
Noisy environment	[38, 54]
Increased psychosocial stressors	[24]
Mental health disorders; schizophrenia, depression, anxiety	[44, 55, 56]
Medical problems; CHF, COPD, sleep apnea, chronic pain, enlarged prostate	[12, 24, 33, 37, 43–45, 57, 58]
Substance abuse	[56]

1044 individuals (age range from 18 to 91 years) were surveyed [59]. Those with severe or very severe stress were twice as likely to report poor sleep quality compared with those with mild or no stress (83 % vs. 35 %). Pain was also associated with poor sleep quality. 65 % of those with no pain reported good sleep quality compared to 45 % with acute pain and 35 % with chronic pain.

Seasonal differences have been reported in patients suffering from chronic insomnia. In Norway a survey of a representative sample of 14,667 adults living in the municipality of Tromso, north of the Arctic Circle, revealed increased incidence of complaints of insomnia during the dark period of the year than during any other time [15] (Table 2.3) [8, 12, 13, 24, 33, 37, 38, 43–45, 53–58].

Psychiatric Disorders

In 1989 Ford and Kamerow surveyed 7954 subjects with standardized questionnaires and then repeated the survey a year later. Of this community 10.2 % had insomnia at baseline. The risk of developing new major depression over the course of 1 year was much higher in those who had insomnia at baseline (odds ratio, 39.8; 95 % confidence interval, 19.8–80.0). The risk was less (odds ratio, 1.6; 95 % confidence interval, 0.5–5.3) in those whose insomnia had resolved by the time of the second visit [60].

In 1997 Chang et al. published a landmark paper on the subject of insomnia and its relation to the development of depression. A total of 1053 men provided information on sleep habits during medical school at The Johns Hopkins University (classes of 1948–1964) and were followed for several years after graduation. During a median follow-up period of 34 years (range 1–45), 101 men developed clinical depression (12.2 %) and 13 committed suicide. A Cox proportional hazard analysis adjusted for age at graduation, class year, parental history of clinical depression, coffee drinking, and measures of temperament revealed that the relative risk of subsequent clinical depression was greater in those who reported insomnia in medical school [61]. In the same year Weissman et al. published a study that reported data from a survey of over 10,000 adults living in three US communities. Psychiatric disorders were assessed utilizing a structured diagnostic interview. The prevalence of insomnia (not due to medical conditions, medication, and drug or alcohol abuse), during the subsequent 1 year of follow-up, was also assessed. The results revealed that 8% of subjects who had primary insomnia had sought psychiatric help at the end of that year for different psychiatric problems vs. 2.5% of the normal controls. Uncomplicated or primary insomnia was also associated with an increase in risk for first onset of major depression, panic disorder, and alcohol abuse over the following year [55]. These, and similar studies, have suggested that insomnia is a risk factor for the development of major depression and other psychiatric disorders [62].

It also appears that individuals who have an anxiety-prone personality and who have a lower ability to manage day-to-day stresses are more prone to insomnia. Le Blanc et al. evaluated 464 good sleepers over 1 year to assess the incidence of developing insomnia and potential risk factors. Five variables were associated with a new onset of insomnia syndrome: (1) previous episode of insomnia, (2) positive family history of insomnia, (3) higher arousability predisposition, (4) poorer self-rated general health, and (5) higher bodily pain. Individuals who developed insomnia also appeared to have a premorbid psychological vulnerability to poor sleep, characterized by higher depressive and anxiety symptoms, lower extraversion, and poorer self-rated mental health at baseline [63]. Individuals with lower extraversion tend to be less outgoing, and are more reserved and less talkative. The activation of the hypothalamic pituitary adrenal axis leads to hyperarousal and sleeplessness in patients with insomnia. Vgontzas showed that plasma ACTH and 24-h serum cortisol in insomniacs were higher compared to controls and the greatest elevation occurred in the evening and the first half of the night [64]. In an excellent review Reimann explores the concept that primary insomnia can be conceptualized as a final common pathway resulting from the interplay between a genetic vulnerability and an imbalance between arousing and sleep-inducing brain activity, psychosocial and medical stresses, and perpetuating mechanisms like dysfunctional sleep-related behavior, learned sleep-preventing associations, and tendency to ruminate [65].

Morbidity and Mortality

A number of studies have demonstrated a decreased quality of life as a direct consequence of the insomnia. Chevalier and colleagues, using the SF-36, demonstrated that the degree of impairment in quality of life was directly proportional to the severity of insomnia. They also demonstrated that individuals with severe insomnia showed a higher level of healthcare utilization [42]. Hajak and the SINE group (Study of Insomnia in Europe) in Germany and Leger and colleagues in France reported very similar results regarding quality of life and health care utilization [39, 66]. Zammit et al. and Hatoum et al., independently, reported similar results in the USA [67, 68]. In a qualitative study individuals with insomnia described feeling isolated and daily difficulties with cognitive emotional and physical functioning and had the cumulative effect of reducing work performance and social participation [69]. Cognitive deficits identified on objective testing have been associated with chronic, persistent, insomnia as well [70, 71]. In a recent study by Fortier-Brochu, individuals with insomnia showed clinically significant alterations in attention and episodic memory. Objective deficits on neuropsychological variables were also more pronounced and appeared to be associated with sleep continuity [72].

In a meta-analysis which summarized the findings of 21 studies, patient with insomnia had a twofold increased risk of developing depression [73].

The limited numbers of studies that have examined the association between insomnia, its treatment, and mortality have been inconsistent. Kripke et al. followed 1.1 million subjects for 6 years and reported that insomnia alone was not associated with increased mortality [74]. However, another study showed that mortality risk over a 6-year follow-up period was significantly elevated in older adults who used medications other than traditional hypnotics for improving sleep [75]. There is an association between difficulties falling asleep and mortality due to coronary artery disease in men [76]. In a study published by Suka M et al. on Japanese middle-aged male workers and after adjusting for all confounders (age, BMI, smoking, alcohol, and job stress), persistent complaints of difficulty initiating and maintaining sleep were associated with an increased risk of hypertension [77]. In another study by Vgontzas et al. chronic insomnia with short sleep duration was associated with increased risk of developing diabetes after adjusting for age, race, sex, BMI, smoking, alcohol use, depression, sleep-disordered breathing, and periodic limb movements [78].

Epidemiology of Hypnotic Use

The use of hypnotics increases with age, particularly among middle-aged and elderly women [79, 80]. Sleeping pill use varies with occupation. According to one study, the rate of frequent or habitual hypnotic use among male gardeners, female social office workers, and male construction workers was higher than the rate in other surveyed occupations [81]. Alcohol is the most commonly used hypnotic among insomniacs (roughly 15 % have reported using alcohol for insomnia) [56, 82]. Between 1987 and 1996 there was a dramatic shift, in the USA, towards the use of antidepressants instead of hypnotics for the symptomatic treatment of insomnia, despite a paucity of data regarding their efficacy, and despite the potential for serious side effects [83]. Antidepressants and over-the-counter sleep aids remain the most commonly recommended and prescribed treatments for insomnia complaints [83]. Despite the favorable safety profile of benzodiazepine receptor agonists they remain less utilized in the USA, possibly owing to concerns regarding their potential for dependence and abuse and their DEA status as "scheduled" agents and, until recently, their cost [84].

Economic Impact of Insomnia

Insomnia costs the American public $92.5 to $107.5 billion annually, in both direct and indirect expenses, due to medical procedures and medications, accidents, and reduced productivity associated with absenteeism and decreased work efficiency [85]. Insomnia sufferers place a significant burden on both the health care system and their employers [86]. Weissman et al. noted that insomnia sufferers were more prone to access medical and psychiatric care providers during a 1-year follow-up period [55]. In 1995 Walsh and Engelhardt reported a total direct cost of $13.9 billion in the USA [87].

Conclusion

Insomnia is a prevalent complaint and often encountered by health care practitioners. It is costly and can cause significant morbidity if not addressed appropriately. Women and the elderly tend to suffer from insomnia more than other groups of the population. Other risk factors include psychosocial stressors, psychiatric and medical problems, low income, unemployment, excessive environmental noise, not having a life partner, and job-related stressors among others.

References

1. Mahowald MW, Kader G, Schenck CH. Clinical categories of sleep disorders I. Continuum. 1997;3:35–65.
2. Young TB. Natural history of chronic insomnia. NIH insomnia abstract. J Clin Sleep Med. 2005;1(Suppl):e466–7.
3. Association of Sleep Disorders Center. Diagnostic classification of sleep and arousal disorders. Sleep. 1979;2:5–122.
4. American Psychiatric Association. Sleep disorders. In: Diagnostic and statistical manual of mental disorders: diagnostic criteria for primary insomnia, 5th ed., text revision. Arlington, VA: American Psychiatric Association; 2013. p. 361.
5. American Academy of Sleep Medicine. The international classification of sleep disorders. 3rd ed. Darien, IL: American Academy of Sleep Medicine; 2014.
6. World Health Organization. The ICD-10 classification of mental and behavioral disorders. Geneva: World Health Organization; 1992.
7. Mellinger GD, Balter MB, Uhlenhuth EH. Insomnia and its treatment: prevalence and correlates. Arch Gen Psychiatry. 1985;42:225–32.
8. Ohayon M. Epidemiological study on insomnia in the general population. Sleep. 1996;19 Suppl 3:7–15.
9. Leger D, Guilleminault C, Dreyfus JP, Delahaye C, Paillard M. Prevalence of insomnia in a survey of 12,778 adults in France. J Sleep Res. 2000;9:35–42.
10. Sutton DA, Moldofsky H, Badley EM. Insomnia and health problems in Canadians. Sleep. 2001;24:665–70.
11. Simen S, Hajak G, Schlaf G, et al. Chronification of sleep disorders. [Chronification of sleep disorders. Results of a representative survey in West Germany]. Nervenarzt. 1995;66:686–95.

12. Ishigooka J, Suzuki M, Isawa S, Muraoka H, Murasaki M, Okawa M. Epidemiological study on sleep habits and insomnia of new outpatients visiting general hospitals in Japan. Psychiatry Clin Neurosci. 1999;53:515–22.
13. Kim K, Uchiyama M, Okawa M, Liu X, Ogihara R. An epidemiological study of insomnia among the Japanese general population. Sleep. 2000;23:41–7.
14. Pallesen S, Nordhus IH, Nielsen GH, et al. Prevalence of insomnia in the adult Norwegian population. Sleep. 2001;24:771–9.
15. Husby R, Lingjaerde O. Prevalence of reported sleeplessness in northern Norway in relation to sex, age and season. Acta Psychiatr Scand. 1990;81:542–7.
16. Zeitlhofer J, Rieder A, Kapfhammer G, et al. Epidemiology of sleep disorders in Austria. Wien Klin Wochenschr. 1994;106:86–8.
17. Ohayon MM, Hong SC. Prevalence of insomnia and associated factors in South Korea. J Psychosom Res. 2002;53:593–600.
18. Lopez AT, Sanchez EG, Torres FG, et al. Habitos y trastornos del dormir en residentes del area metropolitana de Monterrey. Salud Mental. 1995;18:14–22.
19. Yeo BK, Perera IS, Kok LP, Tsoi WF. Insomnia in the community. Singapore Med J. 1996;37:282–4.
20. Hyyppa M, Kronholm E. How does Finland sleep? Sleeping habits of the Finnish adult population and the rehabilitation of sleep disturbances. Publ Soc Ins Inst. 1987;ML(68):1–110.
21. Dixon KN, Monroe LJ, Jakim S. Insomniac children. Sleep. 1981;4:313–8.
22. Archbold KH, Pituch KJ, Panahi P, Chervin RD. Symptoms of sleep disturbances among children at two general pediatric clinics. J Pediatr. 2002;140:97–102.
23. Nevéus T, Cnattingius S, Olsson U, Hetta J. Sleep habits and sleep problems among a community sample of schoolchildren. Acta Paediatr. 2001;90:1450–5.
24. Liu X, Uchiyama M, Okawa M, Kurita H. Prevalence and correlates of self-reported sleep problems among Chinese adolescents. Sleep. 2000;23:27–34.
25. Ohayon MM, Roberts RE, Zulley J, Smirne S, Priest RG. Prevalence and patterns of problematic sleep among older adolescents. J Am Acad Child Adolesc Psychiatry. 2000;39:1549–56.
26. Saarenpää-Heikkilä OA, Rintahaka PJ, Laippala PJ, Koivikko MJ. Sleep habits and disorders in Finnish schoolchildren. J Sleep Res. 1995;4:173–82.
27. Tynjälä J, Kannas L, Välimaa R. How young Europeans sleep. Health Educ Res. 1993;8:69–80.
28. Levy D, Gray-Donald K, Leech J, Zvagulis I, Pless IB. Sleep patterns and problems in adolescents. J Adolesc Health Care. 1986;7:386–9.
29. Price VA, Coates TJ, Thoresen CE, Grinstead OA. Prevalence and correlates of poor sleep among adolescents. Am J Dis Child. 1978;132:583–6.
30. Kirmil-Gray K, Eagleston J, Gibson E. Sleep disturbance in adolescents: sleep quality, sleep habits, beliefs about sleep, and daytime functioning. J Youth Adolesc. 1984;13:375–84.
31. Rimpela A, Ahlstrom S. Health habits among Finnish youth. Helsinki: National Board of Health; 1983. p. 71–83.
32. Ohayon MM. Epidemiology of insomnia: what we know and what we still need to learn. Sleep Med Rev. 2002;6:97–111.
33. Klink ME, Quan SF, Kaltenborn WT, Lebowitz MD. Risk factors associated with complaints of insomnia in a general adult population: influence of previous complaints of insomnia. Arch Intern Med. 1992;152:1634–7.
34. Mitchell ES, Woods NF. Symptom experiences of midlife women: observations from the Seattle Midlife Women's Health Study. Maturitas. 1996;25:1–10.
35. Owens JF, Matthews KA. Sleep disturbance in healthy middle-aged women. Maturitas. 1998;30:41–50.
36. Camhi SL, Morgan WJ, Pernisco N, Quan SF. Factors affecting sleep disturbances in children and adolescents. Sleep Med. 2000;1:117–23.
37. Chiu HF, Leung T, Lam LC, et al. Sleep problems in Chinese elderly in Hong Kong. Sleep. 1999;22:717–26.
38. Li RH, Wing YK, Ho SC, Fong SY. Gender differences in insomnia-a study in the Hong Kong Chinese population. J Psychosom Res. 2002;53:601–9.

39. Hajak G, SINE Study Group. Epidemiology of severe insomnia and its consequences in Germany. Eur Arch Psychiatry Clin Neurosci. 2001;251:49–56.
40. Foley DJ, Monjan AA, Izmirlian G, Hays JC, Blazer DG. Incidence and remission of insomnia among elderly adults in a biracial cohort. Sleep. 1999;22 Suppl 2:373–8.
41. McGhie A, Russell S. The subjective assessment of normal sleep patterns. J Ment Sci. 1962;108:642–54.
42. Chevalier H, Los F, Boichut D, et al. Evaluation of severe insomnia in the general population: results of a European multinational survey. J Psychopharmacol. 1999;13 Suppl 1:21–4.
43. Janson C, Lindberg E, Gislason T, Elmasry A, Boman G. Insomnia in men: a 10-year prospective population-based study. Sleep. 2001;24:425–30.
44. Morgan K, Clarke D. Risk factors for late-life insomnia in a representative general practice sample. Br J Gen Pract. 1997;47:166–9.
45. Foley DJ, Monjan A, Simonsick EM, Wallace RB, Blazer DG. Incidence and remission of insomnia among elderly adults: an epidemiologic study of 6,800 persons over three years. Sleep. 1999;22 Suppl 2:366–72.
46. Ohayon MM, Zulley J, Guilleminault C, Smirne S, Priest RG. How age and daytime activities are related to insomnia in the general population: consequences for older people. J Am Geriatr Soc. 2001;49:360–6.
47. Blazer DG, Hays JC, Foley DJ. Sleep complaints in older adults: a racial comparison. J Gerontol A Biol Sci Med Sci. 1995;50:M280–4.
48. Jean-Louis G, Magai CM, Cohen CI, et al. Ethnic differences in self-reported sleep problems in older adults. Sleep. 2001;24:926–33.
49. 2010 Sleep in America Poll. Sleep and ethnicity. Washington, DC: National Sleep Foundation; 2015. http://sleepfoundation.org/sleep-polls-data/sleep-in-america-poll/2010-sleep-and-ethnicity. Accessed 15 Oct 2015.
50. Ohayon MM, Lemoine P, Arnaud-Briant V, Dreyfus M. Prevalence and consequences of sleep disorders in a shift worker population. J Psychosom Res. 2002;53:577–83.
51. Härmä M, Tenkanen L, Sjöblom T, Alikoski T, Heinsalmi P. Combined effects of shift work and life-style on the prevalence of insomnia, sleep deprivation and daytime sleepiness. Scand J Work Environ Health. 1998;24:300–7.
52. Dumont M, Montplaisir J, Infante-Rivard C. Sleep quality of former night-shift workers. Int J Occup Environ Health. 1997;3 Suppl 2:10–4.
53. Doi Y, Minowa M, Okawa M, Uchiyama M. Prevalence of sleep disturbance and hypnotic medication use in relation to sociodemographic factors in the general Japanese adult population. J Epidemiol. 2000;10:79–86.
54. Kageyama T, Kabuto M, Nitta H, et al. A population study on risk factors for insomnia among adult Japanese women: a possible effect of road traffic volume. Sleep. 1997;20:963–71.
55. Weissman MM, Greenwald S, Niño-Murcia G, Dement WC. The morbidity of insomnia uncomplicated by psychiatric disorders. Gen Hosp Psychiatry. 1997;19:245–50.
56. Costa e Silva JA, Chase M, Sartorius N, Roth T. Special report from a symposium held by the World Health Organization and the World Federation of Sleep Research Societies: an overview of insomnias and related disorders—recognition, epidemiology, and rational management. Sleep. 1996;19:412–6.
57. Dodge R, Cline MG, Quan SF. The natural history of insomnia and its relationship to respiratory symptoms. Arch Intern Med. 1995;155:1797–800.
58. Katz DA, McHorney CA. Clinical correlates of insomnia in patients with chronic illness. Arch Intern Med. 1998;158:1099–107.
59. 2015 Sleep in America Poll. Sleep and pain. Washington, DC: National Sleep Foundation; 2015. http://sleepfoundation.org/sleep-polls-data/2015-sleep-and-pain. Accessed 15 Oct 2015.
60. Ford DE, Kamerow DB. Epidemiologic study of sleep disturbances and psychiatric disorders: an opportunity for prevention? JAMA. 1989;262:1479–84.
61. Chang PP, Ford DE, Mead LA, Cooper-Patrick L, Klag MJ. Insomnia in young men and subsequent depression: the Johns Hopkins Precursors Study. Am J Epidemiol. 1997;146:105–14.
62. Mallon L, Broman JE, Hetta J. Relationship between insomnia, depression, and mortality: a 12-year follow-up of older adults in the community. Int Psychogeriatr. 2000;12:295–306.

63. LeBlanc M, Mérette C, Savard J, Ivers H, Baillargeon L, Morin CM. Incidence and risk factors of insomnia in a population-based sample. Sleep. 2009;32:1027–37.
64. Vgontzas AN, Bixler EO, Lin HM, et al. Chronic insomnia is associated with nyctohemeral activation of the hypothalamic-pituitary-adrenal axis: clinical implications. J Clin Endocrinol Metab. 2001;86:3787–94.
65. Riemann D, Spiegelhadler R, Feige B, et al. The hyperarousal model of insomnia: a review of the concept and its evidence. Sleep Med Rev. 2010;14:19–31.
66. Léger D, Scheuermaier K, Philip P, Paillard M, Guilleminault C. SF-36: evaluation of quality of life in severe and mild insomniacs compared with good sleepers. Psychosom Med. 2001;63:49–55.
67. Hatoum HT, Kong SX, Kania CM, Wong JM, Mendelson WB. Insomnia, health-related quality of life and healthcare resource consumption: a study of managed-care organisation enrollees. Pharmacoeconomics. 1998;14:629–37.
68. Zammit GK, Weiner J, Damato N, Sillup GP, McMillan CA. Quality of life in people with insomnia. Sleep. 1999;22 Suppl 2:379–85.
69. Kyle SD, Espie CA, Morgan K. "… Not just a minor thing, it is something major, which stops you from functioning daily": quality of life and daytime functioning in insomnia. Behav Sleep Med. 2010;8:123–40.
70. Hauri PJ. Cognitive deficits in insomnia patients. Acta Neurol Belg. 1997;97:113–7.
71. Espie CA, Inglis SJ, Harvey L, Tessier S. Insomniacs' attributions. psychometric properties of the Dysfunctional Beliefs and Attitudes about Sleep Scale and the Sleep Disturbance Questionnaire. J Psychosom Res. 2000;48:141–8.
72. Fortier-Brochu E, Morin CM. Cognitive impairment in individuals with insomnia: clinical significance and correlates. Sleep. 2014;37:1787–98.
73. Baglioni C, Battagliese G, Feige B, et al. Insomnia as a predictor of depression: a meta-analytic evaluation of longitudinal epidemiological studies. J Affect Disord. 2011;135:10–9.
74. Kripke DF, Garfinkel L, Wingard DL, Klauber MR, Marler MR. Mortality associated with sleep duration and insomnia. Arch Gen Psychiatry. 2002;59:131–6.
75. Rumble R, Morgan K. Hypnotics, sleep, and mortality in elderly people. J Am Geriatr Soc. 1992;40:787–91.
76. Mallon L, Broman JE, Hetta J. Sleep complaints predict coronary artery disease mortality in males: a 12-year follow-up study of a middle-aged Swedish population. J Intern Med. 2002;251:207–16.
77. Suka M, Yoshida K, Sugimori H. Persistent insomnia is a predictor of hypertension in Japanese male workers. J Occup Health. 2003;45:344–50.
78. Vgontzas AN, Liao D, Pejovic S, Calhoun S, Karataraki M, Bixler EO. Insomnia with objective short sleep duration is associated with type 2 diabetes. Diabetes Care. 2009;32:1980–5.
79. Quera-Salva MA, Orluc A, Goldenberg F, Guilleminault C. Insomnia and use of hypnotics: study of a French population. Sleep. 1991;14:386–91.
80. Asplund R. Sleep and hypnotic use in relation to perceived somatic and mental health among the elderly. Arch Gerontol Geriatr. 2000;31:199–205.
81. Partinen M, Eskelinen L, Tuomi K. Complaints of insomnia in different occupations. Scand J Work Environ Health. 1984;10(6 Spec No):467–9.
82. Johnson EO, Roehrs T, Roth T, Breslau N. Epidemiology of alcohol and medication as aids to sleep in early adulthood. Sleep. 1998;21:178–86.
83. Walsh JK, Schweitzer PK. Ten-year trends in the pharmacological treatment of insomnia. Sleep. 1999;22:371–5.
84. Walsh JK, Roehrs T, Roth T. Pharmacologic treatment of primary insomnia. In: Kryger M, Roth T, Dement W, editors. Principles and practice of sleep medicine. Philadelphia: Saunders; 2005. p. 749–60.
85. Stoller MK. Economic effects of insomnia. Clin Ther. 1994;16:873–97. discussion 854.
86. Léger D, Guilleminault C, Bader G, Lévy E, Paillard M. Medical and socioprofessional impact of insomnia. Sleep. 2002;25:625–9.
87. Walsh JK, Engelhardt CL. The direct economic costs of insomnia in the United States for 1995. Sleep. 1999;22 Suppl 2:386–93.

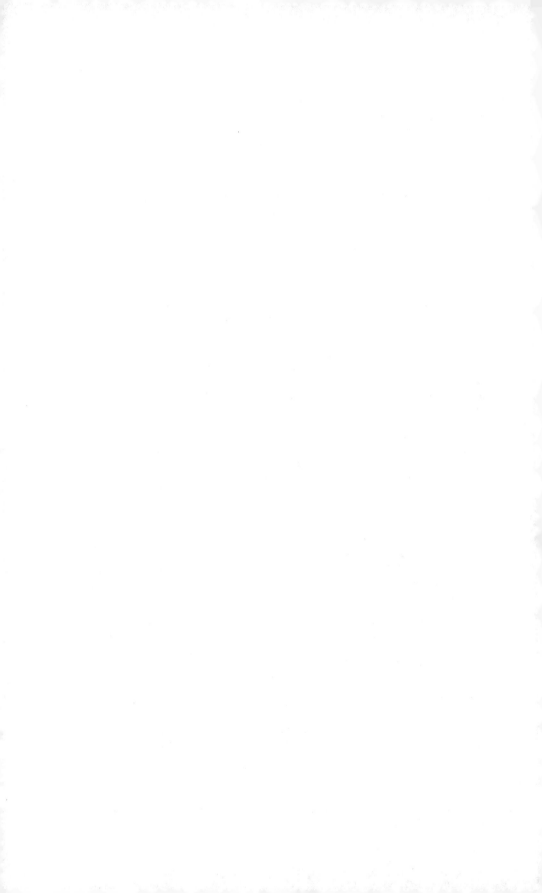

Chapter 3
Clinical Features, Diagnosis, and Differential Diagnosis

Mary B. O'Malley and Edward B. O'Malley

Abstract Chronic insomnia disorders (CID) are often a final common pathway for many people who initially develop sleeplessness in the context of acute stressors (e.g., pain, job loss), but then acquire a form of "learned" sleeplessness as they become increasingly over-concerned about their unsatisfying sleep patterns. Patients report reduced total sleep time, with increased sleep latency (greater than 30 min), or increased wake after sleep onset time, though these findings are not always corroborated on PSG studies. Patients with this form of chronic insomnia are often vexed by its seemingly unpredictable nature from night to night, but to be diagnosed symptoms must be present on three or more nights per week, for more than 3 months (ICSD-3). This chapter summarizes the clinical features of this disorder, the approach to diagnostic assessment, including the use of newer sleep apps and other technologies, and differential diagnosis.

Keywords Chronic insomnia • Psychophysiological insomnia • Diagnostic criteria • Beliefs and attitudes about sleep • Sleep apps

Introduction

Chronic insomnia disorder (CID) in adults is essentially a diagnosis of exclusion though there are many clinically specific findings. The essential feature of CID is a pattern of sleep disturbance that may have a non-determinate beginning but that

M.B. O'Malley, M.D., Ph.D. (✉)
Berkshire Medical Center, Pittsfield, MA, USA
e-mail: momalley@bhs1.org

E.B. O'Malley, Ph.D.
Your Optimal Nature, Great Barrington, MA, USA

© Springer International Publishing Switzerland 2017
H.P. Attarian (ed.), *Clinical Handbook of Insomnia*, Current Clinical Neurology,
DOI 10.1007/978-3-319-41400-3_3

usually evolves over time as a result of psychological distress that triggers unhelpful behaviors and physiological arousal. Patients report reduced total sleep time, with increased sleep latency (greater than 30 min), or increased wake after sleep onset time though these findings are not always corroborated on PSG studies. Patients with this form of chronic insomnia are often plagued by its seemingly unpredictable nature from night tonight, but to be diagnosed symptoms must be present on three or more nights per week for more than 3 months. This chapter summarizes the current understanding of this disorder and the clinical features underlying accurate diagnosis that are crucial for successful treatment. CID diagnosis in children is covered in another chapter in this volume.

Clinical Features

Chronic insomnia is a final common pathway for many people who have experienced a lifelong difficulty obtaining sleep, or initially develop sleeplessness in the context of acute stressors (e.g., pain, job loss). Common to all insomnia subtypes however is the ensuing "learned" helplessness and maladaptive behaviors leading to over-concern about their unsatisfying sleep patterns. The essential feature of chronic insomnia disorder is persistent difficulty with sleep that results in an overall feeling that sleep is unsatisfying (see Table 3.1) [1]. Further, the sleep difficulty is usually experienced as problematic because of its impact on daytime functioning. The distress surrounding poor sleep may be in relation to physical vitality during the day, and impaired functioning at work, social, or family spheres. Further, the sleep difficulty occurs despite having adequate time to devote to sleep. CID may be comorbid with underlying medical illnesses, mental illness, or the effects of substance abuse.

Though the sleep symptoms that patients report are subjective, there are some generally accepted parameters for clinically significant sleep complaints. Delayed sleep onset and wake after sleep onset (WASO) time of 30 min or more is the commonly accepted threshold for a diagnosis of insomnia in middle-aged and older adults [2]. Early awakening is similarly and abnormally "early" if at least 30 min before desired wake time. These values increase in the elderly as sleep generally worsens with age [3]. Complaints about unrefreshing or non-restorative sleep frequently accompany this diagnosis, but are not sufficient to define this disorder alone [4].

Typically, chronic insomnia sufferers present with complaints of daytime impairment [5]. The most common symptoms are fatigue, irritability, problems with concentration or memory, and worry about sleep. In contrast to patients with hypersomnolence, insomnia patients complain that they cannot nap even when they try and rarely have unintentional sleep episodes. Work place and school performance errors are common however, and do place patients with chronic insomnia at some risk [6]. Physical complaints of headaches, gastrointestinal distress, and poor exercise tolerance are often reported, leading to a pervasive feeling of malaise or disability from their sleep

Table 3.1 Diagnostic criteria for chronic insomnia disorder

Criteria A–F must be met	
A. The patient reports, or the patient's parent or caregiver observes, one or more of the following:[a]	1. Difficulty initiating sleep. 2. Difficulty maintaining sleep. 3. Waking up earlier than desired. 4. Resistance to going to bed on appropriate schedule. 5. Difficulty sleeping without parent or caregiver intervention.
B. The patient reports, or the patient's parent or caregiver observes, one or more of the following related to the nighttime sleep difficulty:	1. Fatigue/malaise. 2. Attention, concentration, or memory impairment. 3. Impaired social, family, occupational, or academic performance. 4. Mood disturbance or irritability. 5. Daytime sleepiness. 6. Behavioral problems (e.g., hyperactivity, impulsivity, aggression). 7. Reduced motivation, energy or initiative. 8. Proneness for errors/accidents. 9. Concerns about or dissatisfaction with sleep.
C. The reported sleep-wake complaints cannot be explained purely by inadequate opportunity (i.e., enough time is allotted for sleep) or inadequate circumstances (i.e., the environment is safe, dark, quiet, and comfortable) for sleep.	
D. The sleep disturbance and associated daytime symptoms occur at least three times per week.	
E. The sleep disturbance and associated daytime symptoms have been present for at least 3 months.[b, c]	
F. The sleep-wake difficulty is not better explained by another sleep disorder.[d]	

[a]Reports of difficulties initiating sleep, difficulties maintaining sleep, or waking up too early can be seen in all age groups. Resistance going to bed on an appropriate schedule and difficulty sleeping without parent or caregiver intervention are seen most commonly in children and older adults who require the supervision of a caretaker due to a significant level of functional impairment (e.g., those with dementia)

[b]Some patients with chronic insomnia may show recurrent episodes of sleep-wake difficulties lasting several weeks at a time over several years, yet not meet the 3-month duration criterion for any single such episode. Nonetheless, these patients should be assigned a diagnosis of chronic insomnia disorder, given the persistence of their intermittent sleep difficulties over time

[c]Some patients who use hypnotic medications regularly may sleep well and not meet the criteria for an insomnia disorder when they take such medications. However, in the absence of such medications these same patients may meet the above criteria. This diagnosis would apply to those patients particularly if they present clinically and voice concerns about their inability to sleep without their sleep medications

(continued)

Table 3.1 (continued)

dMany comorbid conditions such as chronic pain disorders or gastroesophageal reflux disease (GERD) may cause the sleep-wake complaints delineated here. When such conditions are the sole cause of the sleep difficulty, a separate insomnia diagnosis may not apply. However, in many patients such conditions are chronic and are not the sole cause of sleep difficulty. Key determining factors in the decision to invoke a separate insomnia diagnosis include the following: "How much of the time does the sleep difficulty arise as a result of factors directly attributable to the comorbid condition (e.g., pain or GERD)?" or "Are there times that the sleep/wake complaints occur in the absence of these factors?" "Have perpetuating cognitive or behavioral factors (e.g., negative expectations, conditioned arousal, sleep-disruptive habits) arisen, suggesting an autonomous aspect to the ongoing insomnia?" If there is evidence that the patient's sleep-wake complaints are not solely caused by the medical condition, and those sleep-wake complaints seem to merit separate treatment attention, then a diagnosis of chronic insomnia disorder should be made

disruption. This fatigue is often not relieved by rest, and must be differentiated from subjective sleepiness or unintentional sleep episodes. Patients with chronic insomnia often report a sense of reduced alertness, sometimes labeled as "brain fog," and a desire for sleep, but inability to sleep and achieve the relief they seek.

The current diagnostic criteria for CID require symptoms to be present three times per week for at least 3 months (see Table 3.1). However, it is clear that many people suffer from more acute and intermittent forms of this disorder that still cause clinically significant distress and impairment. In cases that meet all the criteria except the frequency and duration for the diagnosis of CID, a diagnosis of short-term insomnia disorder should be assigned instead [1].

Clinical Subtype Features

Notably, prior nosologies of sleep disorders have identified significant subtypes that are now grouped together under the CID designation [7]. According to the 2005 National Institutes of Health Consensus Panel on Manifestations and Management of Chronic Insomnia in Adults [8] the primary and secondary/comorbid nomenclature precluded important treatment consideration by non-sleep specialist providers. In part, the direction of causality remains unclear in many comorbid disorders and the underlying assumption that treating the primary condition resolves "secondary" insomnia has not been found in clinical practice. Further, many insomnia conditions share underlying similarities, and may respond to comparable management protocols. Nevertheless, considering the potential for specific treatment protocols and differential diagnosis the authors have included some of the most distinctive features distinguishing subtypes.

Psychophysiological insomnia has been commonly known as "learned" insomnia reflecting the development as this form of insomnia evolves. Important for management is assessment of negative beliefs and attitudes regarding sleep, and the associated maladaptive behaviors that eventually develop and worsen the condition. Cognitive behavioral therapy that specifically targets the psychological domain is potentially most useful.

Idiopathic insomnia subtype differs significantly from psychophysiological insomnia in that there is a lifelong propensity for poor sleep, probably genetically determined or at least anchored physiologically. While there may be negative behaviors that do develop over time, targeting the psychological realm alone is necessary but not sufficient. Therapies directed toward reducing physiologic hyper-arousal are necessary to counter the physical component of this subtype.

Paradoxical insomnia, formerly referred to as "sleep-state misperception," refers to the patient's report of inadequate or unrefreshing sleep, while objectively recorded data indicate "normal" sleep by standard measures. As the non-restorative sleep complaint with confirmed objective data has been found to be rare, this subtype has been subsumed under the general sleep complaint for CID. However, the subjective sense of non-restorative sleep despite lack of objective findings could be indicative of an undetected disorder that warrants further workup. Disease management in this case may require psychological or psychiatric evaluation.

Inadequate sleep hygiene refers to normal environment or daily activities performed at either inopportune times or such close proximity to prevent disturbance of the sleep period. For example, late-afternoon caffeine intake in the elderly is metabolized more slowly than in the past and now delays usual sleep-onset time. Other activities like evening exercise, irregular sleep wake schedules, late-evening work, or bright light exposure may all contribute to initiating or maintaining sleep difficulties. Taking a detailed inventory of waking caffeine, alcohol, and other substance intake and daily timing of activities allow for specific targeting of known sleep offenders and can directly resolve some insomnia issues while improving other strategies in a comprehensive treatment plan.

Insomnia due to (another) mental disorder is considered to be caused by, or a feature of, an underlying comorbid psychiatric illness. Insomnia symptoms are a common manifestation of mood and anxiety disorders, and often herald their development. Similarly, sleep can often be disturbed during episodes of psychotic illness, or exacerbation of many personality disorders. The degree of sleep disturbance often parallels the degree of psychiatric illness, and worsening insomnia is usually considered a risk of impending psychiatric decompensation, for instance indicating an increased risk of suicide.

Insomnia due to a drug or substance is considered to be caused by the use or withdrawal from a drug or substance. Sleep loss may be the side effect of stimulating substances (e.g., street drugs, medications, caffeine), or the consequence of withdrawal from sedating substances (e.g., alcohol, sedative-hypnotics). The features of this subtype are usually more readily identified by the pattern of underlying substance use, but may also be an insidious additional burden to patients with other primary subtypes of chronic insomnia disorder (e.g., alcohol or sedative use in psychophysiologic subtype).

Insomnia due to a medical disorder is thought to be caused by a co-occurring medical disorder. Like psychiatric illnesses or other primary sleep disorders, many medical conditions present with prominent complaints of sleep disturbance. Sleep disturbance is often clearly linked to conditions that cause pain, and disruptions in breathing or movement. A careful history and workup may be needed to identify some underlying medical conditions (e.g., COPD-related hypoxic intervals) which may not clearly present with bodily distress.

As patients often present with several comorbidities in clinical practice, chronic insomnia disorder may have a mix of subtypes. Many of them share common features, such as poor sleep hygiene or conditioned arousal, and underestimating sleep times. In patients with multiple medical conditions it may be impossible to clearly delineate the true cause of insomnia symptoms. No matter what the initial underlying cause, insomnia patterns may continue to evolve and develop into a chronic insomnia disorder that outlives the inciting illness. Fortunately, available treatments for chronic insomnia appear to be effective across a range of subtypes (Table 3.1).

Diagnostic Workup

The most important element in the clinical assessment of individuals with insomnia complaints is a thorough sleep and medical history. Insomnia symptoms may be complex, emerging from different sources from night to night, and across time. Medications, substances, medical disorders, sleep environment, or scheduling issues may add to the symptoms of insomnia the patients present. Features of CID must be discerned between, with, and among all the patients presenting sleep complaints. A systematic clinical assessment to identify intrinsic or extrinsic conditions that may be contributing to sleeplessness is essential, and insomnia secondary to other conditions should be addressed directly.

A history of escalating over-concern regarding sleep is usually able to be identified out right. Indeed, many patients are desperately aware that their anxiety about sleep is effectively sabotaging their ability to sleep. Occasionally, patients may be completely unaware that they are anxious or tense, and misattribute sleeplessness to other causes. A fairly typical history for chronic insomnia disorder is a patient who has had occasional problems initiating sleep in the past when stressed, but always managed to stay asleep once sleep began. Then, during an extended bout of initial insomnia some time ago, the patient became preoccupied with her problems sleeping and began to have trouble returning to sleep after waking to urinate. These normal awakenings were perceived as problematic, and as the patient's focus on sleep intensified, her sleep initiation expanded to include sleep maintenance symptoms.

What makes CID distinct is the essential role of the patient's psychological and physiological arousal levels in the creation of the ongoing symptoms. So, in addition to the routine elements of a sleep and medical history, the clinician should develop a longitudinal picture of the patient's ability to sleep in novel or stressful situations. The patient may recognize themselves as someone who tends to get "revved up" by life events in general, but may observe their trouble unwinding only in relation to their attempt to sleep. Still other patients do not perceive themselves to be anxious or "wound up," but simply "too awake." The clinician should explore whether the sleep complaints arise in the context of background stress reactivity, and how much insight the patient has about this aspect of themselves. Did this patient have difficulty transitioning to sleep as a child? Was this patient a "light" sleeper, sensitive to variations in their sleep environment? Did this patient feel sleep came easily before the problem of insomnia began, or have they always second-guessed their ability to sleep well? How was their sleep affected on nights before stressful or exciting events? Are they aware of the timing for sleep that really suits them (i.e., morning type versus evening type) or do they feel they "never sleep well"? How well did they sleep during their school years? Were they frequently late for the morning school bus, suggesting a longstanding issue that may underscore a circadian or other organic sleep disturbance?

A comprehensive approach to understanding both the behaviors and the attitudes and beliefs around sleep issues has been demonstrated to be very important to adequately address insomnia symptoms [9]. Morin and colleagues have developed a variety of assessment tools (recently abbreviated and updated) that can identify the cognitive distortions (e.g., "if I don't sleep 8 h, I won't be able to function at all"), and misperceptions related to sleep. Most insomniacs carry dysfunctional patterns of thinking and feeling about sleep that represents a real barrier to improved sleep. Informed clinicians can readily identify these patterns, and help patients to change them by using these assessment tools (see Appendix 1 for Dysfunctional Beliefs and Attitudes About Sleep). While this type of history takes less time now with the abbreviated version, not all clinicians may feel able or willing to use this approach. However, the investment of time to identify this information will usually allow the clinician to more quickly and precisely correct the patient's approach to sleep, and developing a more effective treatment plan (Table 3.2).

Table 3.2 Assessment tools

Tool	Utility
Sleep diary	Provides immediate and current perception of sleep pattern, circadian rhythmicity, weekend vs. weekday differences, and other information pertinent to the sleep period.
Epworth Sleepiness Scale (ESS)	Offers an assessment of subjective sleepiness. Note that if scores are subclinical and daytime somnolence is suspected then further evaluation is indicated.
Actigraphy	If circadian sleep issues are suspected, or chronic partial sleep deprivation is in the differential diagnosis.
Screening Questionnaire	Gives an overview of the patient's perceived sleep issues and can be completed by the patient before arriving for evaluation.
Beliefs and Attitudes Questionnaire	Contributes detailed information regarding the cognitive component of sleep disturbance.
Fatigue Severity Scale	Helps differentiate fatigue from sleepiness. Also, as many disorders have a component of fatigue it provides another domain that may require management.

An important element of an insomnia assessment is the use of outpatient self-report forms to document sleep patterns over the 24-h day. Patients may be annoyed by the task, but sleep logs (sleep diaries) are essential to the process of ongoing assessment of their sleep at home, and its response to treatment. There are many formats that can be used; the authors employ a format that shows blocks of sleep visually, and includes a way to indicate what time the patient got into bed relative to when they first attempted to fall asleep (i.e., would show the time spent reading in bed before "lights out"). It is not necessary to have patients complete an exhaustive diary of meals, activities, and mental status; the patient can include relevant details when they recognize the potential to affect their sleep (e.g., "I was very stressed after phone call"). Patient's subjective reporting on sleep logs is well supplemented with actigraphy [10]. Wrist-worn actigraphs are inexpensive, durable, and simple devices that sensitively and continuously record movement activity and rest periods that correspond well to wake and sleep on polysomnography. The patient wears the actigraph on the non-dominant wrist with a wrist watch, and objective measurements of activity levels can be collected for up to 4 weeks, allowing an objective assessment under longitudinal sleep patterns at home. Sleep logs, even without actigraphy, are more accurate and informative than a verbal report of their sleep patterns, particularly because patients tend to overestimate or globalize their lack of sleep (e.g., "it takes me 3 h to fall asleep"). With consistent use, sleep logs will facilitate collecting data on circadian, sleep hygiene, and sleep timing patterns that will guide the treatment process. In fact, weekly logs may initially provide the only "proof" to the patient that there are incremental improvements in his sleep patterns.

In recent years there has been an explosion of interest and corresponding technology to monitor sleep. Most are based on motion detection, similar to actigraphy [11]. A number of sleep applications ("apps") have been designed to be used in concert with smartphones containing native movement indicators, many taking advantage of Bluetooth technology which allows close-proximity transmission of data [12]. The wearable device or smartphone uploads the data to the application for analysis, providing downloadable (in some cases) summary graphs and histograms on a daily and also a cumulative basis. Some offer sleep-staged data, purporting to differentiate not only between sleep and wake, but also light and deep sleep, and even REM sleep. Unfortunately, most head-to-head studies using simultaneous PSG and sleep device/app data collection have failed to confirm accuracy for sleep staging, although some devices are better than others and do a reasonable assessment of sleep vs. wake states [13]. What is useful to consider is that as a result of the nearly ubiquitous availability of this technology more people are paying attention to their sleep patterns, and are attempting to improve sleep [14]. The downside is patients bring in their data to the clinician claiming to have reduced sleep efficiency (determined by an inaccurate device) and ask how they can improve it. Of course, the astute sleep clinician will use this opportunity to explore good sleep hygiene practices regardless of the source of the data!

The role of sleep testing. If the diagnosis of chronic insomnia disorder is clear, a nocturnal polysomnogram is not indicated [10, 15]. However, one may be needed to rule out other underlying sleep disorders. Patients with chronic insomnia are often surprised when they're able to sleep in the testing environment, and this can be a useful outcome measure as well—to reassure them that their brain can generate effective sleep, even under potentially adverse conditions. This information is useful for the clinician as well as CID is generally associated with less difficulty sleeping in new environments. Polysomnography may reveal physiologic clues to the patient's history of sleeplessness: surges in heart rate with awakenings may correspond with anxiety or pain; short and REM sleep-onset latency may be seen in patients with residual (or prodromal) major depression; a relative lack of light (N1 and N2) and REM sleep and excess "spindling" will betray exposure to benzodiazepines. Patients may focus upon the findings for clues that their brain is "not broken," and the clinician should be aware that the patient may really benefit from hearing the good news about a relatively normal polysomnogram.

Finally, if the behavioral treatment program has not produced significant improvement after several weeks of patient-compliant therapy then a polysomnogram would be indicated to rule out underlying organic disturbance that may have been missed or under-reported by the patient. These studies sometimes reveal significant sleep apnea (e.g., upper airway resistance syndrome; [16]) or other primary sleep disorders whose treatment may fully resolve the subjective sleep complaints or accelerate the patient's insomnia therapy.

Differential Diagnosis

Because insomnia presents as a symptomatic complaint, potentially underlying medical, psychiatric, or other primary sleep disorders need to be ruled out. Mood and anxiety disorders commonly present with complaints of insomnia and may initiate, exacerbate, or co-occur independently with CID.

Recent research has shown that chronic insomnia is an independent risk factor for major depression disorder (MDD; [17]) and conversely that MDD is an independent risk factor for chronic insomnia [18]. It is important to note that in the cases where these are comorbid disorders it is recommended that both need to be managed simultaneously [19]. For general anxiety disorder (GAD) recent studies strongly suggest a similar relationship to that of MDD and CID [20]. Clinicians would do well to consider MDD and GAD screening instruments integral to a comprehensive sleep evaluation. Of note, the cycling between manic and depressive phases of bipolar disorder may make it even more difficult to distinguish mood from insomnia symptoms. Patients can report being awake for days at a time, alternating with excessive sleepiness and or fatigue. Consequently, mood disorder instruments and psychological referrals may be indicated for the comprehensive evaluation of such complicated patients.

Insomnia may present as a complaint in the context of other primary sleep disorders which need to be addressed for accurate diagnosis and management considerations. Sleep apnea is a common primary sleep disorder that may present initially as insomnia. While most obstructive sleep apnea patients report hypersomnia, a subset complains of difficulty maintaining sleep, particularly during early stages of the syndrome [21]. Central sleep apnea while less common is more likely to produce repetitive awakenings followed by shortness of breath and associated arousal [22]. Neither disorder is likely to respond to typical insomnia treatment protocols—the alert clinician would do well to consider these potentially comorbid conditions.

Movement disorders such as restless leg disorder (RLS) and periodic limb movement disorder (PLMD) can present with sleep initiation or sleep maintenance complaints, respectively [23]. As there is significant overlap between these disorders, however, sufferers may complain of both symptoms. Their symptoms typically worsen in the evening and when immobile, occurring at bedtime and especially when lying down to sleep. It may take multiple tries with physical activity (e.g., getting up and walking) in between attempts to quiet the motor system sufficiently to allow for sleep to occur. Conversely, those with only PLMD may have limb motor activity of sufficient intensity and frequency to experience repetitive arousals throughout the sleep period, with attendant and negative daytime consequences. Either disorder is sufficient to generate insomnia complaints which are actually due to an organic issue.

Circadian rhythm disorders comprise the other major sleep disorder diagnostic category that could present as CID [24]. Delayed and advanced sleep-wake-phase disorders, and to a lesser degree shift work sleep disorder, can all present as difficulty initiating, maintaining, or waking too early complaints. Paying close attention to sleep pattern and regular sleep-wake schedule as well as work or school hours may serve to clearly differentiate these disorders.

Numerous medical disorders have shown strong relationships, many bidirectional with insomnia [25]. Whether from endogenous symptomatology directly or the medications and protocols employed to treat the disorder all may serve to significantly disturb sleep. Conversely, poor sleep may extend healing time or worsen symptoms of medical disorders. The major comorbid medical conditions are explored in detail in other chapters in this volume.

A point worth noting, hospital stays are notoriously sleep disturbing due to a variety of reasons [26]. The constant noise of monitoring devices, intensely bright lights at all circadian times, and nocturnal medicine checks/administrations routinely and negatively impact sleep. Introducing "sleep protocols" can go a long way toward reducing this potential cause of insomnia [27].

Appendix 1

Dysfunctional Beliefs About Sleep Scale

Please indicate to what extent you personally agree or disagree with each statement by circling a number that indicates where your personal rating falls.

1. I need 8 hours of sleep to feel refreshed and function well during the day.

    Strongly Disagree   1   2   3   4   5   6   7   8   9   10   Strongly Agree

2. When I don't get the proper amount of sleep on a given night, I need to catch up on the next day by napping or on the next night by sleeping longer.

    Strongly Disagree   1   2   3   4   5   6   7   8   9   10   Strongly Agree

3. I am concerned that chronic insomnia may have serious consequences on my physical health.

    Strongly Disagree   1   2   3   4   5   6   7   8   9   10   Strongly Agree

4. I am worried that I may lose control over my ability to sleep.

    Strongly Disagree   1   2   3   4   5   6   7   8   9   10   Strongly Agree

5. After a poor nights sleep, I know that it will interfere with my daily activities on the next day.

    Strongly Disagree   1   2   3   4   5   6   7   8   9   10   Strongly Agree

6. In order to be alert and function well during the day, I am better off taking a sleeping pill rather than having a poor night's sleep.

    Strongly Disagree   1   2   3   4   5   6   7   8   9   10   Strongly Agree

7. When I feel irritated, depressed, or anxious during the day, it is mostly because I did not sleep well the night before.

    Strongly Disagree   1   2   3   4   5   6   7   8   9   10   Strongly Agree

8. When I sleep poorly on one night, I know it will disturb my sleep schedule for the whole week.

    Strongly Disagree   1   2   3   4   5   6   7   8   9   10   Strongly Agree

9. Without an adequate night's sleep, I can hardly function the next day.

    Strongly Disagree   1   2   3   4   5   6   7   8   9   10   Strongly Agree

10. I can't ever predict whether I'll have a good night's sleep.

    Strongly Disagree   1   2   3   4   5   6   7   8   9   10   Strongly Agree

11. I have little ability to manage the negative consequences of disturbed sleep.

    Strongly Disagree   1   2   3   4   5   6   7   8   9   10   Strongly Agree

12. When I feel tired, have no energy, or just seem not to function well during the day, it is generally because I did not sleep well the night before.

    Strongly Disagree   1   2   3   4   5   6   7   8   9   10   Strongly Agree

13. I believe insomnia is essentially the result of a chemical imbalance.

    Strongly Disagree   1   2   3   4   5   6   7   8   9   10   Strongly Agree

14. I feel insomnia is ruining my ability to enjoy life and prevents me from doing what I want.

    Strongly Disagree   1   2   3   4   5   6   7   8   9   10   Strongly Agree

15. A "nightcap" before bedtime is a good solution to sleeplessness.

    Strongly Disagree   1   2   3   4   5   6   7   8   9   10   Strongly Agree

16. It usually shows in my physical appearance when I haven't slept well.

    Strongly Disagree   1   2   3   4   5   6   7   8   9   10   Strongly Agree

References

1. American Academy of Sleep Medicine. International classification of sleep disorders. 3rd ed. Darien, IL: American Academy of Sleep Medicine; 2014. p. 41–5.
2. Lichstein KL, Durrence HH, Taylor DJ, Bush AJ, Riedel BW. Quantitative criteria for insomnia. Behav Res Ther. 2003;41:427–45.
3. Driscoll HC, Serody L, Patrick S, et al. Sleeping well, aging well: a descriptive and cross-sectional study of sleep in "successful agers" 75 and older. Am J Geriatr Psychiatry. 2008;16:74–82.
4. Roth T, Zammit G, Lankford A, Mayleben D, Stern T, Pitman V, Clark D, Werth JL. Nonrestorative sleep as a distinct component of insomnia. Sleep. 2010;33(4):449–58.
5. Fortier-Brochu É, Morin CM. Cognitive impairment in individuals with insomnia: clinical significance and correlates. Sleep. 2014;37:1787–98.
6. Mai E, Buysse DJ. Insomnia: prevalence, impact, pathogenesis, differential diagnosis, and evaluation. Sleep Med Clin. 2008;3:167–74.
7. Sateia MJ. International classification of sleep disorders-third edition. Chest. 2014;146(5):1387–94.
8. NIH State-of-the-Science Conference Statement on manifestations and management of chronic insomnia in adults. NIH Consens State Sci Statements. 2005;22(2):1–30.
9. Morin CM, Vallières A, Ivers H. Dysfunctional Beliefs and Attitudes about Sleep (DBAS): validation of a Brief Version (DBAS-16). Sleep. 2007;30(11):1547–54.
10. Morgenthaler T, Kramer M, Alessi C, et al. Practice parameters for the psychological and behavioral treatment of insomnia: an update. An American Academy of Sleep Medicine report. Sleep. 2006;29(11):1415–9.
11. Meltzer LJ, Hiruma LS, Avis K, Montgomery-Downs H, Valentin J. Comparison of a commercial accelerometer with polysomnography and actigraphy in children and adolescents. Sleep. 2015;38(8):1323–30.
12. Chen Z, Lin M, Chen F, Lane ND, Cardone G, Wang R, Li T, Chen Y, Choudhury T, Campbell AT. Unobtrusive sleep monitoring using smartphones. In Pervasive computing technologies for healthcare (PervasiveHealth), 2013 7th International Conference on Pervasive Computing Technologies for Healthcare and Workshops, pp. 145–152. IEEE, 2013.
13. Winter C. Personal sleep monitors: do they work? 2014; Posted: 02/26/2014 8:41 am EST Updated: 04/28/2014 5:59 am EDT; http://www.huffingtonpost.com/dr-christopher-winter/sleep-tips_b_4792760.html; accessed 10/15/2015
14. Wood M. Bedtime technology for a better night's sleep. 2014; http://www.nytimes.com/2014/12/25/technology/personaltech/bedroom-technology-for-a-better-nights-sleep.html?_r=0; accessed 10/15/2015
15. Suh S, Nowakowski S, Bernert RA, Ong JC, Siebern AT, Dowdle CL, Manber R. Clinical significance of night-to-night sleep variability in insomnia. Sleep Med. 2012;13(5):469–75. Epub 2012 Feb 20.
16. Krakow B, Romero E, Ulibarri VA, Kikta S. Prospective assessment of nocturnal awakenings in a case series of treatment-seeking chronic insomnia patients: a pilot study of subjective and objective causes. Sleep. 2012;35(12):1685–92.
17. Baglioni C, Battagliese G, Feige B, et al. Insomnia as a predictor of depression: a meta-analytic evaluation of longitudinal epidemiological studies. J Affect Disord. 2011;135:10–9.
18. Goldman-Mellor S, Gregory AM, Caspi A, Harrington H, Parsons M, Poulton R, Moffitt TE. Mental health antecedents of early midlife insomnia: evidence from a four-decade longitudinal study. Sleep. 2014;37(11):1767–75.
19. Neckelmann D, Mykletun A, Dahl AA. Chronic insomnia as a risk factor for developing anxiety and depression. Sleep. 2007;30(7):873–80.
20. Manber R, Edinger JD, Gress JL, San Pedro-Salcedo MG, Kuo TF, Kalista T. Cognitive behavioral therapy for insomnia enhances depression outcome in patients with comorbid major depressive disorder and insomnia. Sleep. 2008;31:489–95.

21. Krell SB, Kapur VK. Insomnia complaints in patients evaluated for obstructive sleep apnea. Sleep Breath. 2005;9:104–10.
22. Redeker NS, Jeon S, Muench U, Campbell D, Walsleben J, Rapoport DM. Insomnia symptoms and daytime function in stable heart failure. Sleep. 2010;33(9):1210–6.
23. Allen RP, Picchietti D, Hening WA, Trenkwalder C, Walters AS, Montplaisir J. Restless legs syndrome: diagnostic criteria, special considerations, and epidemiology. A report from the restless legs syndrome diagnosis and epidemiology workshop at the National Institutes of Health. Sleep Med. 2003;4:101–19.
24. Sack RL, Auckley D, Auger RR, Carskadon MA, Wright KP, Vitiello MV, Zhdanova IV. Circadian rhythm sleep disorders: Part I, basic principles, shift work and jet lag disorders. Sleep. 2007;30(11):1460–83.
25. Taylor DJ, Mallory LJ, Lichstein KL, Durrence HH, Riedel BW, Bush AJ. Comorbidity of chronic insomnia with medical problems. Sleep. 2007;30:213–8.
26. Young JS, Bourgeois JA, Hilty DM, Hardin KA. Sleep in hospitalized medical patients, Part 1: factors affecting sleep. J Hosp Med. 2008;3:473–82. doi:10.1002/jhm.372.
27. Bartick MC, Thai X, Schmidt T, Altaye A, Solet JM. Decrease in as-needed sedative use by limiting nighttime sleep disruptions from hospital staff. J Hosp Med. 2010;5:20–4. doi:10.1002/jhm.549.

Chapter 4
Pathophysiology of Insomnia

Michael H. Bonnet and Donna L. Arand

Abstract Primary insomnia has been previously viewed first as a symptom of mental disorders and more recently as a type of behavior disorder. However, increasing evidence has shown that objective primary insomnia is associated with activation or pathology in whole body and brain metabolic systems, the cardiovascular system, and the endocrine system. Data have shown the appearance of pathophysiology prior to and leading to the development of changes in cognitive and mood function. Pathophysiology has also been shown in an animal model that suggested specific brain arousal areas impacted and treatment by modification of those brain arousal sites. Primary objective insomnia is a significant risk for important medical pathology including hypertension, diabetes, depression, and mortality. Recognition of primary insomnia as a significant medical risk means that treatment of insomnia should be directed toward measurement and reduction of this risk. Current data suggest that reduction in risk is best accomplished by increasing total sleep time above 7 h. However, research showing the success of these changes in diagnosis, treatment goals, and treatment outcomes requires significant research emphasis.

Keywords Insomnia • Sleep deprivation • Hyperarousal • Metabolic rate • Heart rate variability • Hypertension • Diabetes

Supported by the Sleep-Wake Disorders Research Institute

M.H. Bonnet, Ph.D. (✉)
Department of Neurology, Wright State Boonshoft School of Medicine, Dayton, OH, USA

Sycamore Kettering Sleep Disorders Center, Miamisburg, OH 45342, USA
e-mail: bonnetmichael@yahoo.com

D.L. Arand
Department of Neurology, Wright State Boonshoft School of Medicine, Dayton, OH, USA

© Springer International Publishing Switzerland 2017
H.P. Attarian (ed.), *Clinical Handbook of Insomnia*, Current Clinical Neurology,
DOI 10.1007/978-3-319-41400-3_4

41

Introduction

Patients with insomnia often have symptoms that include tension, anxiety, depression, fatigue, and irritability [1]. Insomnia frequently begins in conjunction with a significant stress. As a result, many investigators have hypothesized that insomnia is the result of internalization of emotions producing emotional arousal. Others have hypothesized that insomnia can develop entirely from physiological activation, as in phase-shift insomnia or use of stimulant medication. More recently, it has become evident that insomnia often begins in individuals with a physiological disposition who experience stress. This chapter examines evidence for physiological activation in patients with primary insomnia and describes research that implicates physiological activation as a key in the expression of insomnia and the medical risks associated with this abnormal physiological activation. Appropriate treatment of insomnia should be directed toward reduction in these risks.

Historical Studies of Insomnia

Following the development of modern recording methods, many studies reported comparisons of poor sleepers or insomnia patients with controls on a range of physiological measures with studies frequently showing increased rectal temperature, heart rate, basal skin resistance, frontalis and mentalis EMG, beta and less alpha frequencies in the EEG, and phasic vasoconstrictions prior to and during sleep in poor sleepers and insomnia patients. However, results were not consistent across studies. The fact that results were inconsistent was taken to indicate that either physiological activation was not a major factor in all patients [2] or that wide variability and small sample sizes may have made it difficult to show clear physiological differences. The lack of control of daytime activity in the studies might also have obscured differences. It was also possible that the involved physiological system(s) differed from patient to patient or in different classes of patients, and that more global measures, such as whole-body oxygen use, heart rate variability, or brain metabolic activity in arousal areas, would more consistently show differences. Finally, it was possible that physiological differences would be more apparent in insomnia patients who were documented to have objective decrease in total sleep time rather than those with only a subjective complaint.

Carefully controlled studies where psychophysiological insomnia patients were required to demonstrate decreased sleep time based upon EEG criteria and were carefully matched with objectively identified normal sleeping controls based on age, sex, and weight [3] began to appear about 20 years ago. Whole-body metabolic data collected for each minute across the night and for 20-min resting wake periods following MSLT across the day showed that patients with objective insomnia had significantly increased VO_2 both during sleep at night and during the day. VO_2 was also significantly increased when data associated with awakenings, movements, and arousals was eliminated, and even when only SWS was examined. Whole-body metabolic rate was also found to be significantly increased in patients with paradoxical insomnia (despite no difference in sleep stage amounts) compared with controls [4], although the difference was not as great as that seen in psychophysiological insomnia patients. These physiological findings were supported by spectral analysis of EEG that showed increased higher frequency EEG in the paradoxical insomnia patients [5].

More recently, patients with insomnia have been shown to have specific changes in brain metabolism that are consistent with their insomnia complaint. A study using positron emission tomography (PET) showed that insomnia patients had higher glucose metabolism during sleep and wakefulness. Of equal importance, insomnia patients had a smaller decrease in glucose metabolism compared with controls in arousal areas of the brain during NREM sleep [6]. The same authors have reported more recently that both subjective and objective wake time during sleep is significantly correlated with brain glucose metabolism in several pontine and thalamocortical areas [7].

Similar careful studies of patients with psychophysiological insomnia and matched normal sleepers who did not differ in age, weight, or usual time in bed at night [8] have also been done to examine heart rate and heat rate variability. Nocturnal heart data examined in 5-min blocks based upon sleep stage showed that heart rate was lower and the variability was greater in the normal Ss as compared to the insomnia patients. These results replicated higher heart rates found in a number of earlier studies [9–11]. Varkevisser more recently reported a nonsignificant 4.1 BPM increase in insomnia patients compared to normal sleepers.

These same 5-min blocks of digitized heart data were analyzed by spectral analysis to provide estimates of low-frequency and high-frequency spectral power. These data were used to construct low-frequency power (LFP) and high-frequency power (HFP) ratios that are, respectively, associated with sympathetic and parasympathetic nervous system activity. LFP was significantly increased and HFP was significantly decreased in insomnia patients as compared to normals across all sleep stages.

Other research has examined daytime function in insomnia patients to verify their subjectively reported deficits in performance, mood, and alertness. The cumulative partial sleep deprivation assumed to occur in chronic insomnia should produce daytime sleepiness or increased susceptibility to acute sleep loss in insomnia patients. However, studies consistently found that these patients were not sleepier than normal controls on multiple sleep latency tests (MSLT) and actually had longer MSLT latencies (see review in [12]). Studies did find that insomnia patients made more errors on a line tracing task, produced fewer responses in a word category test, or performed worse on the Romberg (balance) test, but these results may be viewed as demonstrating that patients have poor performance on tests where too much arousal reduces steadiness or blocks higher order associates. Studies comparing daytime performance in insomnia patients to normal controls generally did not find differences on tests that are sensitive to sleep loss [13]. Based upon these results and patient reports that they were fatigued or "washed out" during the day, it was hypothesized that standard sleep and sleep loss tests were confounded in that they "simultaneously measure sleep need and hyperarousal, which is interfering with sleep onset" ([14], p. 59).

In addition to the traditional MSLT, numerous studies have shown significant positive correlations between physiological activation and sleep variables, usually measured by heart rate and sleep latency [15–17]. Studies have shown that sleep latency is reliably increased for up to 90 min in normal young adults after brief physiological arousal (5 min of normal walking) and that increases in MSLT are paralleled by increased heart rate [18, 19]. Patients with insomnia tested in this model had significantly longer sleep latencies than normals after rest (10.5 vs. 6.7 min), after a brief walk to produce state arousal (16.2 vs. 13.0 min), and after the walk compared to their own resting baseline [17]. The implication is that the insomnia patients have chronic increased physiological activation accounting for the resting differences in sleep latency but also continue to respond with additional state physiological activation that produces a further increase in sleep latency after a walk. These sleep latency results were corroborated by heart rate, which increased from 59 bpm at rest to 62 bpm at the beginning of the MSLT after activity in the normals while increasing from 63 to 65 bpm in the insomnia patients in the same conditions. These studies directly support the concept of elevated trait physiological arousal directly associated with sleep latency in daytime naps in the insomnia patients.

Modeling Studies of Insomnia and Physiological Activation

In addition to poor sleep, it has been established that many patients with insomnia will (a) report daytime fatigue or dysphoria; (b) have normal or longer than normal MSLT values; (c) report increased stress; (d) have abnormal Minnesota Multiphasic Personality Inventory (MMPI) values; and (e) subjectively misperceive their sleep process. These findings are summarized in Table 4.1 (left column).

Because insomnia patients typically display both mood alteration and evidence of physiological activation, differentiation of cognitive versus physiological pathology as the primary causal factor has been difficult. Production of consistent and long-lasting mood changes in normal individuals to test the effect of mood change on sleep and daytime function is difficult. However, it is possible to produce a state of chronic physiological activation and to follow these hyperaroused normals for the development of both nocturnal and daytime symptoms of insomnia.

Caffeine 400 mg TID was given to 12 normal young adult sleepers for a week as a means of increasing physiological arousal [20], and standard insomnia outcome variables were measured. As expected, the chronic use of caffeine significantly increased whole-body metabolic rate, which was used as the objective measure of arousal level, and sleep efficiency was found to decline significantly. Responses from the Profile of Mood States (POMS) suggested increasing dysphoria as caffeine administration progressed (see Table 4.1, center column, for a summary of caffeine effects). Initial caffeine administration produced an immediate significant increase in vigor and tension (anxiety) followed by a decrease as caffeine administration

Table 4.1 Variables that differentiate insomnia patients versus normal sleepers given caffeine 400 mg TID or the sleep on an insomnia patient. Data from normal sleepers who had situational insomnia are also reported

	True insomnia	Hyperaroused normals	"Yoke" insomnia normals	Situational insomnia
MSLT	Increased	Increased[a]	Decreased[b]	Increased[c]
Metabolic rate	Increased	Increased[a]	Increase PM[b] Decrease AM	No difference
Heart rate	Increased	Not measured	Not measured	Increased[c]
Body temperature	Increased	Increased	Decreased[b]	Not measured
Mood (tension, confusion)	Increased	Increased[a]	Decreased[b]	No change
Mood (vigor)	Decreased	Decreased[a]	Decreased[b]	No change
Personality disturbance	Increased	Increased MMPI PT	No change	No change
Subjective sleep Latency/wake	Overestimated	Mild overestimation	No change	No change

[a]Significant differences reported in [20]
[b]Significant differences reported in [21]
[c]Significant differences reported in [28]

continued (significant for vigor). Fatigue was significantly increased at the end of caffeine administration compared to placebo. These results were of interest because they showed that the chronic daytime dysphoria and fatigue reported by insomnia patients could be paradoxically produced by unrelenting physiological arousal.

The MSLT data revealed that sleep latencies were significantly increased throughout caffeine administration as compared to baseline and withdrawal, which did not differ. The mean latency after early caffeine use was significantly longer than the latency after chronic caffeine use. Respective means for baseline, early caffeine, late caffeine, and withdrawal were 10.7, 17.9, 13.4, and 11.3 min. Again, these increased sleep latencies were similar to those seen in insomnia patients rather than normals.

The MMPI is a nontransparent measure of relatively stable personality characteristics. At baseline, as expected, all of the MMPI values were characteristic of normal young adults. However, after a week of caffeine administration, there was movement toward increased pathology on all the clinical scales except MF, and the change was statistically significant for the PT (anxiety) scale. These findings indicated that even stable aspects of personality could shift significantly towards pathology in a short time secondary to relatively simple physiological activation.

As can be seen from Table 4.1, Ss given caffeine had significant changes in the direction of chronic insomnia patients on MSLT, metabolic rate, negative moods, and personality. The data indicate that chronic hyperarousal with no predisposing psychological component produced the typical pattern of poor sleep, mood change, and personality change commonly seen in patients with psychophysiologic insomnia. However, it could not be determined from this data if the mood and personality symptoms were produced by the hyperarousal or secondarily from the poor sleep that was also produced.

The Effects of Poor Sleep

It has been implied that increased physiological arousal, possibly even as an innate phenomenon, produces an environment in which an individual is prone to report insomnia. Many insomnia patients, however, feel that their sleep is the central problem and that the poor sleep leads to their symptoms of fatigue and dysphoria. To test whether the insomnia sleep pattern by itself could produce hyperarousal and the other symptoms of primary insomnia, the poor sleep found in insomnia patients was produced for a week in normal young adults, and subjects were followed for the development of insomnia symptoms [21]. Primary insomnia patients were identified by the standard sleep criteria mentioned earlier, and the sleep parameters of those patients were used in a yoke-control fashion to produce comparable sleep in a group of matched normal sleepers. It was hypothesized that if the yoked normal sleepers developed the spectrum of secondary symptoms seen in the "true" insomnia patients after sleeping like the patients, then those symptoms could be seen as secondary to the poor sleep. On the other hand, if the yoked normal sleepers did not develop the symptoms seen in the "true" insomnia patients, then some factor other than poor sleep itself would be responsible for those secondary symptoms.

In this study, the EEG sleep characteristics of primary insomnia patients were reproduced in matched normal sleepers for a week. Sleep patterns were matched by making experimental arousals and awakenings throughout the night in normal sleepers to match the pattern of wake time and arousals seen in the patients with insomnia. Since the EEG sleep produced in the study was similar to that found in patients reporting insomnia, changes in the outcome variables should have reflected the consequences of pure "insomnia" sleep. Table 4.1 provides a summary of typical findings in patients with insomnia and compares those findings with the results of this yoke-control study (right column). Changes secondary to the poor sleep produced in the yoke-control study were clearly different from the symptoms most frequently reported by insomnia patients. Insomnia patients typically have difficulty falling asleep both at night and during the MSLT. However, both sleep latency and MSLT data from the yoke-control study supported significantly increasing ease of falling asleep as the nights of insomnia increased. Insomnia patients frequently have elevated body temperature and whole-body metabolic rate. Except for an increase in nocturnal metabolic rate probably associated with the experimental sleep disturbance itself [22], the trends in the yoke-control study showed lower metabolic rate and decreased body temperature during the day (both of these are increased in insomnia patients). Insomnia patients typically report increased stress, anxiety, or depression. However, in the yoke-control study, the state measures of tension and depression decreased significantly during the study. Insomnia patients typically have elevated MMPI scales, but the MMPI measures were unchanged in this study. Insomnia patients report increased fatigue and decreased vigor, and similar changes were found in the yoke-control study. However, these changes are also found during simple sleep deprivation. Finally, insomnia patients overestimate their time spent awake during the night. Despite increased awakenings and wake time in the yoke-control study, the normal sleepers continued to estimate their wake time during the night correctly.

The most parsimonious explanation for the results was that the insomnia sleep pattern resulted only in partial sleep deprivation when imposed upon normal sleepers. This interpretation is supported by rebounds of REM and SWS during the recovery night after the seven nights of yoke-insomnia along with decreasing MSLT values. These changes are classic signs of sleep loss. Decreases in vigor and body temperature also suggested simple sleep loss. Since total sleep time in the study was reduced to 6 h for a week, this could easily have resulted in partial sleep deprivation. For example, a study by Rosenthal et al. [23] has shown increased sleepiness on the MSLT after just one night of 5.6 h of sleep.

The data from this study showing that normal sleepers with the insomnia sleep pattern became sleepier suggest that some patients with insomnia may suffer from mild partial sleep deprivation. As in normal subjects, however, the degree of deficit should be related to the amount of sleep lost and should typically recover after an occasional night of improved sleep. In fact, one could hypothesize that poor sleep in response to hyperarousal is an adaptive response that acts as a homeostatic mechanism to cause partial sleep deprivation and reduce the impact of hyperarousal. Unfortunately, in patients with chronic insomnia, a night of relatively good sleep would remove a portion of the chronic partial sleep deprivation and leave the patient more susceptible to the effect of hyperarousal on the next day. This situation leaves patients in the uncomfortable situation of either suffering from hyperarousal or from hyperarousal masked by sleep deprivation.

If the poor sleep of insomnia patients produces only mild sleep loss in matched normal sleepers, how does one explain the consistent secondary symptoms reported by insomnia patients? As can be seen from Table 4.1, the secondary symptoms of insomnia patients appear in normal sleepers who are hyperaroused [20] but not in normal sleepers actually given the poor sleep experienced by patients with insomnia. The major implication of such data is that it is the increased arousal and not the poor sleep per se that is responsible for the symptoms. Another possibility is that the development of these insomnia symptoms in patients is actually dependent upon poor sleep interacting with personality variables in the insomnia patient. If this is the case, then one would expect that insomnia patients having particularly poor nights of sleep would experience an exacerbation of their insomnia symptoms.

Poor Sleep in Insomnia Patients

In a following study [24], it was hypothesized that if nocturnal sleep parameters produced the daytime dysphoria reported by patients with insomnia, then sleep maintenance insomnia patients who were kept awake even longer than usual during the night should have had increased dysphoria during the following day. To test this hypothesis, patients with sleep maintenance insomnia were allowed only 80 % of their already reduced total sleep each night for seven consecutive nights. This sleep reduction was accomplished by waking patients at the end of each quarter of the night if they accumulated more than 80 % of their baseline sleep for that quarter of the night (while holding time in bed for the entire night at the baseline level). This paradigm produced very poor sleep (average total sleep of 4.2 h on each night for the week).

This reduction of total sleep time by experimental awakenings resulted in a significant decrease in daytime MSLT values in these insomnia patients. After seven nights of 4.2 h of sleep, MSLT values had decreased from 15.6 to 11.1 min. While this reduction was statistically significant, the 11.1-min value was still within the normal range for the MSLT. In comparison, when total sleep was reduced to 5 h per night in normal young adults [25], sleep latency on the MSLT was reduced to 41 % of baseline compared to a reduction to 71 % of baseline in our insomnia patients. These results indicated that while the insomnia patients did show a small increase in sleepiness after sleep restriction, the change was not consistent with the change in normal sleepers after similar sleep restriction. In fact, the insomnia patients did not become pathologically sleepy on the MSLT, and this probably indicated the degree to which their hyperarousal was successful in masking their sleep tendency. Of equal interest, patients did not report significant decreases in their sleep quality or show changes in their personality or physiological parameters consistent with more severe insomnia when their wake time during the night was increased by 2 h. One conclusion from such data is that the reports of poor sleep quality and daytime dysphoria from insomnia patients are not directly related to their EEG sleep at all but rather to their level of arousal [26]. In support of these results, Chambers and Kim [27] reported a significant negative correlation between state anxiety at bedtime and reports of feeling rested the next day in insomnia patients despite the fact that neither anxiety nor reports of feeling rested were significantly correlated with sleep values.

The Development of Insomnia

It is well known that the incidence of insomnia increases with age. This increase could be associated with increasing sympathetic nervous system dominance that is also associated with age, or the increased insomnia could be associated with cognitive or behavioral changes. Unfortunately, little empirical work has examined how insomnia starts or develops. One theory holds that individuals placed in a situation of temporary stress develop poor sleep hygiene or inappropriate conditioned responses to their sleep environment. Then, the poor hygiene or inappropriate responses continue to produce poor sleep after the period of stress passes.

One study exposed 50 normal young adults to a series of stressful experiences including first night in a sleep laboratory, 3-h phase advance of sleep time, 6-h advance of sleep time, and sleep following administration of caffeine 400 mg 30 min prior to bedtime [28] to look at individual responses to temporary stress.

It was found that some Ss continued to have nearly normal nights of sleep even after a 6-h phase advance of bedtime or significant caffeine while other Ss had poor sleep following all of the stresses. A large number of Ss participated in this study so that it was possible to form "extreme" groups—in this case the 25 % of the population that slept best on the first night in the laboratory (good sleepers) and the 25 % who had the worst sleep on that night (situational insomnia). Subjects who had poor sleep on their laboratory adaptation night (and were therefore called the "situational insomnia" or SI group) also had increased MSLT latencies on the day that followed. They then had normal sleep on the baseline night that followed (adaptation to the first-night stress) but then had significantly worse sleep on the phase advance nights and after caffeine administration. The SI group also had very poor sleep after caffeine administration but surprisingly, their MSLT after caffeine administration was significantly increased. The good-sleep group did not have any significant changes in their MSLT throughout the study. The implication is that the SI group was both more sensitive to all of the stresses in terms of the production of poor sleep and more sensitive to the arousing effect of caffeine.

This study also examined other differences between the SI and good-sleeping groups (see Table 4.1, far right column). No significant differences were found on the MMPI or mood measures. Whole-body metabolic rate was nonsignificantly increased in the SI group. The SI group was found to have increased heart rate, increased low-frequency EKG spectral power, and decreased high-frequency EKG spectral power compared to the good sleepers. These physiological findings in "pre-insomnia" patients suggest that their existing hyper-reactivity to sleep-related stress and caffeine could be secondary to elevated sympathetic nervous system activity and that this could be a marker for the development of chronic insomnia at a later date. The finding of elevated physiological activity prior to mood change, personality change, or complaint of chronic insomnia provides another clue that underlying physiology could also be the key to the later development of psychological and behavioral insomnia symptoms.

A recent animal study has taken this approach of producing situational insomnia a step further. In this study, male rats were placed in a cage previously occupied by a male rat, which produces a stress response (anticipating the return of an outsider) [29] to produce an acute stress response. Rats exposed to this stress took longer to fall asleep (59 min vs. 32 min in controls) and had increased wakefulness during sleep. The rats were sacrificed 5.5 h later, and Fos expression was found to be significantly elevated in the cerebral cortex, limbic system, and parts of the arousal (specifically locus coeruleus) and autonomic systems compared with controls. However, Fos expression was also found in the sleep-promoting areas of the brain. These dual findings suggested that the rats were showing "simultaneous activation of the sleep and arousal systems" [29] (p. 10173). Other data showed that lesions in the limbic system or arousal system at the identified sites of similarly stressed rates were associated with improved sleep. The finding of activation in brain sleep centers is an indicator that the poor sleep was not secondary to reduced drive for sleep but rather to abnormal activation in arousal systems when sleep was attempted. Human physiology is different from the rat, but this study shows the value of an animal model for understanding the neurophysiological impact of insomnia, identifying sites of arousal/activation and the potential for development of agents to target specific brain arousal sites.

Altered regional brain function has also been found in human neuroimaging studies. Initial studies showed that primary insomnia patients had less decline in metabolism during sleep in the reticular system, hypothalamus, thalamus, insular cortex, amygdala, and hippocampus compared with controls. This suggested increased general arousal and increased activity in the "emotional arousal areas" of the brain [6]. In another study, positive correlations between wake time during sleep and brain metabolic rate in areas associated with emotion were found [7]. In addition, treatment with eszopiclone in primary insomnia patients reduced NREM metabolism in brainstem arousal centers, thalamus, and parietal cortex [30]. Other studies have shown reduced GABA in insomnia patients [31] (and see review in [32]). Inconsistent changes have been reported in hippocampal volume [32], and more consistent reductions have been seen in gray matter in the left orbitofrontal cortex [32].

Medical Implications of These Physiological Arousal Data

Recent reviews have summarized the current knowledge of significant alterations in cardiac measures, hormone measures, metabolic measures, and EEG measures seen in patients with insomnia as compared with controls [12, 33]. However, of more importance, recent work has also begun to show how the abnormal arousal associated with insomnia is related to specific medical risk.

Elevated Blood Pressure/Hypertension

It would be expected that increased sympathetic activation in insomnia patients associated with increased heart rate and altered heart rate variability would also have an impact on blood pressure. Lanfranchi et al. [34] documented significantly higher systolic blood pressure and decreased systolic pressure dipping across the night in primary insomnia patients compared with controls. The difference in systolic blood pressure of 9 mmHg was significant despite the fact that there were no sleep-stage differences between the groups. This suggests that it was not differences in EEG sleep, such as increased wake time or arousals, that caused the blood pressure difference. It also suggests that nocturnal blood pressure could be even more abnormal in insomnia patients with objective sleep deficits.

Many studies have shown an association between insomnia and elevated cardiovascular risk (see meta-analysis by Schwartz et al.) [35]. In a large study including PSG recordings, Vgontzas et al. [36] have shown an elevated risk for hypertension in patients with insomnia who also slept for 6 h or less on their PSG but not for insomnia patients who slept more than 6 h on their PSG or normal subjects who slept less than 5 h on their PSG. The most significant hypertension risk was in insomnia patients with a PSG sleep time of 5 h or less. These data show that hypertension risk increases as PSG total sleep time decreases in patients with insomnia. This study was the first to suggest that medical risk for insomnia patients is dependent upon the severity of the insomnia [36]. It is also one of few studies to classify severity of insomnia based upon an objective measure of total sleep time. Risk data such as these suggest for the first time that the major goal for the treatment of insomnia should be directed toward reduction in medical risk and that the appropriate mechanism is by increasing total sleep time above set amounts, such as 7 h per night. One study in patients with treated hypertension showed that many continued to have poor sleep and a non-dipping blood pressure pattern at night. The abnormal non-dipping blood pressure (and sleep) was significantly improved when patients with poor sleep were treated with zolpidem 10 mg at bed time [37].

Glycemic Control/Diabetes

Several studies have shown an association between insomnia and elevated diabetes risk (see review in [38]). Patients with diabetes and insomnia have elevated insulin, IP-10, and leptin compared with diabetes patients without insomnia [39]. Vgontzas et al. [40] found that patients with objective insomnia who slept 6 h or less were at increased risk for diabetes while patients with insomnia who slept for more than 6 h were not. Normal sleepers who slept less than 5 h in the lab were not at risk. Again, the data consistently suggest that the risk for diabetes or abnormal glycemic control increases as insomnia severity increases, as measured by complaint of insomnia and total sleep time reduction, and these are both necessary for the increased risk. Treatment with 2 mg of prolonged-release melatonin administered to type 2 diabetes patients with subjective insomnia significantly improved sleep efficiency and glycemic control as measured by HbA1c [41].

Depression

Insomnia is known to be a strong predictor for the later development of depression, as shown in a recent meta-analysis [42]. One study that included both PSG and subjective data in a sample of 711 patients with depression found that 73% of patients reported insomnia symptoms and concluded that objectively measured prolonged sleep latency and short sleep duration independently or in conjunction with subjective insomnia were risk factors for poor depression treatment outcome [43]. Another study with PSG data from a large sample has shown that the odds of developing depression 7.5 years after PSG were highest (also significant) based upon short sleep time at baseline [44]. Persistence of insomnia and worsening of poor sleep into insomnia also significantly increased the odds of depression at follow-up [44]. Several studies have also shown that concomitant treatment of insomnia and depression results in both improved sleep and a more rapid clinical response with lower doses of antidepressant medication compared with only antidepressant therapy [45, 46].

Immune Function

Reduced sleep impacts the immune system. Two studies have directly examined immunity in primary insomnia patients and controls and have shown significant decreases in the numbers of CD3+,CD4+ and CD8+ T cells [47] and with reduced NK-cell responses [48] in patients compared with controls. Other large studies have shown a relationship between poor sleep and infection, specifically upper respiratory infection [49], response to viral challenge [50], and pneumonia risk [51]. However, insomnia treatment studies to examine improvement in immune function with increased total sleep have not been done.

Mortality

Questionnaire studies looking for links between insomnia and mortality have been inconsistent (see review in [38]). Three recent studies found an increased risk for all-cause death for patients reporting nearly everyday insomnia [52]; decreased survival for patients with insomnia and COPD [53]; and increased mortality within a year of inpatient re-habilitation in relation to Pittsburgh Sleep Quality Index scores [54]. Unfortunately, all studies were limited by inability to actually diagnose insomnia or differentiate it from poor sleep caused by other sleep disorders. A large-scale PSG study [55] that controlled for sleep-disordered breathing (and age, race, education, BMI, smoking status, alcohol-use depression, hypertension, and diabetes) showed a significantly increased risk of mortality in males with insomnia with objective sleep time of less than 6 h, but not for males with insomnia who slept longer or normal males who slept less than 5 h. A recent study examined risk of mortality at a 20-year follow-up from patients earlier classified as having no insomnia, intermittent insomnia, or persistent insomnia and found an increased risk of all-cause mortality and specific cardiopulmonary mortality in patients who had earlier reported persistent insomnia [56]. These latter patients also had higher CRP levels at baseline and a more rapid increase in CRP over time indicating a possible role for inflammation in the development of cardiopulmonary diseases [56]. Another study has shown that CBTI without sleep restriction was associated with reduced risk of a high CRP level [57].

Discussion

It is generally accepted that there are changes in several physiological systems in association with primary insomnia. Current research has attempted to refine our understanding of the relationship between physiological arousal, poor EEG sleep, psychological status, and subjective report of insomnia. The finding that experimentally produced chronic physiological arousal in normal young adults produces the mood and personality changes seen in insomnia patients provides a compelling description of how chronic insomnia could develop in physiologically susceptible individuals. The studies showing that the poor sleep of insomnia patients by itself does not produce the arousal, mood, and personality characteristics of patients and that the production of much worse EEG sleep in insomnia patients does not magnify symptoms lead to the conclusions that (1) the symptoms produced by chronic physiological arousal were not mediated by the poor sleep that was produced and (2) the symptom complex that was associated with psychophysiological insomnia is not really a sleep disorder but rather an arousal disorder. Finally, the importance of physiological arousal as the harbinger of insomnia was enhanced by the finding of elevated heart rate and cardiac spectral activity in normal subjects with no sleep complaint who were found to have EEG-defined situational insomnia and specific physiological activation. These data have been extended by rat studies identifying activation in specific brain sites during sleep. These research findings have set the stage for our current understanding of insomnia as a physiological hyperarousal disorder that increases the risk for significant medical sequelae.

We have recognized for many years that some patients have lifelong problems with excessive sleepiness secondary to disorders such as narcolepsy or idiopathic hypersomnolence. The extent to which these disorders demonstrate a failure of the sleep system versus a failure of the arousal system can be debated. Certainly, these disorders are commonly treated with medications that have direct impact by increasing CNS arousal. Recognition that another group of patients suffer from the opposite lifelong problem (hyposomnolence or hyperarousal) has been more difficult. At this point, much work has identified the physiological markers of chronic hyperarousal in insomnia patients. What is left is changing how we identify insomnia and choose our treatment goals.

Insomnia has always been diagnosed based upon subjective report of long sleep latency or increased wake time during sleep. Treatment has always been directed toward improving these subjective symptoms. Unfortunately, symptomatic relief may not always offer sufficient treatment for the real medical risks associated with insomnia. For example, sleep restriction therapy, which has strong efficacy because it significantly reduces time in bed and total sleep time with the goal of improving sleep latency and sleep efficiency, does produce sleepiness and degraded performance [58] and may also increase medical risks associated with further reduction in objective total sleep time in insomnia patients [59].

Recent findings of an association of insomnia with risk of significant medical consequences and specifically a dose–response relationship between objective total sleep time and risk for hypertension, diabetes, depression, and mortality for the first time provide empirical support that insomnia should be identified based upon objective total sleep time and treated specifically to increase objective total sleep time above 7 h per night because sleeping for 7 h or longer, even with a patient complaint of poor sleep, was not associated with increased risk of significant medical consequences. Important data showing that improvement of objective total sleep time above specific cutoffs actually results in reduced risk of medical consequences remain to be shown conclusively, although studies do support increased total sleep time in some areas [38, 57]. However, the association of insomnia, defined as short objective total sleep time, with medical consequences is not surprising in light of large accumulating knowledge that partial sleep deprivation for only a few days in normal individuals is associated with significant movement toward medical pathology in several dimensions including hypertension, glycemic control, hormone levels (particularly leptin, ghrelin, and cortisol), inflammation, and immune function (see [59] for review).

A recent review [38] suggests that an insomnia consult needs to look much more like a primary care consult. Medical history including measurement and history of blood pressure and a number of clinical values including thyroid levels, blood chemistry, CRP, HbA1c, and CRP are needed. A measure of objective total sleep time can provide a baseline and determine the level of risk. Treatment directed to increase objective total sleep time should reduce risk, and follow-up measurement of objective sleep and clinical lab results should show improvement in medical risk areas. Periodic review of objective sleep times with yearly clinical labs would support continuing clinical efficacy of treatment.

Diagnosis and treatment of insomnia have often been neglected, and many patients have not received diagnosis or treatment because the risk associated with reported long sleep latency or wake during sleep did not seem as great as the potential risks of treatment with hypnotics. Understanding the physiological basis of insomnia and the resulting multiple medical risks fundamentally changes our understanding of this disorder. Appropriate treatment holds the potential to reduce risk in several core clinical areas and changes the risk/benefit ratio so that identification and treatment of insomnia at the primary care level is now an important goal.

References

1. Kales JD, Kales A, Bixler EO, Soldatos CR, Cadieux RJ, Kashurba GJ, et al. Biopsychobehavioral correlates of insomnia, V: clinical characteristics and behavioral correlates. Am J Psychiatry. 1984;141(11):1371–6.
2. Borkovec TD. Insomnia. J Cons Clin Psychol. 1982;50(6):880–95.
3. Bonnet MH, Arand DL. 24-Hour metabolic rate in insomniacs and matched normal sleepers. Sleep. 1995;18:581–8.
4. Bonnet MH, Arand DL. Physiological activation in patients with sleep state misperception. Psychosomatic Med. 1997;59:533–40.
5. Ad K, Edinger JD, Wohlgemuth WK, March GR. Non-REM sleep EEG frequency spectral correlates of sleep complaints in primary insomnia subtypes. Sleep. 2002;25:630–40.
6. Nofzinger EA, Buysse DJ, Germain A, Price JC, Miewald JM, Kupfer DJ. Functional neuroimaging evidence for hyperarousal in insomnia. Am J Psychiatry. 2004;161(11):2126–8.
7. Nofzinger EA, Nissen C, Germain A, Moul D, Hall M, Price JC, et al. Regional cerebral metabolic correlates of WASO during NREM sleep in insomnia. J Clin Sleep Med. 2006;2(3):316–22.
8. Bonnet MH, Arand DL. Heart rate variability in insomniacs and matched normal sleepers. Psychosomatic Med. 1998;60:610–5.
9. Monroe LJ. Psychological and physiological differences between good and poor sleepers. J Abnorm Psychol. 1967;72:255–64.

10. Stepanski E, Glinn M, Zorick F, Roehrs T, Roth T. Heart rate changes in chronic insomnia. Stress Med. 1994;10:261–6.
11. Haynes SN, Adams A, Franzen M. The effects of presleep stress on sleep-onset insomnia. J Abnorm Psychol. 1981;90(6):601–6.
12. Bonnet MH, Arand DL. Hyperarousal and insomnia: state of the science. Sleep Med Rev. 2010;14:9–15.
13. Mendelson WB, Garnett D, Linnoila M. Do insomniacs have impaired daytime functioning? Biol Psychiatry. 1984;19(8):1261–4.
14. Stepanski E, Zorick F, Roehrs T, Young D, Roth T. Daytime alertness in patients with chronic insomnia compared with asymptomatic control subjects. Sleep. 1988;11(1):54–60.
15. Johns MW, Thornton C, Dore C. Heart rate and sleep latency in young men. J Psychosom Med. 1976;20:549–53.
16. Bonnet MH, Arand DL. The use of lorazepam TID for chronic insomnia. Int Clin Psychopharmacol. 1999;14:81–90.
17. Bonnet MH, Arand DL. Activity, arousal, and the MSLT in patients with insomnia. Sleep. 2000;23(2):205–12.
18. Bonnet MH, Arand DL. Sleepiness as measured by the MSLT varies as a function of preceding activity. Sleep. 1998;21(5):477–83.
19. Bonnet MH, Arand DL. Sleep latency testing as a time course measure of state arousal. J Sleep Res. 2005;14:387–92.
20. Bonnet MH, Arand DL. Caffeine use as a model of acute and chronic insomnia. Sleep. 1992;15:526–36.
21. Bonnet MH, Arand DL. The consequences of a week of insomnia. Sleep. 1996;19:453–61.
22. Bonnet MH, Berry RB, Arand DL. Metabolism during normal sleep, fragmented sleep, and recovery sleep. J Appl Physiol. 1991;71:1112–8.
23. Rosenthal L, Roehrs TA, Rosen A, Roth T. Level of sleepiness and total sleep time following various time in bed conditions. Sleep. 1993;16:226–32.
24. Bonnet MH, Arand DL. The consequences of a week of insomnia II: patients with insomnia. Sleep. 1998;21:359–78.
25. Carskadon MA, Dement WC. Cumulative effects of sleep restriction on daytime sleepiness. Psychophysiology. 1981;18:107–13.
26. Bonnet MH. The perception of sleep onset in normals and insomniacs. In: Bootzin R, Kihlstrom J, Schacter D, editors. Sleep and cognition. Washington, DC: American Psychological Association; 1990. p. 148–59.
27. Chambers MJ, Kim JY. The role of state-trait anxiety in insomnia and daytime restedness. Behav Med. 1993;19:42–6.
28. Bonnet MH, Arand DL. Situational insomnia: consistency, predictors, and outcomes. Sleep. 2003;26:1029–36.
29. Cano G, Mochizuki T, Saper CB. Neural circuitry of stress-induced insomnia in rats. J Neurosci. 2008;28(40):10167–84.
30. Nofzinger E, Buysse D, Moul D, Hall M, Germain A, Julie P. Eszopiclone reverses brain hyperarousal in insomnia: evidence from [18]-FDG PET. Sleep. 2008;31(abstract):A232.
31. Winkelman JW, Buxton OM, Jensen JE, Benson KL, O'Connor SP, Wang W, et al. Reduced brain GABA in primary insomnia: preliminary data from 4T proton magnetic resonance spectroscopy (1H-MRS). Sleep. 2008;31(11):1499–506.
32. Spiegelhalder K, Regen W, Baglioni C, Riemann D, Winkelman J. Neuroimaging studies in insomnia. Curr Psychiatry Rep. 2013;15:405.
33. Riemann D, Spiegelhalder K, Feige B, Voderholzer U, Berger M, Perlis M, et al. The hyperarousal model of insomnia: a review of the concept and its evidence. Sleep Med Rev. 2010;14(1):19–31.
34. Lanfranchi PA, Pennestri M, Fradette L, Dumont M, Morin CM, Montplaisir J. Nighttime blood pressure in normotensive subjects with chronic insomnia: implications for cardiovascular risk. Sleep. 2009;32:760–6.

35. Schwartz S, Anderson WM, Cole SR, Cornoni-Huntley J, Hays JC, Blazer D. Insomnia and heart disease: a review of epidemiologic studies. J Psychosom Res. 1999;47:313–33.
36. Vgontzas AN, Liao D, Bixler EO, Chrousos GP, Vela-Bueno A. Insomnia with objective short sleep duration is associated with a high risk for hypertension. Sleep. 2009;32:491–7.
37. Huang Y, Mai W, Cai X, Hu Y, Song Y, Qiu R, et al. The effect of zolpidem on sleep quality, stress status, and nondipping hypertension. Sleep Med. 2012;13(3):263–8.
38. Bonnet M, Burton G, Arand D. Physiological and medical findings in insomnia: implications for diagnosis and care. Sleep Med Rev. 2014;18:111–22.
39. Jain S, Kahlon G, Morehead L, Lieblong B, Stapleton T, Hoeldtke R, et al. The effect of sleep apnea and insomnia on blood levels of leptin, insulin resistance, IP-10, and hydrogen sulfide in type 2 diabetic patients. Metab Syndr Relat Disord. 2012;10:331–6.
40. Vgontzas AN, Liao D, Pejovic S, Calhoun S, Karataraki M, Bixler EO. Insomnia with objective short sleep duration is associated with type 2 diabetes: a population-based study. Diabetes Care. 2009;32:1980–5.
41. Garfinkel D, Zorin M, Wainstein J, Matas Z, Laudon M, Zisapel N. Efficacy and safety of prolonged-release melatonin in insomnia patients with diabetes: a randomized, double-blind, crossover study. Diabetes Metab Syndr Obes. 2011;4:307–13.
42. Baglioni C, Battagliese G, Feige B, Spiegelhalder K, Nissen C, Voderholzer U, et al. Insomnia as a predictor of depression: a meta-analytic evaluation of longitudinal epidemiological studies. J Affect Disord. 2011;135:10–9.
43. Troxel W, Kupfer D, Reynolds C, Frank E, Thase M, Miewald J, et al. Insomnia and objectively measured sleep disturbances predict treatment outcome in depressed patients treated with psychotherapy or psychotherapy-pharmacotherapy combinations. J Clin Psychiatry. 2012;73:478–85.
44. Fernandez-Mendoza J, Shea S, Vgontzas A, Calhoun S, Liao D, Bixler E. Insomnia and incident depression: role of objective sleep duration and natural history. J Sleep Res. 2015;24:390–8.
45. Fava M, McCall WV, Krystal A, Wessel T, Rubens R, Caron J, et al. Eszopiclone co-administered with fluoxetine in patients with insomnia coexisting with major depressive disorder. Biol Psychiatry. 2006;59:1052–60.
46. Riemann D, Participants W. Does effective management of sleep disorders reduce depressive symptoms and the risk of depression? Drugs. 2009;69 Suppl 2:43–64.
47. Savard J, Laroche L, Simard S, Ivers H, Morin CM. Chronic insomnia and immune functioning. Psychosom Med. 2003;65:211–21.
48. Irwin M, Clark C, Kennedy B, Gillin CJ, Ziegler M. Nocturnal catecholamines and immune function in insomniacs, depressed patients, and control subjects. Brain Behav Immun. 2003;17:365–72.
49. Cohen S, Doyle W, Skoner D, Rabin B, Gwaltney JJ. Social ties and susceptibility to the common cold. JAMA. 1997;277:1940–4.
50. Cohen S, Doyle W, Alper C, Janicki-Deverts D, Turner R. Sleep habits and susceptibility to the common cold. Arch Intern Med. 2009;169:62–7.
51. Patel S, Malhotra A, Gao X, Hu F, Neuman M, Fawzi WW. A prospective study of sleep duration and pneumonia risk in women. Sleep. 2012;35:97–101.
52. Chien K, Chen P, Hsu H, Su T, Sung F, Chen M, et al. Habitual sleep duration and insomnia and the risk of cardiovascular events and all-cause death: report from a community-based cohort. Sleep. 2010;33:177–84.
53. Omachi T, Blanc P, Claman D, Chen H, Yelin E, Julian L, et al. Disturbed sleep among COPD patients is longitudinally associated with mortality and adverse COPD outcomes. Sleep Med. 2012;13:476–83.
54. Martin J, Fiorentino L, Jouldjian S, Mitchell M, Josephson K, Alessi C. Poor self-reported sleep quality predicts mortality within one year of inpatient post-acute rehabilitation among older adults. Sleep. 2011;34:1715–21.
55. Vgontzas AN, Liao D, Pejovic S, Calhoun S, Karataraki M, Basta M, et al. Insomnia with short sleep duration and mortality: the Penn State cohort. Sleep. 2010;33(9):1159–64.

56. Parthasarathy S, Vasquez M, Halonen M, Bootzin R, Quan S, Martinez F, et al. Persistent insomnia is associated with mortality risk. Am J Med. 2015;128(3):268–75.
57. Carroll J, Seeman T, Olmstead R, Melendez G, Sadakane R, Bootzin R, et al. Improved sleep quality in older adults with insomnia reduces biomarkers of disease risk: pilot results from a randomized controlled comparative efficacy trial. Psychoneuroendocrinology. 2015;55:184–92.
58. Kyle S, Miller C, Rogers Z, Siriwardena A, MacMahon K, Espie C. Sleep restriction therapy for insomnia is associated with reduced objective total sleep time, increased daytime somnolence, and objectively-impaired vigilance: implications for the clinical management of insomnia disorder. Sleep. 2014;37:229–37.
59. Bonnet MH, Arand DL. The implications of sleep restriction research for insomnia diagnosis and treatment. In: Winston T, editor. Handbook on burnout and sleep deprivation. Hauppauge, NY: Nova; 2015. p. 1–28.

Chapter 5
Prognosis and Complications

Ramadevi Gourineni

Abstract Chronic insomnia is a persistent disorder with periods of remissions and relapses. Persistence rates vary between 40 and 75 % over 1–20 years and are higher in women and older adults. Initial insomnia severity can predict the longitudinal course of this disorder and subjects with severe symptoms are three times more likely to have persistent insomnia with relapses. When left untreated, it is associated with negative psychiatric and medical outcomes, although the bidirectional relation between insomnia and these disorders is difficult to understand. Insomnia is associated with a two- to fourfold increased risk of developing depression, and this risk can be seen even up to 30 years later. Persistent insomnia can be associated with negative treatment outcomes during depression therapy, and is a risk factor for increased episodes of depression relapse and suicidal behavior. Insomnia is also associated with neurocognitive impairment, but its role as a risk factor for dementia is less clear. Insomnia is a risk factor for obesity, diabetes, hypertension, cardiac disease, and stroke, particularly when associated with short sleep duration. Insomnia is also a major public health issue and is associated with absenteeism, reduced work productivity, and increased disability, accidents, and health care costs. The indirect costs of untreated insomnia clearly outweigh the potential direct costs of treating it. Therefore, insomnia should be recognized and managed early in its course.

Keywords Insomnia • Depression • Neurocognitive impairment • Obesity • Diabetes • Hypertension • Cardiovascular disease • Absenteeism

Prognosis and Complications

The prognosis of insomnia is difficult to discuss due to the sparsity of studies evaluating its longitudinal course. Chronic insomnia is however known to fluctuate over time, with periods of remissions and relapses [1–4]. Available studies show that the rate of insomnia persistence varies between 40 and 75 % over 1–20 years and is

R. Gourineni, M.D. (✉)
Department of Neurology, Northwestern Feinberg Hospital, Northwestern Feinberg School of Medicine, Chicago, IL, USA
e-mail: ramagourineni@gmail.com

© Springer International Publishing Switzerland 2017
H.P. Attarian (ed.), *Clinical Handbook of Insomnia*, Current Clinical Neurology,
DOI 10.1007/978-3-319-41400-3_5

Table 5.1 Psychiatric and medical consequences of insomnia

Consequences of insomnia	
Psychiatric illness	Depression, anxiety, substance abuse
Neurocognitive function	Cognitive impairment, dementia
Metabolic disorders	Diabetes, dyslipidemia, and obesity
Cardiovascular disease	Coronary heart disease, congestive heart failure, hypertension, stroke
Burden of illness	Absenteeism, presenteeism, reduced work performance, health care utilization, quality of life, and nursing home placement

higher in women and older adults [1–3, 5, 6]. Initial insomnia severity can predict the longitudinal course of insomnia, and individuals with severe insomnia symptoms are three times more likely to have persistent insomnia with relapses [1]. There is an association between insomnia and mortality, particularly in men with short sleep duration [7, 8]. It can also predict premature death in young adults and is associated with shorter survival in older adults during the post-acute rehabilitation period [9, 10].

Keeping the high rate of insomnia persistence in mind, treatment should be initiated after initial evaluation. When left untreated, insomnia is associated with negative health outcomes (see Table 5.1) and mortality. The negative health outcomes of insomnia, as well as its burden on the industrial sector, health care system, and society are discussed in this chapter.

Psychiatric Disorders

- Insomnia is a core symptom of psychiatric illness.
- People with insomnia have a two- to fourfold increased risk of developing depression.
- Persistent insomnia during depression treatment predicts poor treatment response, increase in depression relapses, and increase in suicidal behavior.
- Insomnia is associated with substance abuse.

There is a strong link between insomnia and psychiatric illness. Insomnia may be a symptom of or a risk factor for psychiatric disorders. The bidirectional relationship between the two makes it difficult to understand which is the cause and effect. In addition, when present, insomnia may affect the course and effectiveness in treatment of these disorders.

Insomnia is a core symptom of psychiatric illness, particularly depression and anxiety disorders. Up to two-thirds of subjects report insomnia complaints during a major depressive episode [10, 11]. In addition, 30–60 % of patients with insomnia will have an underlying psychiatric illness [6, 12–16].

People with insomnia have a two- to fourfold increased risk of developing depression [6, 17–21]. This vulnerability is seen throughout the lifecycle from adolescence to elderly adulthood [18, 22, 23]. The John Hopkins Precursors study followed 1053 young men who provided information about sleep habits during medical school. During the median follow-up of 34 years, the relative risk (RR) of developing subsequent clinical depression was two times higher in subjects who reported insomnia in medical school [18]. In addition insomnia can be associated with self-harm and suicidal behavior in both adolescents and adults [22, 24–26]. Of all the risk factors studied, the strongest predictor of depression is the presence of a current sleep disturbance [21, 27]. When the frequency and severity of insomnia symptoms are greater, the association with depression is stronger [28]. The use of sleep medication also independently predicts depression [23, 29]. Although the cause is not clear, the observed associations may reflect a common vulnerability in individuals for both insomnia and depression.

Insomnia is one of the most persistent symptoms in people with depression. When present, it is associated with increased severity and duration of depressive symptoms, poorer response to treatment, and an increased rate of depression relapses [30–34]. Among elderly people with major depressive disorder those with insomnia symptoms were 1.8–3.5 times more likely to remain depressed than those without them [35]. Outcomes of depression treatment with psychotherapy, pharmacotherapy, and combination psycho-pharmacotherapy were worse in individuals with persistent insomnia [30]. In summary, insomnia may not respond to standard depression management and needs to be treated independently. In addition, early management of insomnia symptoms in depressed patients may help improve depression treatment outcomes and prevent recurrence of depressive episodes.

In a study looking at the effect of early insomnia treatment in depressed individuals, eszopiclone/fluoxetine cotherapy showed an improvement in measures of sleep and depression, compared to placebo [36, 37]. Although both groups received fluoxetine, the eszopiclone group demonstrated a significantly greater improvement in depressive symptoms [37]. These findings further emphasize the need for early management of insomnia, but more trials are needed to study the effects of other insomnia therapies for longer periods of time.

Insomnia symptoms are also associated with substance abuse [22, 38–40]. Adolescents with insomnia, short sleep duration, and large weekday-weekend bedtime differences have higher odds of using alcohol and other drugs [38]. Heavy drinking is linked to the frequency of insomnia symptoms and veterans who misuse alcohol are more likely to endorse suicidal ideation [39, 41]. Careful screening for potential alcohol and substance abuse should be part of insomnia evaluation.

Neurocognitive Function

Most studies support a link between insomnia and cognitive decline. The association with cognitive decline is seen in both middle-aged and older adults and is stronger in men than women [42–48]. There is however a study which shows increased cognitive impairment in elderly women reporting regular difficulty with sleep compared to those without [49]. Insomnia in special populations such as congestive heart failure may also be associated with impaired cognition [50]. Both subjective and objective measures of sleep initiation and maintenance were associated with cognitive impairment [45, 47–49, 51]. People with insomnia performed worse on tests of attention, abstract problem solving, visuospatial reasoning, and memory including working, episodic, long-term, and verbal memory [43, 51, 52]. They also had problems with processing speed and inhibitory function [52]. However, the studies discussed are cross sectional or retrospective in nature and lasted no longer than 2–3 years. The bidirectional relation between insomnia and cognitive impairment is therefore difficult to understand.

Unlike with cognitive impairment, most studies do not support an association between insomnia and dementia [53]. However the study results are mixed and one study did show a strong association, particularly when hypnotic medications are used [54]. Use of hypnotic medications is associated with a twofold greater risk of developing dementia, regardless of the type of hypnotic used [54]. In addition, the association is stronger in the 50–65-year age group, and when higher doses or medications with longer half-life are used [54]. The effect was likely more difficult to see after the age of 65, since dementia becomes more common then. For this reason, hypnotic medications should be used sparingly in middle-aged to older adults with cognitive impairment. Cognitive and behavioral therapies should be tried first in this age group.

Structural brain changes may be seen in patients with insomnia, but results from studies are not consistent. Brain imaging studies in patients with primary insomnia have shown reduced hippocampal volume bilaterally, smaller volumes of CA3 and dentate subfields, and reduced gray matter in the left orbitofrontal cortex (LOFC) [55–58]. Other studies were unable to replicate these findings [59, 60]. When changes were found, they were associated strongly with the severity of insomnia symptoms [56, 57].

Metabolic Disorders

The relation between short sleep duration and to a lesser extent long sleep duration with obesity and diabetes has been reported [61–65]. Insomnia symptoms and insomnia disorder are also associated with these and other metabolic conditions. Body mass index (BMI) has been associated with persistent and increasing insomnia symptoms including difficulties with sleep initiation and maintenance [66, 67]. These associations are also seen in children and adolescents. Frequent nocturnal awakenings in children are associated with childhood obesity odds ratio (OR = 1.7), and teens with difficulty falling asleep have higher BMIs ranging from 0.86 to 1.41 units [68, 69]. Poor sleep quality is shown to be related to increased nighttime eating, and this may partly explain the relationship between sleep quality and obesity [63].

Chronic insomnia is associated with a high risk of diabetes and the risk is highest in individuals who sleep 5 h or less (OR = 2.95), and between 5 and 6 h (OR = 2.07) [70]. Chronic insomnia with short sleep duration is likely a more pathological form of insomnia [71] (Table 5.2). Individuals with insomnia symptoms such as difficulty

Table 5.2 Medical consequences of chronic insomnia with short sleep duration

Author, year	Variable	Study type	Findings
Vgontzas, 2010	Mortality	Longitudinal	Mortality was significantly increased in men with chronic insomnia with <6 h of sleep (OR = 4.33), compared to insomnia with longer sleep duration and GS.
Fernandez-Mendoza, 2010	Neuropsychological performance	Cross sectional	Chronic insomnia with <6 h sleep showed poorer performance in processing speed, set-switching attention, and visual memory errors/omissions compared to insomnia with longer sleep duration and GS.
Vgontzas, 2013	Obesity	Longitudinal	Highest incidence of obesity (BMI ≥ 30) (OR = 2.18) was seen in poor sleepers with <5 h sleep and second highest with 5–6 and 6–7 h of sleep (OR = 1.18–1.19) compared to longer sleep duration and GS.
Vgontzas, 2009	Diabetes	Cross sectional	Highest association with diabetes was seen in subjects with chronic insomnia with ≤5 h of sleep (OR = 2.95) and 5–6 h (OR = 2.07) compared to longer duration and GS.
Vgontzas, 2009	Hypertension	Cross sectional	Highest association of HTN was seen in chronic insomnia with <5 h sleep (OR = 5.1) and second highest with 5–6 h (OR = 3.5) compared to longer duration and GS.
Fernandez-Mendoza, 2012	Hypertension	Longitudinal	Highest risk of HTN was seen in chronic insomnia with <6 h sleep (OR = 3.8), compared to 6 h or more and GS.

OR odds ratio, *GS* good sleepers, *BMI* body mass index, *HTN* hypertension

maintaining sleep and early-morning awakenings lasting longer than 2 weeks were also found to have elevated HbA1c levels in a dose–response fashion [72]. In addition, diabetic individuals with insomnia have a 23 % higher fasting glucose level, a 48 % higher fasting insulin level, and an 82 % higher homeostatic model assessment (HOMA) level [73]. In summary, insomnia symptoms are associated with obesity and diabetes and the risk of diabetes is particularly high in chronic insomniacs with short sleep duration. Insomnia in diabetics may also contribute to poorer glucose control.

Cardiovascular Disease

It is well know that sleep-disordered breathing is linked to hypertension (HTN) and cardiovascular disease (CVD) [74–76]. Although insomnia was previously not considered a risk factor, it is being increasingly linked to these disorders. Insomnia is associated with a high risk of HTN, particularly when associated with short sleep duration [77–80]. The risk is highest in insomniacs with less than 5 h of sleep and second highest with 5–6 h of sleep, compared to insomnia with longer sleep duration and good sleepers [77]. A study using MSLT as a measure of physiological hyperarousal found that insomnia with hyperarousal (MSLT > 14 min) is associated with a significantly higher risk of developing hypertension in a dose–response manner [81]. The risk of HTN is related proportionately to the frequency of insomnia symptoms, based on medication prescription data [82]. Although most of these studies are cross-sectional, a longitudinal study was performed demonstrating that chronic insomnia with objectively measured short sleep duration (OSSD) is a significant risk factor for incident HTN [83]. Individuals with chronic insomnia who sleep less than 6 h had 3.8 times higher odds of developing HTN than those who slept 6 h or more [83]. Presence of insomnia may also effect the treatment of hypertension. Poor sleep quality is shown to be more prevalent in women with treatment-resistant hypertension than those without it [84].

Insomnia is associated with an overall 45 % increased risk of developing or dying of cardiovascular disease [85]. Insomnia itself may not be related to cardiovascular disease, unless associated with short sleep duration. Short sleepers reporting insomnia symptoms had the highest risk of overall cardiovascular events [86–90]. This relation was seen among various ethnic groups, including older American-Indians and people of Chinese origin in Taiwan [88, 89]. A dose-dependent effect was also seen between the number of insomnia symptoms and the risk of heart failure [91]. Nightshift workers with insomnia during daytime and nighttime had a 3.07-fold increased risk of developing CVD, compared to those without insomnia [92]. A 2.79-fold increase risk of developing CVD was also seen in day workers with insomnia. These results suggest that insomnia accentuates the cardiovascular risk reported with nightshift work [92].

One study also reported a 54 % increased risk of developing ischemic stroke in subjects with insomnia, compared to those without insomnia [93]. Subjects with persistent insomnia also have a higher 3-year cumulative incidence rate of stroke compared to subjects in remission [93]. Although these findings are impressive, more studies need to be conducted to better understand the relation between insomnia and stroke.

Higher nighttime systolic blood pressure (SBP), as well as blunted daytime-to-nighttime dipping of SBP, is seen in normotensive subjects with chronic insomnia [94]. Although these findings are in normotensive subjects, they suggest a possible mechanism that links insomnia with HTN and CVD [94]. In addition, insomnia with OSSD may be a more severe phenotype of the disorder [71]. Unlike insomnia with normal sleep duration, insomnia with OSSD is associated with medical comorbidity including obesity, diabetes, dyslipidemia, HTN, and CVD [70, 77, 83, 86, 95, 96]. Studies have shown that chronic insomnia with OSSD is associated with activation of both limbs of the stress system including the hypothalamic pituitary adrenal (HPA) axis and the sympatho-adrenal-medullary (sympathetic) axis, which correlates positively with objective measures of sleep continuity including total wake time (TWT) and wake after sleep onset (WASO) during overnight polysomnography

[97, 98]. Elevations of cortisol, norepinephrine, and catecholamine metabolites are seen not only at night, but also during the entire 24-h period, suggesting 24-h activation of the stress system [97]. The greatest 24-h elevation of cortisol and adrenocorticotrophic hormone (ACTH) is seen in the evening and first half of the night [98]. In summary, insomnia with OSSD is associated with activation of the stress system and this activation correlates positively with objectively measured sleep disturbances during overnight polysomnography [97, 98]. This phenotype of insomnia is important to recognize, since it is associated with higher medical consequences.

Burden of Illness

Insomnia is a major public health issue and a burden to society. It contributes to absenteeism, reduced work productivity, and increased disability, accidents, and health care costs. Insomnia is a significant predictor of sick leave and insomniacs miss work almost twice as often as individuals without insomnia [99–101]. One study showed that insomnia is the strongest predictor of sick leave among 36 variables studied [102, 103]. The level of absenteeism is also linked to the severity of insomnia symptoms, but the degree varies between studies [102, 104]. In a detailed evaluation, the mean number of hours absent from work for 3 months was the highest in subjects with insomnia syndrome, compared to subjects with insomnia symptoms and good sleepers [104]. A report of sleep disturbance also predicted the increased likelihood of taking long-term sickness leave (≥90 days) 2 years later [105].

A study across job categories found a higher level of absenteeism among blue-collar workers with insomnia compared to white-collar workers (64 % vs. 54 %), and the duration of absence was the longest in women and workers in managerial roles [100]. Sleep complaints are also associated with increased school absenteeism in adolescents between the ages of 16 and 19 years (OR = 3.26) [106]. Large differences between weekday and weekend bedtimes and daytime tiredness contribute to this [106]. Two studies looked at the long-term cost-effectiveness of treating primary insomnia with eszopiclone and showed reduced costs associated with worker absenteeism [107, 108]. In summary, insomnia is associated with short-term and long-term sickness absence, as well as school nonattendance. The level of absenteeism is also linked to the severity of insomnia. Treating insomnia may reduce the costs associated with worker absenteeism, but this needs to be studied further.

Workplace performance and productivity are also affected by insomnia [104]. Workers with poor sleep are 2.5 times more likely than good sleepers to report difficulty with occupational activities [109]. When the work productivity and activity impairment (WPAI) questionnaire developed by Bolge was administered, subjects with insomnia were found to have a 13 % higher score for presenteeism (impairment at work/reduced on the job effectiveness) and a 10.3 % greater work productivity loss (combination of absenteeism and presenteeism) than subjects without insomnia [110]. Menopausal women with chronic sleep maintenance insomnia did not show increased absenteeism, but after administering the WPAI, 17.3 % greater productivity impairment was seen compared to women without insomnia [111]. A greater number of subjects with severe insomnia report being less energetic and efficient at work, as well as difficulty with completing complicated tasks, compared to good sleepers [112]. They also report making errors at work, which may have resulted in serious consequences (15 % vs. 6 %) [100].

Perception of poor career progression and poor job satisfaction is also linked to insomnia [113]. Significantly lower job performance scores were found in white-collar workers with insomnia compared to good sleepers in a study using a six-item job performance scale to measure job performance [114]. A study in navy seamen showed that poor sleepers performed less effectively in all measures of navy performance and showed poor career advancement in the navy [115]. Another study however failed to show differences between insomniacs and good sleepers when asked to rate achievement of their annual objectives [114]. While insomnia seems to be linked to absenteeism, work productivity, and job satisfaction, it is not clear if these factors are eventually related to the achievement of long-term goals and career advancement in jobs, and this should be further studied.

In addition to its effect on work productivity, insomnia is also a strong predictor of permanent work disability, though the extent varies between studies (OR = 1.66–4.56) [116]. Also, out of the subjects receiving disability pension (DP), 33 % of men and 41 % of women report insomnia symptoms [117]. Insomnia also plays a stronger role in DP when it is comorbid with pain [118].

Most studies show that insomnia is associated with an increased risk of accidents. Work-related accidents are higher in subjects with insomnia [112]. The National Sleep Foundation poll found a significantly higher rate of work-related accidents and injuries in subjects who reported a sleep latency of >30 min [119]. Motor vehicle accidents due to sleep disturbance are usually the result of sleep apnea, daytime sleepiness, or insufficient sleep, but insomnia may also play a role [120]. Subjects with insomnia reported a two- to threefold increased risk of having 2–3 serious road accidents compared to good sleepers in a study of insomnia in the workforce [100]. There is also a strong association between hypnotic medication use and motor vehicle accidents [121].

Insomnia is associated with both direct and indirect costs which cause significant burden to the society (Table 5.3). Subjects with insomnia utilize the health care system to a greater degree than good sleepers [104, 122]. Direct costs include health care consultations, transportation, hospitalization, prescription, and over-the-counter medication and alcohol used as a sleep aid. Middle- and older aged adults with insomnia show greater odds of hospitalization, home health service use, and nursing home placement [123]. In men, insomnia is the strongest predictor of nursing home placement, which exceeds even cognitive impairment [124].

Indirect costs of insomnia include money lost due to absenteeism, lost work productivity, and accidents. Several studies tried to systematically calculate these costs. Daley's study from 2009 studied 948 randomly selected subjects from the Quebec province [125]. They were divided into insomnia syndrome (SYND), insomnia symptoms (SYMPT), and good sleepers (GS) based on the presence and frequency

Table 5.3 Direct and indirect costs of insomnia

Direct costs of treating insomnia	Indirect costs of untreated insomnia
• Health care consultations	• Absenteeism
• Hospitalization	• Reduced work productivity
• Home health services	• School nonattendance
• Prescription and OTC medications	• Long-term and permanent work disability
• Alcohol as sleep aid	• Workplace and motor vehicle accidents

of insomnia symptoms. The annual per person insomnia-related costs in Canadian dollars (direct and indirect) were $5010 ($293 and $4717) for SYND and $1413 ($160 and $1271) for SYMPT and even GS had $421 ($45 and $376). Based on this the total annual cost of insomnia in the Quebec province is $6.6 billion. The highest direct costs were spent for alcohol (58%) and health consultations (33%). These costs are higher than previous studies, particularly in the SYND group due to the time period in which the study was conducted and the further division of insomnia subjects SYND and SYMPT. In previous studies the analyses were conducted on all insomnia subjects, regardless of insomnia severity, diluting the findings. This alone shows that subjects with more severe insomnia symptoms are a higher burden to society. The cost of medications is lower in the Quebec province since benzodiazepines and zopiclone are the most prescribed medications, and both are present in generic forms. In addition, the overall health care costs are less in the Quebec province. Kessler in 2011 also reported an annual cost of insomnia of $63.2 billion, for the entire US workforce, based on individual-level human capital value estimate of $2280 for lost work productivity. Based on these findings, it is clear that the indirect costs of insomnia clearly outweigh the direct costs. We can therefore clearly conclude that the cost of not treating insomnia is greater than the cost of treating it.

In summary, insomnia is a chronic and persistent condition, which should be evaluated and managed early in its course. When left untreated, insomnia is associated with significant psychiatric and medical consequences. In addition, it is associated with absenteeism and reduced productivity, which are a great burden to society.

References

1. Morin CM, Belanger L, LeBlanc M, Ivers H, Savard J, Espie CA, et al. The natural history of insomnia: a population-based 3-year longitudinal study. Arch Intern Med. 2009;169(5):447–53.
2. Foley DJ, Monjan A, Simonsick EM, Wallace RB, Blazer DG. Incidence and remission of insomnia among elderly adults: an epidemiologic study of 6,800 persons over three years. Sleep. 1999;22 Suppl 2:S366–72.
3. Foley DJ, Monjan AA, Izmirlian G, Hays JC, Blazer DG. Incidence and remission of insomnia among elderly adults in a biracial cohort. Sleep. 1999;22 Suppl 2:S373–8.
4. Mendelson WB. Long-term follow-up of chronic insomnia. Sleep. 1995;18(8):698–701.
5. Morphy H, Dunn KM, Lewis M, Boardman HF, Croft PR. Epidemiology of insomnia: a longitudinal study in a UK population. Sleep. 2007;30(3):274–80.
6. Buysse DJ, Angst J, Gamma A, Ajdacic V, Eich D, Rossler W. Prevalence, course, and comorbidity of insomnia and depression in young adults. Sleep. 2008;31(4):473–80.

7. Vgontzas AN, Liao D, Pejovic S, Calhoun S, Karataraki M, Basta M, et al. Insomnia with short sleep duration and mortality: the Penn State cohort. Sleep. 2010;33(9):1159–64.
8. Sivertsen B, Pallesen S, Glozier N, Bjorvatn B, Salo P, Tell GS, et al. Midlife insomnia and subsequent mortality: the Hordaland health study. BMC Public Health. 2014;14:720.
9. Martin JL, Fiorentino L, Jouldjian S, Mitchell M, Josephson KR, Alessi CA. Poor self-reported sleep quality predicts mortality within one year of inpatient post-acute rehabilitation among older adults. Sleep. 2011;34(12):1715–21.
10. Hamilton M. Frequency of symptoms in melancholia (depressive illness). Br J Psychiatry. 1989;154:201–6.
11. Perlis ML, Giles DE, Buysse DJ, Thase ME, Tu X, Kupfer DJ. Which depressive symptoms are related to which sleep electroencephalographic variables? Biol Psychiatry. 1997;42(10):904–13.
12. Buysse DJ, Reynolds 3rd CF, Hauri PJ, Roth T, Stepanski EJ, Thorpy MJ, et al. Diagnostic concordance for DSM-IV sleep disorders: a report from the APA/NIMH DSM-IV field trial. Am J Psychiatry. 1994;151(9):1351–60.
13. Ohayon MM. Prevalence of DSM-IV diagnostic criteria of insomnia: distinguishing insomnia related to mental disorders from sleep disorders. J Psychiatr Res. 1997;31(3):333–46.
14. Ohayon MM, Smirne S. Prevalence and consequences of insomnia disorders in the general population of Italy. Sleep Med. 2002;3(2):115–20.
15. Ohayon MM. Epidemiology of insomnia: what we know and what we still need to learn. Sleep Med Rev. 2002;6(2):97–111.
16. Roth T, Jaeger S, Jin R, Kalsekar A, Stang PE, Kessler RC. Sleep problems, comorbid mental disorders, and role functioning in the national comorbidity survey replication. Biol Psychiatry. 2006;60(12):1364–71.
17. Baglioni C, Battagliese G, Feige B, Spiegelhalder K, Nissen C, Voderholzer U, et al. Insomnia as a predictor of depression: a meta-analytic evaluation of longitudinal epidemiological studies. J Affect Disord. 2011;135(1–3):10–9.
18. Chang PP, Ford DE, Mead LA, Cooper-Patrick L, Klag MJ. Insomnia in young men and subsequent depression. The Johns Hopkins Precursors Study. Am J Epidemiol. 1997;146(2):105–14.
19. Neckelmann D, Mykletun A, Dahl AA. Chronic insomnia as a risk factor for developing anxiety and depression. Sleep. 2007;30(7):873–80.
20. Riemann D, Voderholzer U. Primary insomnia: a risk factor to develop depression? J Affect Disord. 2003;76(1–3):255–9.
21. Breslau N, Roth T, Rosenthal L, Andreski P. Sleep disturbance and psychiatric disorders: a longitudinal epidemiological study of young adults. Biol Psychiatry. 1996;39(6):411–8.
22. Roane BM, Taylor DJ. Adolescent insomnia as a risk factor for early adult depression and substance abuse. Sleep. 2008;31(10):1351–6.
23. Jaussent I, Bouyer J, Ancelin ML, Akbaraly T, Peres K, Ritchie K, et al. Insomnia and daytime sleepiness are risk factors for depressive symptoms in the elderly. Sleep. 2011;34(8):1103–10.
24. Hysing M, Sivertsen B, Stormark KM, O'Connor RC. Sleep problems and self-harm in adolescence. Br J Psychiatry. 2015.
25. Liu X. Sleep and adolescent suicidal behavior. Sleep. 2004;27(7):1351–8.
26. Sun L, Zhang J, Liu X. Insomnia symptom, mental disorder and suicide: a case-control study in Chinese rural youths. Sleep Biol Rhythms. 2015;13(2):181–8.
27. Livingston G, Blizard B, Mann A. Does sleep disturbance predict depression in elderly people? A study in inner London. Br J Gen Pract. 1993;43(376):445–8.
28. Taylor DJ, Lichstein KL, Durrence HH, Reidel BW, Bush AJ. Epidemiology of insomnia, depression, and anxiety. Sleep. 2005;28(11):1457–64.
29. Potvin O, Lorrain D, Belleville G, Grenier S, Preville M. Subjective sleep characteristics associated with anxiety and depression in older adults: a population-based study. Int J Geriatr Psychiatry. 2014;29(12):1262–70.

30. Troxel WM, Kupfer DJ, Reynolds 3rd CF, Frank E, Thase ME, Miewald JM, et al. Insomnia and objectively measured sleep disturbances predict treatment outcome in depressed patients treated with psychotherapy or psychotherapy-pharmacotherapy combinations. J Clin Psychiatry. 2012;73(4):478–85.
31. Fava M. Daytime sleepiness and insomnia as correlates of depression. J Clin Psychiatry. 2004;65 Suppl 16:27–32.
32. Salo P, Sivertsen B, Oksanen T, Sjosten N, Pentti J, Virtanen M, et al. Insomnia symptoms as a predictor of incident treatment for depression: prospective cohort study of 40,791 men and women. Sleep Med. 2012;13(3):278–84.
33. Gulec M, Selvi Y, Boysan M, Aydin A, Besiroglu L, Agargun MY. Ongoing or re-emerging subjective insomnia symptoms after full/partial remission or recovery of major depressive disorder mainly with the selective serotonin reuptake inhibitors and risk of relapse or recurrence: a 52-week follow-up study. J Affect Disord. 2011;134(1–3):257–65.
34. Manglick M, Rajaratnam SM, Taffe J, Tonge B, Melvin G. Persistent sleep disturbance is associated with treatment response in adolescents with depression. Aust N Z J Psychiatry. 2013;47(6):556–63.
35. Pigeon WR, Hegel M, Unutzer J, Fan MY, Sateia MJ, Lyness JM, et al. Is insomnia a perpetuating factor for late-life depression in the IMPACT cohort? Sleep. 2008;31(4):481–8.
36. Soares CN, Joffe H, Rubens R, Caron J, Roth T, Cohen L. Eszopiclone in patients with insomnia during perimenopause and early postmenopause: a randomized controlled trial. Obstet Gynecol. 2006;108(6):1402–10.
37. Fava M, McCall WV, Krystal A, Wessel T, Rubens R, Caron J, et al. Eszopiclone co-administered with fluoxetine in patients with insomnia coexisting with major depressive disorder. Biol Psychiatry. 2006;59(11):1052–60.
38. Sivertsen B, Skogen JC, Jakobsen R, Hysing M. Sleep and use of alcohol and drug in adolescence. A large population-based study of Norwegian adolescents aged 16 to 19 years. Drug Alcohol Depend. 2015;149:180–6.
39. Chakravorty S, Grandner MA, Mavandadi S, Perlis ML, Sturgis EB, Oslin DW. Suicidal ideation in veterans misusing alcohol: relationships with insomnia symptoms and sleep duration. Addict Behav. 2014;39(2):399–405.
40. Babson KA, Boden MT, Bonn-Miller MO. Sleep quality moderates the relation between depression symptoms and problematic cannabis use among medical cannabis users. Am J Drug Alcohol abuse. 2013;39(3):211–6.
41. Haario P, Rahkonen O, Laaksonen M, Lahelma E, Lallukka T. Bidirectional associations between insomnia symptoms and unhealthy behaviours. J Sleep Res. 2013;22(1):89–95.
42. Fortier-Brochu E, Beaulieu-Bonneau S, Ivers H, Morin CM. Insomnia and daytime cognitive performance: a meta-analysis. Sleep Med Rev. 2012;16(1):83–94.
43. Fortier-Brochu E, Morin CM. Cognitive impairment in individuals with insomnia: clinical significance and correlates. Sleep. 2014;37(11):1787–98.
44. Jelicic M, Bosma H, Ponds RW, Van Boxtel MP, Houx PJ, Jolles J. Subjective sleep problems in later life as predictors of cognitive decline. Report from the Maastricht Ageing Study (MAAS). Int J Geriatr Psychiatry. 2002;17(1):73–7.
45. Miyata S, Noda A, Iwamoto K, Kawano N, Okuda M, Ozaki N. Poor sleep quality impairs cognitive performance in older adults. J Sleep Res. 2013;22(5):535–41.
46. Cricco M, Simonsick EM, Foley DJ. The impact of insomnia on cognitive functioning in older adults. J Am Geriatr Soc. 2001;49(9):1185–9.
47. Blackwell T, Yaffe K, Ancoli-Israel S, Redline S, Ensrud KE, Stefanick ML, et al. Association of sleep characteristics and cognition in older community-dwelling men: the MrOS sleep study. Sleep. 2011;34(10):1347–56.
48. Potvin O, Lorrain D, Forget H, Dube M, Grenier S, Preville M, et al. Sleep quality and 1-year incident cognitive impairment in community-dwelling older adults. Sleep. 2012;35(4):491–9.
49. Tworoger SS, Lee S, Schernhammer ES, Grodstein F. The association of self-reported sleep duration, difficulty sleeping, and snoring with cognitive function in older women. Alzheimer Dis Assoc Disord. 2006;20(1):41–8.

50. Hjelm C, Stromberg A, Arestedt K, Brostrom A. Association between sleep-disordered breathing, sleep-wake pattern, and cognitive impairment among patients with chronic heart failure. Eur J Heart Fail. 2013;15(5):496–504.
51. Schmutte T, Harris S, Levin R, Zweig R, Katz M, Lipton R. The relation between cognitive functioning and self-reported sleep complaints in nondemented older adults: results from the Bronx aging study. Behav Sleep Med. 2007;5(1):39–56.
52. Nebes RD, Buysse DJ, Halligan EM, Houck PR, Monk TH. Self-reported sleep quality predicts poor cognitive performance in healthy older adults. J Gerontol Ser B Psychol Sci Soc Sci. 2009;64(2):180–7.
53. Merlino G, Piani A, Gigli GL, Cancelli I, Rinaldi A, Baroselli A, et al. Daytime sleepiness is associated with dementia and cognitive decline in older Italian adults: a population-based study. Sleep Med. 2010;11(4):372–7.
54. Chen PL, Lee WJ, Sun WZ, Oyang YJ, Fuh JL. Risk of dementia in patients with insomnia and long-term use of hypnotics: a population-based retrospective cohort study. PLoS One. 2012;7(11), e49113.
55. Riemann D, Voderholzer U, Spiegelhalder K, Hornyak M, Buysse DJ, Nissen C, et al. Chronic insomnia and MRI-measured hippocampal volumes: a pilot study. Sleep. 2007;30(8):955–8.
56. Neylan TC, Mueller SG, Wang Z, Metzler TJ, Lenoci M, Truran D, et al. Insomnia severity is associated with a decreased volume of the CA3/dentate gyrus hippocampal subfield. Biol Psychiatry. 2010;68(5):494–6.
57. Altena E, Vrenken H, Van Der Werf YD, van den Heuvel OA, Van Someren EJ. Reduced orbitofrontal and parietal gray matter in chronic insomnia: a voxel-based morphometric study. Biol Psychiatry. 2010;67(2):182–5.
58. Joo EY, Kim H, Suh S, Hong SB. Hippocampal substructural vulnerability to sleep disturbance and cognitive impairment in patients with chronic primary insomnia: magnetic resonance imaging morphometry. Sleep. 2014;37(7):1189–98.
59. Winkelman JW, Benson KL, Buxton OM, Lyoo IK, Yoon S, O'Connor S, et al. Lack of hippocampal volume differences in primary insomnia and good sleeper controls: an MRI volumetric study at 3 Tesla. Sleep Med. 2010;11(6):576–82.
60. Spiegelhalder K, Regen W, Baglioni C, Kloppel S, Abdulkadir A, Hennig J, et al. Insomnia does not appear to be associated with substantial structural brain changes. Sleep. 2013;36(5):731–7.
61. Gangwisch JE, Malaspina D, Boden-Albala B, Heymsfield SB. Inadequate sleep as a risk factor for obesity: analyses of the NHANES I. Sleep. 2005;28(10):1289–96.
62. Patel SR, Blackwell T, Redline S, Ancoli-Israel S, Cauley JA, Hillier TA, et al. The association between sleep duration and obesity in older adults. Int J Obes. 2008;32(12):1825–34.
63. Yeh SS, Brown RF. Disordered eating partly mediates the relationship between poor sleep quality and high body mass index. Eat Behav. 2014;15(2):291–7.
64. Hsieh SD, Muto T, Murase T, Tsuji H, Arase Y. Association of short sleep duration with obesity, diabetes, fatty liver and behavioral factors in Japanese men. Intern Med. 2011;50(21):2499–502.
65. Gottlieb DJ, Punjabi NM, Newman AB, Resnick HE, Redline S, Baldwin CM, et al. Association of sleep time with diabetes mellitus and impaired glucose tolerance. Arch Intern Med. 2005;165(8):863–7.
66. Lallukka T, Haario P, Lahelma E, Rahkonen O. Associations of relative weight with subsequent changes over time in insomnia symptoms: a follow-up study among middle-aged women and men. Sleep Med. 2012;13(10):1271–9.
67. Meyer KA, Wall MM, Larson NI, Laska MN, Neumark-Sztainer D. Sleep duration and BMI in a sample of young adults. Obesity. 2012;20(6):1279–87.
68. Li L, Ren J, Shi L, Jin X, Yan C, Jiang F, et al. Frequent nocturnal awakening in children: prevalence, risk factors, and associations with subjective sleep perception and daytime sleepiness. BMC Psychiatry. 2014;14:204.

69. Chen DR, Truong KD, Tsai MJ. Prevalence of poor sleep quality and its relationship with body mass index among teenagers: evidence from Taiwan. J School Health. 2013;83(8):582–8.
70. Vgontzas AN, Liao D, Pejovic S, Calhoun S, Karataraki M, Bixler EO. Insomnia with objective short sleep duration is associated with type 2 diabetes: a population-based study. Diabetes Care. 2009;32(11):1980–5.
71. Vgontzas AN, Fernandez-Mendoza J, Liao D, Bixler EO. Insomnia with objective short sleep duration: the most biologically severe phenotype of the disorder. Sleep Med Rev. 2013;17(4):241–54.
72. Kachi Y, Nakao M, Takeuchi T, Yano E. Association between insomnia symptoms and hemoglobin A1c level in Japanese men. PLoS One. 2011;6(7), e21420.
73. Knutson KL, Van Cauter E, Zee P, Liu K, Lauderdale DS. Cross-sectional associations between measures of sleep and markers of glucose metabolism among subjects with and without diabetes: the Coronary Artery Risk Development in Young Adults (CARDIA) Sleep Study. Diabetes Care. 2011;34(5):1171–6.
74. Young T, Peppard P, Palta M, Hla KM, Finn L, Morgan B, et al. Population-based study of sleep-disordered breathing as a risk factor for hypertension. Arch Intern Med. 1997;157(15):1746–52.
75. Bixler EO, Vgontzas AN, Lin HM, Ten Have T, Leiby BE, Vela-Bueno A, et al. Association of hypertension and sleep-disordered breathing. Arch Intern Med. 2000;160(15):2289–95.
76. Nieto FJ, Young TB, Lind BK, Shahar E, Samet JM, Redline S, et al. Association of sleep-disordered breathing, sleep apnea, and hypertension in a large community-based study. Sleep Heart Health Study. JAMA. 2000;283(14):1829–36.
77. Vgontzas AN, Liao D, Bixler EO, Chrousos GP, Vela-Bueno A. Insomnia with objective short sleep duration is associated with a high risk for hypertension. Sleep. 2009;32(4):491–7.
78. Vgontzas AN, Liao D, Bixler EO. Insomnia and hypertension. Sleep. 2009;32(12):1547.
79. Vozoris NT. Insomnia symptom frequency and hypertension risk: a population-based study. J Clin Psychiatry. 2014;75(6):616–23.
80. Meng L, Zheng Y, Hui R. The relationship of sleep duration and insomnia to risk of hypertension incidence: a meta-analysis of prospective cohort studies. Hypertens Res. 2013;36(11):985–95.
81. Li Y, Vgontzas AN, Fernandez-Mendoza J, Bixler EO, Sun Y, Zhou J, et al. Insomnia with physiological hyperarousal is associated with hypertension. Hypertension. 2015;65(3):644–50.
82. Haaramo P, Rahkonen O, Hublin C, Laatikainen T, Lahelma E, Lallukka T. Insomnia symptoms and subsequent cardiovascular medication: a register-linked follow-up study among middle-aged employees. J Sleep Res. 2014;23(3):281–9.
83. Fernandez-Mendoza J, Vgontzas AN, Liao D, Shaffer ML, Vela-Bueno A, Basta M, et al. Insomnia with objective short sleep duration and incident hypertension: the Penn State Cohort. Hypertension. 2012;60(4):929–35.
84. Bruno RM, Palagini L, Gemignani A, Virdis A, Di Giulio A, Ghiadoni L, et al. Poor sleep quality and resistant hypertension. Sleep Med. 2013;14(11):1157–63.
85. Sofi F, Cesari F, Casini A, Macchi C, Abbate R, Gensini GF. Insomnia and risk of cardiovascular disease: a meta-analysis. Eur J Prev Cardiol. 2014;21(1):57–64.
86. Westerlund A, Bellocco R, Sundstrom J, Adami HO, Akerstedt T, Trolle LY. Sleep characteristics and cardiovascular events in a large Swedish cohort. Eur J Epidemiol. 2013;28(6):463–73.
87. Canivet C, Nilsson PM, Lindeberg SI, Karasek R, Ostergren PO. Insomnia increases risk for cardiovascular events in women and in men with low socioeconomic status: a longitudinal, register-based study. J Psychosom Res. 2014;76(4):292–9.
88. Sabanayagam C, Shankar A, Buchwald D, Goins RT. Insomnia symptoms and cardiovascular disease among older American Indians: the Native Elder Care Study. J Environ Public Health. 2011;2011:964617.
89. Chien KL, Chen PC, Hsu HC, Su TC, Sung FC, Chen MF, et al. Habitual sleep duration and insomnia and the risk of cardiovascular events and all-cause death: report from a community-based cohort. Sleep. 2010;33(2):177–84.

90. Laugsand LE, Vatten LJ, Platou C, Janszky I. Insomnia and the risk of acute myocardial infarction: a population study. Circulation. 2011;124(19):2073–81.
91. Laugsand LE, Strand LB, Platou C, Vatten LJ, Janszky I. Insomnia and the risk of incident heart failure: a population study. Eur Heart J. 2014;35(21):1382–93.
92. Silva-Costa A, Griep RH, Rotenberg L. Disentangling the effects of insomnia and night work on cardiovascular diseases: a study in nursing professionals. Braz J Med Biol Res. 2015;48(2):120–7.
93. Wu MP, Lin HJ, Weng SF, Ho CH, Wang JJ, Hsu YW. Insomnia subtypes and the subsequent risks of stroke: report from a nationally representative cohort. Stroke. 2014;45(5):1349–54.
94. Lanfranchi PA, Pennestri MH, Fradette L, Dumont M, Morin CM, Montplaisir J. Nighttime blood pressure in normotensive subjects with chronic insomnia: implications for cardiovascular risk. Sleep. 2009;32(6):760–6.
95. Vgontzas AN, Lin HM, Papaliaga M, Calhoun S, Vela-Bueno A, Chrousos GP, et al. Short sleep duration and obesity: the role of emotional stress and sleep disturbances. Int J Obes. 2008;32(5):801–9.
96. Vgontzas AN, Fernandez-Mendoza J, Miksiewicz T, Kritikou I, Shaffer ML, Liao D, et al. Unveiling the longitudinal association between short sleep duration and the incidence of obesity: the Penn State Cohort. Int J Obes. 2014;38(6):825–32.
97. Vgontzas AN, Tsigos C, Bixler EO, Stratakis CA, Zachman K, Kales A, et al. Chronic insomnia and activity of the stress system: a preliminary study. J Psychosom Res. 1998;45(1):21–31.
98. Vgontzas AN, Bixler EO, Lin HM, Prolo P, Mastorakos G, Vela-Bueno A, et al. Chronic insomnia is associated with nyctohemeral activation of the hypothalamic-pituitary-adrenal axis: clinical implications. J Clin Endocrinol Metab. 2001;86(8):3787–94.
99. Sivertsen B, Overland S, Bjorvatn B, Maeland JG, Mykletun A. Does insomnia predict sick leave? The Hordaland Health Study. J Psychosom Res. 2009;66(1):67–74.
100. Leger D, Massuel MA, Metlaine A, Group SS. Professional correlates of insomnia. Sleep. 2006;29(2):171–8.
101. Godet-Cayre V, Pelletier-Fleury N, Le Vaillant M, Dinet J, Massuel MA, Leger D. Insomnia and absenteeism at work. Who pays the cost? Sleep. 2006;29(2):179–84.
102. Leigh JP. Employee and job attributes as predictors of absenteeism in a national sample of workers: the importance of health and dangerous working conditions. Soc Sci Med. 1991;33(2):127–37.
103. Leger D, Bayon V. Societal costs of insomnia. Sleep Med Rev. 2010;14(6):379–89.
104. Daley M, Morin CM, LeBlanc M, Gregoire JP, Savard J, Baillargeon L. Insomnia and its relationship to health-care utilization, work absenteeism, productivity and accidents. Sleep Med. 2009;10(4):427–38.
105. Akerstedt T, Kecklund G, Alfredsson L, Selen J. Predicting long-term sickness absence from sleep and fatigue. J Sleep Res. 2007;16(4):341–5.
106. Hysing M, Haugland S, Stormark KM, Boe T, Sivertsen B. Sleep and school attendance in adolescence: results from a large population-based study. Scand J Public Health. 2015;43(1):2–9.
107. Botteman MF, Ozminkowski RJ, Wang S, Pashos CL, Schaefer K, Foley DJ. Cost effectiveness of long-term treatment with eszopiclone for primary insomnia in adults: a decision analytical model. CNS Drugs. 2007;21(4):319–34.
108. Snedecor SJ, Botteman MF, Bojke C, Schaefer K, Barry N, Pickard AS. Cost-effectiveness of eszopiclone for the treatment of adults with primary chronic insomnia. Sleep. 2009;32(6):817–24.
109. Doi Y, Minowa M, Tango T. Impact and correlates of poor sleep quality in Japanese white-collar employees. Sleep. 2003;26(4):467–71.
110. Bolge SC, Doan JF, Kannan H, Baran RW. Association of insomnia with quality of life, work productivity, and activity impairment. Qual Life Res. 2009;18(4):415–22.
111. Bolge SC, Balkrishnan R, Kannan H, Seal B, Drake CL. Burden associated with chronic sleep maintenance insomnia characterized by nighttime awakenings among women with menopausal symptoms. Menopause. 2010;17(1):80–6.

112. Leger D, Guilleminault C, Bader G, Levy E, Paillard M. Medical and socio-professional impact of insomnia. Sleep. 2002;25(6):625–9.
113. Kucharczyk ER, Morgan K, Hall AP. The occupational impact of sleep quality and insomnia symptoms. Sleep Med Rev. 2012;16(6):547–59.
114. Kuppermann M, Lubeck DP, Mazonson PD, Patrick DL, Stewart AL, Buesching DP, et al. Sleep problems and their correlates in a working population. J Gen Intern Med. 1995;10(1):25–32.
115. Johnson LC, Spinweber CL. Good and poor sleepers differ in Navy performance. Mil Med. 1983;148(9):727–31.
116. Sivertsen B, Overland S, Pallesen S, Bjorvatn B, Nordhus IH, Maeland JG, et al. Insomnia and long sleep duration are risk factors for later work disability. The Hordaland Health Study. J Sleep Res. 2009;18(1):122–8.
117. Canivet C, Staland-Nyman C, Lindeberg SI, Karasek R, Moghaddassi M, Ostergren PO. Insomnia symptoms, sleep duration, and disability pensions: a prospective study of Swedish workers. Int J Behav Med. 2014;21(2):319–28.
118. Lallukka T, Overland S, Haaramo P, Saastamoinen P, Bjorvatn B, Sivertsen B. The joint contribution of pain and insomnia to sickness absence and disability retirement: a register-linkage study among Norwegian and Finnish employees. Eur J Pain. 2014;18(6):883–92.
119. National Sleep Foundation. Gallup poll on sleep, performance and the workplace. Washington DC. 2008.
120. Karimi M, Eder DN, Eskandari D, Zou D, Hedner JA, Grote L. Impaired vigilance and increased accident rate in public transport operators is associated with sleep disorders. Accid Anal Prev. 2013;51:208–14.
121. Gustavsen I, Bramness JG, Skurtveit S, Engeland A, Neutel I, Morland J. Road traffic accident risk related to prescriptions of the hypnotics zopiclone, zolpidem, flunitrazepam and nitrazepam. Sleep Med. 2008;9(8):818–22.
122. Sivertsen B, Krokstad S, Mykletun A, Overland S. Insomnia symptoms and use of health care services and medications: the HUNT-2 study. Behav Sleep Med. 2009;7(4):210–22.
123. Kaufmann CN, Canham SL, Mojtabai R, Gum AM, Dautovich ND, Kohn R, et al. Insomnia and health services utilization in middle-aged and older adults: results from the Health and Retirement Study. J Gerontol A Biol Sci Med Sci. 2013;68(12):1512–7.
124. Pollak CP, Perlick D, Linsner JP, Wenston J, Hsieh F. Sleep problems in the community elderly as predictors of death and nursing home placement. J Community Health. 1990;15(2):123–35.
125. Daley M, Morin CM, LeBlanc M, Gregoire JP, Savard J. The economic burden of insomnia: direct and indirect costs for individuals with insomnia syndrome, insomnia symptoms, and good sleepers. Sleep. 2009;32(1):55–64.

Chapter 6
Cognitive Behavioral Therapy for Insomnia

Kelly Glazer Baron, Michael L. Perlis, Sara Nowakowski, Michael T. Smith Jr., Carla R. Jungquist, and Henry J. Orff

Abstract In this chapter we provide an overview of how chronic insomnia is assessed and treated using cognitive behavioral treatments. In addition, we provide some (1) "information" which reviews the cognitive and behavioral theories regarding the etiology of chronic insomnia that set up the rationale for treatment approaches and (2) information on the efficacy of cognitive behavioral therapy (CBT) for insomnia and (3) recent innovations in the delivery of CBT for insomnia, such as brief interventions developed for medical and community settings and use of technology. The former is provided so that the reader may appreciate the principles on which CBT is founded. The latter is provided so that the reader may appreciate the extent to which CBT for insomnia has been empirically validated, studied, and disseminated.

Keywords Insomnia • Sleep • Cognitive behavioral therapy • Actigraphy • Polysomnography • Stimulus control • Sleep restriction

K.G. Baron, Ph.D., M.P.H., C.B.S.M. (✉)
Department of Neurology, Feinberg School of Medicine, Rush University,
710 N Lake Shore Dr., Room 523, Abbott Hall, Chicago, IL 60657, USA
e-mail: kgbaron@rush.edu

M.L. Perlis, Ph.D.
Department of Psychiatry and School of Nursing, UPENN Behavioral Sleep Medicine Program, University of Pennsylvania, Philadelphia, PA, USA
e-mail: mperlis@upenn.edu

S. Nowakowski, Ph.D.
Department of Obstetrics and Gynecology, University of Texas Medical Branch, Galveston, TX, USA
e-mail: sanowako@utmb.edu

M.T. Smith Jr. , Ph.D.
Department of Psychiatry, Johns Hopkins School of Medicine, Baltimore, MD, USA
e-mail: msmith62@jhmi.edu

C.R. Jungquist, A.N.P., Ph.D.
School of Nursing, University of Buffalo, Buffalo, NY, USA
e-mail: carlajun@buffalo.edu

H.J. Orff, Ph.D.
Department of Psychology, VA San Diego Healthcare System, San Diego, CA, USA
e-mail: horff@ucsd.edu

© Springer International Publishing Switzerland 2017
H.P. Attarian (ed.), *Clinical Handbook of Insomnia*, Current Clinical Neurology,
DOI 10.1007/978-3-319-41400-3_6

Theoretical Perspectives on Insomnia

Behavioral Perspective

Since the late 1980s, insomnia has largely been conceptualized from within a behavioral framework. The original model was proposed by Spielman and colleagues and it continues to be the leading theory for both sleep medicine and the subspecialty area of behavioral sleep medicine [1]. As illustrated in Fig. 6.1, the behavioral model posits that insomnia occurs acutely in relation to both predisposing (trait) and precipitating (state) factors and occurs chronically in relation to perpetuating or maintaining factors. Thus, an individual may be prone to insomnia due to trait characteristics, experience acute episodes because of precipitating events, and have chronic insomnia owing to a variety of perpetuating factors.

With respect to trait factors, personality characteristics [2], physiologic arousal [3], and genetic predisposition [4, 5] are thought to contribute to predispose the individual to acute episodes of insomnia. Typical precipitating events (which represent stressors within the larger stress diathesis model of disease) include situational stress [6], acute injury or pain, and bereavement. Perpetuating factors, as the term implies, maintain the chronic form of the disorder even after the precipitating events have either been stabilized or resolved. Perpetuating factors are any of a variety of compensatory strategies in which the patient engages in an attempt to cope with insomnia symptoms. Typical examples of such factors include excessive daytime napping, extending sleep opportunity, keeping variable sleep-wake schedules, using alcohol as a hypnotic, spending excessive time awake in bed, and diminishing daily activity level due to fatigue.

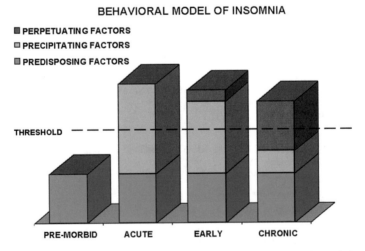

Fig. 6.1 A schematic of the differential diagnosis process for the diagnosis of chronic insomnia

Central to the behavioral model of chronic insomnia is the role of classical conditioning as the primary maintaining factor. It is hypothesized that, over time, insomnia becomes a conditioned response to the bed and bedroom environment. This process presumably occurs via traditional principles of classical conditioning, due to repeated parings of the bed and bedroom (conditioned stimuli) with states of psychophysiologic hyperarousal (unconditioned stimuli) that are thought to interfere with the normal biologic processes of sleep initiation and maintenance.

Cognitive Perspective

A number of authors have stressed the importance of cognitive factors in chronic insomnia [7]. Given their emphasis on the role of cognition, they and others have developed interventions, which provide for the cognitive component of the more broad-based cognitive-behavioral approach. Within this perspective, two related types of cognitions are thought to be operational: one set is related to the patient's beliefs about their disorder; the other set is related to cognitive processes like intrusive thoughts and worry.

Morin et al., for example, have found that patients with chronic insomnia have a number of maladaptive beliefs about sleep, including unrealistic views about what constitutes adequate sleep and catastrophic beliefs about the consequences of insomnia. Such beliefs presumably contribute to insomnia via (1) increasing sleep-related performance anxiety and (2) by prompting and promoting maladaptive compensatory behaviors. Support for the role of such factors derives from data showing that successful cognitive-behavioral treatment of insomnia is associated with a reduction in negative beliefs and attitudes about sleep [8, 9]. While this is suggestive, more work is needed to demonstrate the "insomnogenic" potential of such cognitions. This is so, because one can easily imagine that successful therapy may change one's thoughts and beliefs, but also that such changes may not be responsible for the treatment gains.

Other researchers have focused more on cognitive process (vs. content) issues. Central to this area is that patients with insomnia often complain that they are unable to sleep because of intrusive thoughts or excessive worry. These thoughts and images are characterized as being "intrusive" and may occur in isolation or as unwanted perseverative-type problem solving (worry). The content of the "thoughts and worry" may be centered on the kind of dysfunctional attitudes and beliefs described above, but they are often more general in content. The ideation and imagery that occur as intrusive thoughts are often related to mundane daily activities and/or work or relationship issues. As with dysfunctional attitudes and beliefs, intrusive thoughts and perseverative thinking (from within the radical cognitive perspective) are thought to be responsible for the occurrence and severity of insomnia. The more moderate view is that these phenomena are, along with behavioral and conditioning factors, contributory.

Support for the cognitive perspective comes from a variety of studies which have found that patients with chronic insomnia complain of higher levels of pre-sleep rumination compared to normal controls [10, 11]. Investigations of pre-sleep thought content have found that the pre-sleep cognitions of patients with chronic insomnia tend to be more negatively toned, and that patients report increased general problem solving and thoughts pertaining to environmental stimuli at or around sleep onset [12–14].

Neurocognitive Perspective

In sharp contrast to the cognitive model, the neurocognitive perspective all but suggests that dysfunctional beliefs and worry are epiphenomena. It is posited that cognitive factors are likely to mediate the occurrence and severity of insomnia when the disorder is acute. When, however, the disorder is chronic, cognition occurs secondary to conditioned arousal. Put differently, patients with chronic insomnia are not awake because they are given to rumination and worry, but rather ruminate because they are awake.

The neurocognitive perspective [1, 2] is an extension of the traditional behavioral model. As laid out by Spielman and colleagues [1], the behavioral model allows for a compelling conceptualization regarding how maladaptive behaviors lead to conditioned arousal and chronic insomnia. The Spielman model does not, however, spell out what the conditioned arousal is, or why and how "arousal" interferes with sleep initiation and/or maintenance and/or the perception of sleep. These latter issues are precisely the province of the neurocognitive model which defines "arousal" as conditioned cortical arousal. This form of arousal may be observed in patients with chronic insomnia as high-frequency EEG activity (14–45 Hz) at or around sleep onset and during NREM sleep [15]. High-frequency EEG activity, it is hypothesized, allows for abnormal levels of sensory and information processing and long-term memory formation. Increased sensory processing is thought to interfere with the ability to initiate sleep (as measured by traditional PSG measures). Increased information processing during PSG-defined sleep is thought to interfere with the patient's ability to perceive PSG sleep as "sleep." Increased long-term memory formation (attenuation of the normal mesograde amnesia of sleep) is thought to interfere with the patient's morning judgments about sleep quality and quantity.

Support for the neurocognitive perspective [16] comes from a variety of studies which have found Beta EEG (14–45 Hz) to (1) be elevated in patients with insomnia [15, 17–21], (2) be positively associated with patient perceptions of sleep quality [22], (3) be positively associated with sleep-state misperception (the degree of discrepancy between subjective and objective measures of sleep) [15, 23], and (4) vary with successful CBT treatment for insomnia [24].

Assessment and Measurement

Self-Report Assessment

Behavioral sleep medicine specialists often utilize a number of retrospective assessment tools to gather more precise diagnostic information. In addition, behavioral sleep medicine specialists utilize daily sleep diaries [25, 26] to prospectively monitor sleep complaints. Prospective assessment is important for (1) evaluating the severity of insomnia complaints on a day-to-day basis, (2) identifying the behaviors that maintain the insomnia, (3) determining to what extent circadian dysrhythmia is present, and (4) gathering the data needed to measure and guide treatment response.

The sleep component of sleep–wake diaries is typically completed after waking and obtains information on time to bed, wake time, sleep latency (SL), frequency of nightly awakenings (FNA), wake time after sleep onset (WASO), total sleep time (TST), early morning awakenings (EMA), medication/substances taken before bed, and subjective assessments of sleep quality. The daytime measures, which are completed prior to going to bed include, nap frequency and duration, fatigue ratings, stimulant consumption, and medication usage.

Objective Assessment

In current clinical practice, the diagnosis of chronic insomnia does not require an in-laboratory, polysomnographic (PSG) study to substantiate the diagnosis. This is true for three reasons. First, there is enough of a general correspondence between the subjective complaint and objective measures that PSG assessment is not required to verify the sleep continuity disturbance. Second, traditional polysomnography does not reveal, or allow for the quantification of, the underlying sleep pathophysiology that presumably gives rise to the patient's complaints. Third, and most pragmatically, third-party payers will not reimburse for sleep studies on patients with likely chronic insomnia. Sleep studies are, however, indicated if the patient demonstrates symptoms consistent with other intrinsic sleep disorders and/or fails to respond to treatment.

When assessed with polysomnography, patients with chronic insomnia reliably exhibit increased sleep latency, increased frequency of nightly awakenings, increased wake after sleep onset time, and decreased total sleep relative to good sleeper controls. PSG findings, however, do not correspond in a one-to-one fashion to patient perceptions of sleep continuity. Patients with insomnia routinely report more severe sleep disturbance than is evident on traditional PSG measures [27–29]. Some have argued that this discrepancy might be explained by the findings that patients with chronic insomnia show a greater degree of psychopathology, including tendencies to somatize internal conflicts and exaggerate symptoms [30, 31]. Others have argued that the subjective-objective discrepancy findings reflect a cardinal feature of the disorder, that is, the persistence of sensory and information processing into NREM sleep. The continuance of such processes into PSG-defined sleep is thought to be the basis for patient difficulties distinguishing between wakefulness and sleep. The extent to which one or both of these factors contributes to the discrepancies between subjective and objective measures of sleep in insomnia continues to be a matter of ongoing debate.

Actigraphs may be used as another method of collecting objective sleep data regarding the sleep–wake patterns of patients with insomnia. Actigraphs are wristwatch-like devices that utilize sophisticated movement detectors to estimate the traditional sleep continuity parameters (e.g., SL, WASO, FNA, and TST). This information may, in turn, be compared to the self-report data to assess the pattern of insomnia and compare objective with self-report data. At the level of self-report, extreme values (gathered retrospectively or prospectively) may suggest that there is a sleep-state misperception component of the insomnia (e.g., sleep latencies of greater than 2 h, wake after sleep onset of greater than 2 h, or a total sleep time of equal to or less than 4 h). The extent to which subjective/objective discrepancies can be resolved using actigraphy has not been subjected to empirical validation. In our clinical practice, however, we have found that actigraphy can be used to assess for sleep-state misperception as well as adherence to behavioral recommendations and evaluate for the presence of comorbid circadian rhythm disorders.

Cognitive-Behavioral Treatment

The most common treatment approach for chronic insomnia is multicomponent CBT, which typically involves sleep hygiene education, stimulus control, sleep restriction, and cognitive therapy. Relaxation training is a component of some but not all multicomponent regimens. For a detailed explanation of each of these therapies the reader is referred to the following books "Insomnia: Psychological Assessment and Management" by Charles Morin [32] and "Cognitive Behavioral Therapy for Insomnia: A Session by Session Guide" by Michael Perlis and colleagues [33].

Of all the available psychological treatments, stimulus control therapy is the best validated and is considered "the gold standard" for the behavioral treatment of insomnia. There is also high-quality evidence to support the use of relaxation [34, 35] and sleep restriction [34, 36]. At this time, most behavioral sleep medicine clinicians adopt a multicomponent approach that typically contains stimulus control, sleep restriction, and sleep hygiene education [8, 32, 37, 38]. Relaxation and cognitive therapy may or may not be included in such protocols.

Therapeutic Regimen

The cognitive-behavioral treatment of insomnia generally requires 4–8 weeks' time with once-a-week face-to-face meetings with the clinical provider. Sessions range from 30 to 90 min depending on the stage of treatment and the degree of patient compliance. Intake sessions are usually 60–90 min in duration. During this session, the clinical history is obtained and the patient is instructed in the use of sleep diaries. No intervention is provided during the first week. This time frame is used to collect the baseline sleep–wake data that will guide treatment for the balance of therapy. The primary interventions (stimulus control and sleep restriction) are deployed over the course of the next 1–2, 30–60-min sessions. Once these treatments are delivered, the patient enters into a phase of treatment where total sleep time is upwardly titrated over the course of the next two to five visits. These follow-up sessions require about 30 min unless additional interventions are being integrated into the treatment program or extra effort is required to gain the patient compliance. Adjunctive treatments include cognitive therapy, relaxation training, and relapse prevention.

First-Line Interventions

Stimulus Control Therapy

Stimulus control therapy (SCT) is recommended for both sleep initiation and maintenance problems. The therapy is generally considered to be the first-line behavioral treatment for chronic insomnia because it has the most research support [39, 40]. Stimulus control instructions limit the amount of time patients spend awake in the bed/bedroom, and are designed to decondition pre-sleep arousal and re-associate the bed/bedroom environment with rapid, well-consolidated sleep. Typical instructions include the following: (1) keep a fixed wake time 7 days per week, irrespective of how much sleep you got during the night; (2) avoid any behavior in the bed or bedroom other than sleep or sexual activity; (3) sleep only in the bedroom; (4) leave the bedroom when awake for approximately 15–20 min; and (5) return only when sleepy. Some clinicians, in an effort to prevent "clock watching" behavior, encourage patients to leave the bedroom as soon as they feel "clearly awake" or experience annoyance and irritation over the fact that they're awake. The combination of these instructions re-establishes the bed and bedroom as strong cues for sleep, and entrains the circadian sleep–wake cycle to the desired phase.

Sleep Restriction

Sleep restriction therapy (SRT) is recommended for both sleep initiation and maintenance problems. The therapy requires patients to limit the amount of time they spend in bed to an amount equal to their average total sleep time. In order to accomplish this, the clinician works with the patient to (1) establish a fixed wake time and (2) decrease sleep opportunity by limiting the patient's time in bed (TIB) to an amount that equals their average total sleep time (TST) as ascertained by baseline sleep diary measures. Once a target amount of time in bed is set, the patient's bedtime is delayed to later in the night so that the TIB and average TST are the same.

Initially, this intervention results in a reduction in total sleep time, such that the patient gets less total sleep than they are accustomed to. This controlled form of sleep loss usually corresponds to a decrease in sleep latency and wake after sleep onset time. Thus, during the acute phase of treatment, the patient gets less sleep, but sleeps in a more consolidated fashion (i.e., they fall asleep more quickly and stay asleep for longer periods of time). The increase in consolidated sleep is formally represented as sleep efficiency (TST/TIB).

The patient's sleep efficiency is monitored on a weekly basis. If the patient's average weekly sleep efficiency reaches 85–90 % (depending on age), then the patient's sleep opportunity is incrementally increased by 15 min. The increase in sleep opportunity is accomplished by having the patient retire 15 min earlier for the next week of treatment. The upward titration process is usually continued for about 4 weeks, thus allowing for an increase of about 1 h in sleep opportunity. When the patient does not reach the 85–90 % benchmark, some clinicians reduce the total sleep opportunity to the previous "set point," others maintain the patient's total sleep opportunity until adequate sleep efficiency is observed, while still others combine these approaches. With respect to the last possibility, the clinician may maintain the patient's total sleep opportunity for 2–3 weeks and then downwardly titrate the TIB when there is clear evidence that the patient cannot sustain their clinical gains.

This therapy is thought to be effective for two reasons. First, it prevents the patient from coping with their insomnia by extending sleep opportunity. This strategy, while increasing the opportunity to get more sleep, produces a form of sleep that is shallow and fragmented. Second, the initial sleep loss that occurs with SRT is thought to increase the "pressure for sleep" which in turn produces quicker sleep latencies, less wake after sleep onset, and more efficient sleep.

Three points merit further comment. First, total time in bed is manipulated by delaying the patient's sleep period. This, along with keeping a fixed wake time, results in sleep restriction. It is plausible having the patient wake up at an earlier time could alter total time in bed. This approach is not typically adopted for the following reasons: fixing "wakeup time" at an early hour:

- Does not capitalize on the fact that extending wakefulness is easier to tolerate than curtailing sleep
- Delays the initial increase in time awake before sleep for 24 h (and thus delays the clinical effect)
- May reinforce the tendency for early morning awakenings
- Undermines the opportunity to pair "sleep" with the bed/bedroom

Second, it should be noted that SRT has a couple of paradoxical aspects to it. One paradox is that patients who report being unable to sleep are in essence being told to sleep less. The other paradox occurs over the course of treatment. With therapy, patients find that it is difficult to stay awake until the prescribed hour. This, if not paradoxical, is at least ironic for the patient that initially presents with sleep-onset difficulties. Finally, it should be noted that Sleep restriction may be contraindicated in patients with histories of mania or seizure disorder, because it may aggravate these conditions.

Sleep Hygiene Education

Sleep hygiene education is not recommended as a monotherapy but is typically used along with SRT and STC. Sleep hygiene education addresses a variety of behaviors that may influence sleep quality and quantity. The intervention most often involves providing the patient with a handout and then reviewing the items and the rationales for them. Table 6.1 contains a set of sleep hygiene instructions. It should be noted that in this formulation, several aspects of other therapies are adopted [41]. For example, items 1, 2, 12, 13, and 15 are traditionally considered part of stimulus control and/or sleep restriction therapy.

Sleep hygiene education is most helpful when tailored to a behavioral analysis of the patient's sleep–wake behaviors. The tailoring process allows the clinician (1) to demonstrate the extent to which they comprehend the patient's individual circumstances (by knowing which items do and do not apply) and (2) the opportunity to suggest modifications to the rules, which at times are too absolutistic or rigid for individual patients. Examples include the following:

- The admonishment to avoid caffeinated products may be, in general, too simply construed. A reasonable number (1–3 servings) of caffeinated beverages early to midday may be used to combat daytime fatigue (especially during acute therapy).
- The prohibition against napping may not be practical. Elderly patient or patients with extreme work performance demands may indeed need to compensate for sleep loss. A more considerate approach to napping may entail taking into account the time of the nap, the duration of the nap, and how nocturnal sleep is handled on days when patients nap. Napping earlier in the day will allow for more homeostatic pressure for nocturnal sleep. Limiting the duration of the nap will allow for less of a discharge of the homeostat and enhance the patient's sensation of feeling rested from the nap (by avoiding awakening from slow-wave sleep). Going to bed later, when one naps during the day, may minimize the effects of the nap on nocturnal sleep.
- Recommendations to avoid watching TV in bed may be difficult to adhere to early in therapy. Patients who are unable to fall asleep without the use of the television may have anxiety about sleeping without it. The discussion of this rule to remove the TV from the bedroom may involve a gradual change (e.g., turning off the TV before attempting to sleep) rather than abruptly removing it. By demanding removal of the TV in the first few sessions, it may be damaging to the patient's engagement in the treatment because the therapist is perceived as removing something that is helpful and pleasurable.

It can be argued that the most important aspect of sleep hygiene education derives not so much from the "tips" provided, but from allowing the clinician the opportunity to demonstrate their knowledge. Patients often come to treatment with a laundry list of behavioral changes they have tried to no avail and there is little empirical evidence that poor sleep hygiene causes insomnia. However, these types of changes are often "low-hanging fruit" in terms of treatment goals. Patients must

Table 6.1 Sleep hygiene instructions

1. *Sleep only as much as you need to feel refreshed during the following day.* Restricting your time in bed helps to consolidate and deepen your sleep. Excessively long times in bed lead to fragmented and shallow sleep. Get up at your regular time the next day, no matter how little you slept
2. *Get up at the same time each day, 7 days a week.* A regular wake time in the morning leads to regular times of sleep onset, and helps to set your "biological clock"
3. *Exercise regularly.* Schedule exercise times so that they do not occur within 3 h of when you intend to go to bed. Exercise makes it easier to initiate sleep and deepen sleep
4. *Make sure that your bedroom is comfortable and free from light and noise.* A comfortable, noise-free sleep environment will reduce the likelihood that you will wake up during the night. Noise that does not awaken you may also disturb the quality of your sleep. Carpeting, insulated curtains, and closing the door may help
5. *Make sure that your bedroom is at a comfortable temperature during the night.* Excessively warm or cold sleep environments may disturb sleep
6. *Eat regular meals and do not go to bed hungry.* Hunger may disturb sleep. A light snack at bedtime (especially carbohydrates) may help sleep, but avoid greasy or "heavy" foods
7. *Avoid excessive liquids in the evening.* Reducing liquid intake will minimize the need for nighttime trips to the bathroom
8. *Cut down on all caffeine products.* Caffeinated beverages and foods (coffee, tea, cola, chocolate) can cause difficulty falling asleep, awakenings during the night, and shallow sleep. Even caffeine early in the day can disrupt nighttime sleep
9. *Avoid alcohol, especially in the evening.* Although alcohol helps tense people fall asleep more easily, it causes awakenings later in the night
10. *Smoking may disturb sleep.* Nicotine is a stimulant. Try not to smoke during the night when you have trouble sleeping
11. *Don't take your problems to bed.* Plan some time earlier in the evening for working on your problems or planning the next day's activities. Worrying may interfere with initiating sleep and produce shallow sleep
12. *Train yourself to use the bedroom only for sleeping and sexual activity.* This will help condition your brain to see bed as the place for sleeping. Do *not* read, watch TV, or eat in bed
13. *Do not try to fall asleep.* This only makes the problem worse. Instead, turn on the light, leave the bedroom, and do something different like reading a book. Don't engage in stimulating activity. Return to bed only when you are sleepy
14. *Put the clock under the bed or turn it so that you can't see it.* Clock watching may lead to frustration, anger, and worry, which interfere with sleep
15. *Avoid naps.* Staying awake during the day helps you to fall asleep at night

The above list includes the usual practices described as "good sleep hygiene," but it also includes some principles subsumed under "stimulus control therapy" [2, 12, 13], "sleep restriction therapy" [1, 2, 15], and "relaxation" [11, 13]

have realistic expectations for the impact of these changes however. Furthermore, a thoughtful and elaborate review may enhance the patient's confidence in their therapist and in the treatment regimen. Such enhanced confidence may, in turn, lead to greater adherence/compliance with the more difficult aspects of therapy.

Cognitive Therapy

Several forms of cognitive therapy for insomnia have been developed. Some have a didactic focus [32], others use paradoxical intention [42], and others employ "distraction and imagery" [43]. While the approaches differ in procedure, all are based on the observation that patients with insomnia have negative thoughts and beliefs about their condition and its consequences. Helping patients to challenge the veracity of these beliefs is thought to decrease the anxiety and arousal associated with insomnia. The cognitive restructuring approach, adapted from the procedure used for panic disorder [44–46], is illustrated below.

Cognitive restructuring focuses upon catastrophic thinking and the belief that poor sleep is likely to have devastating consequences. While psychoeducation may also address these kinds of issues, the more important ingredient of cognitive restructuring lies not in disabusing the patient of erroneous information, but rather in having them discover that their estimates are ridiculously inaccurate (a testament to the tendency to think in less than clear terms in the middle of the night). When undertaking this exercise with a patient, it needs to be introduced in a considerate way, one which avoids any hint that the therapist is being pedantic, patronizing, or condescending.

The following are examples of the catastrophic thinking that occurs when the patient is lying in bed trying to sleep. "If I don't get a good night's sleep",

- "I'll be in a bad mood tomorrow. If my mood is poor tomorrow, I will—yet again—be short with my wife. If I'm irritable with my wife (again), she may start thinking about not putting up with this anymore. If she thinks about not putting up with this anymore, she'll consider leaving me …" [get divorced].
- "I won't be able to stay awake or concentrate when I'm driving to work. If I don't stay awake or concentrate when I'm driving, I may get into an accident …" [wreck the car].
- "I won't be able to function tomorrow at work. If I am not able to function at work, I may get a reprimand. If I get reprimanded …" [get fired].

The first step in the cognitive restructuring process is to have patients discuss and make a list of the kinds of negative things they think can happen when their sleep is poor. Usually, the list is constructed with the patient and placed on the cognitive therapist's ever-present in-office chalkboard. Column 1 is the list of catastrophic events. Please note that the patient may need to be prompted to identify the underlying and most catastrophic thought. For example, he/she may say "I worry about not being able to fall sleep" when what he/she is primarily worried about is the extreme version of this proposition: spending the entire night awake.

Once the list is compiled (5–10 things constitutes a reasonable list), patients are then asked how likely they think each of the events are, given a night of poor sleep. For instance, the therapist may ask "When you are lying in bed imagining being so tired tomorrow that you might perform badly at work, at that moment how certain are you that your work will be 'substandard', how certain are you that you'll be 'reprimanded'," etc. These data are represented in column 2. Next, the patient is asked how frequently their sleep is poor, and for how many years they have been suffering from insomnia. This number is coded as the "number of days with insomnia" and is set to the side of the table (to be coded later in column 3). The final data needed from the patient is an estimate of how frequently each of the catastrophic events has occurred. These are coded into the fourth column. The combination of these four sources of data is then used to show the patient that there is a substantial mismatch between their degree of certainty and the number of times the negative events have actually transpired.

For example, the clinician might observe, "You have suffered from insomnia for five nights a week for the last three years. This means that you have had about 800 really bad nights. You also said that when you're thinking about what might happen if you don't fall asleep, you are 90% certain that on the next day you are going to perform so badly that you'll be reprimanded. If it happened 90% of the time and you've had 800 bad nights, then you should have been reprimanded about 700—let's say 500—times." These data are represented in column 5. The last column of data is then compared to the list in column 4, so that the patient can see the mismatch between the number of instances that should have occurred and the number of instances that actually occurred, in reality. For an example of the chart described above, see Table 6.2.

Relaxation Training

Different relaxation techniques target different physiological systems. Progressive muscle relaxation is used to diminish skeletal muscle tension [34, 47–49]. Diaphragmatic breathing is used to make respiration slower, deeper, and mechanically driven from the abdomen as opposed to the thorax. (It is interesting to note that this form of respiration resembles what occurs naturally at sleep onset.) Autogenic training focuses on increasing peripheral blood flow by having patients imagine, in a systematic way, that each of their extremities feels warm. There have also been investigations into yoga [50, 51], tai chi [52], and mindfulness [53] in the treatment of insomnia.

Table 6.2 Cognitive restructuring worksheet

1	2	3	4	5
Event	Certainty when lying awake and unable to sleep	# Days with insomnia	# of event occurrences	# of event occurrences given certainty
Get reprimanded	90 %	800	5	620 (500)
Get fired				
Get divorced				
Wreck the car				
Be awake all night				

Most practitioners select the optimal relaxation method based upon which technique is easiest for the patient to learn and most consistent with how the patient manifests arousal. Like cognitive techniques, learning to effectively use relaxation training often requires substantial practice. Many clinicians recommend the patient rehearse the skill during the day in addition to practicing prior to sleep. When integrating into stimulus control instructions, if relaxation training causes some initial "performance anxiety," it may be best to have the patient practice in a room other than the bedroom. It also should be borne in mind that some patients, especially those with a history of panic disorder, may experience a paradoxical response to relaxation techniques.

Phototherapy

While many may not consider phototherapy a behavioral intervention, the use of bright light is often important to integrate into the treatment regimen. This is especially true when circadian factors appear to substantially contribute to the insomnia complaint [54]. There is substantial empirical evidence that timed bright light has effects on circadian rhythm disturbances that may underlie some insomnia symptoms [55].

In the case where the patient's insomnia has a phase delay component (i.e., the patient prefers to go to bed late and wake up late), bright light exposure in the morning for a period of 30 min or more may enable them to "feel sleepy" at an earlier time in the evening. In the case where the patient's insomnia has a phase advance component (i.e., the patient prefers to go to bed early and wake up early), bright light exposure in the late evening/early night may enable them to stay awake until a later hour. Phototherapy is often accomplished via a "light box" which typically generates white light, or more selectively blue spectrum light at 5000–10,000 lx. The dose is adjusted by altering the distance and duration of light exposure. It is generally assumed that phototherapy has no significant side effects, but this is not always the case. Mania may be triggered by bright light, but rarely, if ever, in patients not previously diagnosed with bipolar mood disorder. Other side effects are insomnia, hypomania, agitation, visual blurring, eye strain, and headaches. Light boxes may not be recommended for individuals with certain eye conditions, including retinopathy secondary to diabetes. In some cases, equivalent or better phase shifting properties may be accomplished by scheduling time outdoors by taking early morning walks, for example.

The sleep-promoting effects of bright light may occur via several mechanisms, including shifting the circadian system, enhancement of the amplitude of the circadian pacemaker, promoting wakefulness during the day and sleep at night, or indirectly via its antidepressant effects.

Although timed bright light treatment is recommended as a practice parameter for circadian rhythm disorders, there is little evidence that bright light improves sleep in insomnia. Two trials have failed to demonstrate a benefit of bright light (morning or evening) to improve objective or self-reported sleep quality among older adults with insomnia [56, 57].

Complicating Factors

There are a number of potential complicating factors that require continuous monitoring and evaluation throughout the course of treatment, particularly if the patient fails to show expected clinical gains after 2–4 sessions of active treatment. The most common complicating factors are poor treatment compliance, issues related to comorbid psychiatric and medical disorders, and the simultaneous use of sedative hypnotics.

Treatment Compliance

The single-most important complicating factor is poor treatment compliance. At the beginning of treatment, the clinician should proactively address the fact that the prescriptions may seem counterintuitive and that adhering to the treatment will be difficult. Providing the patient with a complete and thoughtful rationale for each aspect of the treatment, managing the patient expectations, and encouraging an active self-management approach are essential. Providing the rationale for treatment is likely to gain compliance in at least two ways. First, the effort to explain therapy is less imperative, and thereby makes the patient an active partner in the treatment process and less resistant or reactive to the prescriptions. Second, a fluid, interesting, and compelling explanation will support and enhance the patient's perception of the clinician as a competent authority.

With respect to expectation, patients should not anticipate that the results will be immediate. In fact, patients should be cautioned that their sleep problem is likely to briefly "get worse before it gets better." Sometimes an appeal to the research literature, demonstrating that treatment gains are maintained and often continue to improve in the long term, may help maintain their motivation despite the short-term difficulty adjusting to the procedures by demonstrating that for a large number of patients it is worth the effort. However, patients should be aware that CBT does have short-term negative effects on some patients. In particularly, sleep restriction reduces sleep duration for the first 2 weeks, which may cause negative effects. One study reported negative side effects in $\geq 50\%$ of patients including daytime sleepiness and fatigue as well as frustration/boredom associated with delaying their bedtime [58, 59]. Patients starting sleep restriction treatment may voice concerns about sleep restriction given the research demonstrating health effects of short sleep duration, such as weight gain and metabolic dysfunction, which often are part of their catastrophic beliefs [60, 61]. It should be noted that trials report no adverse events associated with CBT for insomnia and there are no known long-term negative effects of sleep restriction reported. However, some patients may choose to avoid driving in the first week or two of sleep restriction if they feel drowsy and are concerned about drowsy driving.

Another consideration is the role of "active self-management." It is important to remember that the treatment alternative to CBT is medication and that this requires very little in the way of lifestyle change. Thus, the clinician must spend a considerable amount of time working with the patient to "make and stay with the investment." Patients who attend treatment have often tried and failed to benefit from hypnotic medications or continue to report insomnia despite taking medications or escalating the dose. Therefore, it's useful to negotiate a reasonable time period for the patient to determine if their investment of time and effort into the treatment has an opportunity to improve their sleep, typically 12 weeks.

Comorbidity of Mental and Medical Disorders

Many patients with chronic insomnia report mild or subthreshold levels of depressive symptoms. When depressive symptoms become severe, they may interfere with the patient's ability and motivation to successfully follow the recommended protocol. If medical factors become exacerbated, expectations for clinical gains need to be tempered until there is stabilization. Throughout the course of treatment both medical and psychiatric factors should be monitored and consideration given for the need for further evaluation and intervention. Evidence supports simultaneously treating insomnia as well as depression. Many studies have demonstrated that improvements in sleep may contribute to reductions in depressive symptoms [62]. Further, directly addressing insomnia symptoms leads to greater insomnia reduction than targeting depression alone [63]. There is also some evidence to suggest that cognitive behavioral treatment of insomnia may lead to faster remission of depressive symptoms when starting an SSRI [64].

CBT and Sedative Hypnotics

Many of the patients referred for cognitive-behavioral treatment have been taking sedative hypnotics for years and are very apprehensive about discontinuing treatment. Often the initial phases of treatment involve collaboration with the referring physician to assist the patient in the weaning process. Use of sleep diaries to provide feedback about sleep continuity during the withdrawal process and education about rebound insomnia and the medication itself are important for this kind of intervention. As noted previously in this chapter, the natural assumption during the withdrawal from medication is "This is how I will sleep without medications from now on." In combination with a careful weaning process, sleep diaries may serve as the "hard data" to demonstrate to the patient that this assumption is not true. Several studies have demonstrated that planned taper schedules and planned taper schedules plus multicomponent CBT for insomnia are effective at reducing hypnotic medication use and improving sleep quality [65, 66].

There is a growing literature demonstrating that combining hypnotics with CBT for insomnia does not appear to interfere with treatment outcome. Although initial studies were mixed [67–69], later research demonstrated the promise of this approach [70–72]. These studies suggest that the benefit of combined therapy is a more rapid reduction of symptoms. The risk of combining pharmacotherapy with behavioral treatment, however, is that once patients start using medications, they may be less inclined to adopt or tolerate the behavioral interventions. Data suggest that long-term outcomes are better for patients who are given hypnotic medications for short-term use and then tapered off during sessions of CBT [70]. Therefore, it is best to consider time-limited use of hypnotics with a plan to taper while starting CBT.

The Efficacy of CBT

There is a robust body of research supporting the efficacy of multicomponent CBT in the treatment of chronic insomnia [73–78]. Results from these quantitative reviews demonstrate that 70–80 % of patients have clinically meaningful improvement in their insomnia symptoms. Quantitative analysis revealed that sleep latency was reduced by 39.5–43 % (effect sizes: 0.87–0.88), number of intermittent awakenings was reduced by 30–73 % (effect sizes: 0.53–0.63), duration of intermittent awakenings was reduced by 46 % (effect size: 0.65), and total sleep time was increased by 8–9.4 % (effect size: 0.42). In actual minutes, pre-post measures revealed that patients fell asleep 19–28 min sooner, had 0.5–1.2 fewer awakenings, and obtained about 7–32 more minutes of sleep a night. Comparative data showed that sleep restriction therapy or stimulus control yielded the greatest improvement, followed by multicomponent therapies. Treatment gains were maintained or enhanced over follow-up periods ranging from 3 weeks to 3 years.

The large number of insomnia trials have provided the opportunity to analyze the effectiveness of CBT for insomnia in subpopulations and treatment types. For example, analysis of group CBT for insomnia (eight studies met criteria) demonstrated large effect size for subjective and objective measures of sleep, on par with individual treatment [79]. An analysis of CBT for insomnia in medical and psychiatric populations demonstrated improvement in 36 % of those who received CBT versus 17 % in the control conditions, with greater improvement in psychiatric populations compared with medical populations. Results were also sustained (12–18 months) in many trials [80, 81].

Studies have demonstrated efficacy of CBT in patients with chronic pain [82], cancer [77, 83], cardiovascular and pulmonary disease [84], and depression [63, 64, 85].

A major accomplishment in the history of insomnia treatment is the development and roll out of a CBT for insomnia training program within the Veterans Health Administration system (VA) [86, 87]. This program involved the development of a 3-day CBT for insomnia workshop for licensed mental health practitioners within the VA system (psychologists, psychiatrists, nurses, and social workers). Results of this training demonstrate that licensed professionals can acquire skills needed to meet competency criteria in the treatment of insomnia, even for those who do not have a general training in CBT. There are two published reports demonstrating high levels of therapist adherence to the treatment manual among therapists trained in the

VA insomnia training. Furthermore, patients' symptom ratings on the Insomnia Severity Index (ISI) improved ($d=2.3$) as well as measures of depression and quality of life [86, 88].

Abbreviated Versions of CBT-I

Several studies have designed abbreviated versions of CBT for insomnia, typically focusing on behavioral components. These studies have demonstrated that brief protocols have the potential to reduce insomnia symptoms but effect sizes tend to be smaller than the full 6–8 session protocols. Edinger and colleagues created a "primary care-friendly" version of CBT which included 2, 35-min sessions by a psychologist with sleep training [89]. Buysse and colleagues developed a brief CBT intervention that was administered by a nurse over 4 weeks, with two face-to-face sessions (weeks 1, 60 min and 3, 30 min) and two brief telephone follow-ups (weeks 2 and 4, <20 min) [90–92]. These two abbreviated protocols demonstrate that a substantial portion of patients have clinically significant improvement with abbreviated treatment (50–65 %) and treatments can be effectively administered by a non-psychologist with brief training.

A recent study evaluated a single-session CBT ("single shot") among patients with acute insomnia (symptoms ≤1 month) and reported remission of insomnia symptoms among a significant proportion of patients with one 75-min visit [93]. This suggests that brief training may be able to prevent acute insomnia from developing into chronic insomnia. Further research is needed to determine if stepped care or matching approaches can be effectively used to reduce healthcare costs and patient burden in treatment.

Technology and CBT

Over the past few years, emphasis has grown on the use of technology-based interventions for behavioral interventions for various health and psychological conditions, including insomnia [94]. The goal of technology-based treatments is to increase dissemination and availability of insomnia treatment, which is an issue in much of the country due to low numbers of trained providers. There is evidence to support the use of CBT for insomnia via video conferencing [95] and the use of interactive websites [96–98]. A meta-analysis evaluating the effects of media-based CBT for insomnia demonstrated significant improvements in some areas with treatment (sleep quality, sleep efficiency, the number of arousals, sleep-onset latency, and on the Insomnia Severity Index) but not others (WASO, TST) [99]. A recent study compared face-to-face group CBT for insomnia to Internet-based treatment and found that outcomes were not different between groups (i.e., equivalence trial) [63]. These studies demonstrate a growing literature supporting the use of technology in the dissemination of cognitive behavioral treatments for insomnia. Much research is needed to determine which patients will do best with this treatment but these results provide strong support that Web-based treatment is feasible and beneficial to many patients.

Summary

- CBT is designed to address problematic behavioral in chronic insomnia as well as cognitive hyperarousal and learned associations that develop in patients with chronic insomnia.
- Neurocognitive mechanisms may underlie the development of insomnia as well as response to treatment.
- Multicomponent CBT for insomnia demonstrates efficacy in chronic insomnia among patients with and without comorbid mental and physical conditions.
- Recent innovations in delivery of CBT for insomnia include the development of brief CBT versions designed for use in community and medical settings and technology-based interventions.

References

1. Spielman AJ, Caruso LS, Glovinsky PB. A behavioral perspective on insomnia treatment. Psychiatr Clin North Am. 1987;10(4):541–53.
2. Perlis ML, Giles DE, Mendelson WB, Bootzin RR, Wyatt JK. Psychophysiological insomnia: the behavioural model and a neurocognitive perspective. J Sleep Res. 1997;6(3):179–88.
3. Bonnet MH, Arand DL. Hyperarousal and insomnia: state of the science. Sleep Med Rev. 2010;14(1):9–15.
4. Harvey CJ, Gehrman P, Espie CA. Who is predisposed to insomnia: a review of familial aggregation, stress-reactivity, personality and coping style. Sleep Med Rev. 2014;18(3):237–47.
5. Drake CL, Friedman NP, Wright Jr KP, Roth T. Sleep reactivity and insomnia: genetic and environmental influences. Sleep. 2011;34(9):1179–88.
6. Hall M, Buysse DJ, Dew MA, Prigerson HG, Kupfer DJ, Reynolds 3rd CF. Intrusive thoughts and avoidance behaviors are associated with sleep disturbances in bereavement-related depression. Depress Anxiety. 1997;6(3):106–12.
7. Harvey AG. A cognitive model of insomnia. Behav Res Ther. 2002;40(8):869–93.
8. Edinger JD, Wohlgemuth WK, Radtke RA, Marsh GR, Quillian RE. Cognitive behavioral therapy for treatment of chronic primary insomnia: a randomized controlled trial. JAMA. 2001;285(14):1856–64.
9. Morin CM, Blais F, Savard J. Are changes in beliefs and attitudes about sleep related to sleep improvements in the treatment of insomnia? Behav Res Ther. 2002;40(7):741–52.
10. Lichstein KL, Rosenthal TL. Insomniacs' perceptions of cognitive versus somatic determinants of sleep disturbance. J Abnorm Psychol. 1980;89(1):105–7.
11. Nicassio PM, Mendlowitz DR, Fussell JJ, Petras L. The phenomenology of the pre-sleep state: the development of the pre-sleep arousal scale. Behav Res Ther. 1985;23(3):263–71.
12. Van Egeren L, Haynes SN, Franzen M, Hamilton J. Presleep cognitions and attributions in sleep-onset insomnia. J Behav Med. 1983;6(2):217–32.

13. Kuisk LA, Bertelson AD, Walsh JK. Presleep cognitive hyperarousal and affect as factors in objective and subjective insomnia. Percept Mot Skills. 1989;69(3 Pt 2):1219–25.
14. Watts FN, Coyle K, East MP. The contribution of worry to insomnia. Br J Clin Psychol. 1994;33(Pt 2):211–20.
15. Perlis ML, Smith MT, Andrews PJ, Orff H, Giles DE. Beta/gamma EEG activity in patients with primary and secondary insomnia and good sleeper controls. Sleep. 2001;24(1):110–7.
16. Perlis ML, Merica H, Smith MT, Giles DE. Beta EEG activity and insomnia. Sleep Med Rev. 2001;5(5):363–74.
17. Perlis ML, Kehr EL, Smith MT, Andrews PJ, Orff H, Giles DE. Temporal and stagewise distribution of high frequency EEG activity in patients with primary and secondary insomnia and in good sleeper controls. J Sleep Res. 2001;10(2):93–104.
18. Merica H, Gaillard JM. The EEG of the sleep onset period in insomnia: a discriminant analysis. Physiol Behav. 1992;52(2):199–204.
19. Merica H, Blois R, Gaillard JM. Spectral characteristics of sleep EEG in chronic insomnia. Eur J Neurosci. 1998;10(5):1826–34.
20. Freedman RR. EEG power spectra in sleep-onset insomnia. Electroencephalogr Clin Neurophysiol. 1986;63(5):408–13.
21. Lamarche CH, Ogilvie RD. Electrophysiological changes during the sleep onset period of psychophysiological insomniacs, psychiatric insomniacs, and normal sleepers. Sleep. 1997;20(9):724–33.
22. Wu YM, Pietrone R, Cashmere JD, et al. EEG power during waking and NREM sleep in primary insomnia. J Clin Sleep Med. 2013;9(10):1031–7.
23. Krystal AD, Edinger JD, Wohlgemuth WK, Marsh GR. NREM sleep EEG frequency spectral correlates of sleep complaints in primary insomnia subtypes. Sleep. 2002;25(6):630–40.
24. Krystal AD, Edinger JD. Sleep EEG predictors and correlates of the response to cognitive behavioral therapy for insomnia. Sleep. 2010;33(5):669–77.
25. Monk TH, Reynolds CF, Kupfer DJ, et al. The Pittsburgh sleep diary. J Sleep Res. 1994;3(2):111–20.
26. Carney CE, Buysse DJ, Ancoli-Israel S, et al. The consensus sleep diary: standardizing prospective sleep self-monitoring. Sleep. 2012;35(2):287–302.
27. Carskadon MA, Dement WC, Mitler MM, Guilleminault C, Zarcone VP, Spiegel R. Self-reports versus sleep laboratory findings in 122 drug-free subjects with complaints of chronic insomnia. Am J Psychiatry. 1976;133(12):1382–8.
28. Frankel BL, Coursey RD, Buchbinder R, Snyder F. Recorded and reported sleep in chronic primary insomnia. Arch Gen Psychiatry. 1976;33(5):615–23.
29. Coates TJ, Killen JD, George J, Marchini E, Silverman S, Thoresen C. Estimating sleep parameters: a multitrait—multimethod analysis. J Consult Clin Psychol. 1982;50(3):345–52.
30. Kales A, Bixler EO, Vela-Bueno A, Cadieux RJ, Soldatos CR, Kales JD. Biopsychobehavioral correlates of insomnia, III: polygraphic findings of sleep difficulty and their relationship to psychopathology. Int J Neurosci. 1984;23(1):43–55.
31. Kales A, Caldwell AB, Preston TA, Healey S, Kales JD. Personality patterns in insomnia. Theoretical implications. Arch Gen Psychiatry. 1976;33(9):1128–34.
32. Morin CM. Insomnia: psychological assessment and management. New York: Guilford Press; 1993.
33. Perlis M, Jungquist C, Smith MT, Posner D. Cognitive behavioral treatment of insomnia: a session by session guide. New York, NY: Springer; 2005.
34. Lichstein KL, Riedel BW, Wilson NM, Lester KW, Aguillard RN. Relaxation and sleep compression for late-life insomnia: a placebo-controlled trial. J Consult Clin Psychol. 2001;69(2):227–39.
35. Means MK, Lichstein KL, Epperson MT, Johnson CT. Relaxation therapy for insomnia: night-time and day time effects. Behav Res Ther. 2000;38(7):665–78.
36. Friedman L, Benson K, Noda A, et al. An actigraphic comparison of sleep restriction and sleep hygiene treatments for insomnia in older adults. J Geriatr Psychiatry Neurol. 2000;13(1):17–27.

37. Lichstein KL, Wilson NM, Johnson CT. Psychological treatment of secondary insomnia. Psychol Aging. 2000;15(2):232–40.
38. Espie CA, Inglis SJ, Tessier S, Harvey L. The clinical effectiveness of cognitive behaviour therapy for chronic insomnia: implementation and evaluation of a sleep clinic in general medical practice. Behav Res Ther. 2001;39(1):45–60.
39. Chesson Jr AL, Anderson WM, Littner M, et al. Practice parameters for the nonpharmacologic treatment of chronic insomnia. An American Academy of Sleep Medicine report. Standards of Practice Committee of the American Academy of Sleep Medicine. Sleep. 1999;22(8): 1128–33.
40. Schutte-Rodin S, Broch L, Buysse D, Dorsey C, Sateia M. Clinical guideline for the evaluation and management of chronic insomnia in adults. J Clin Sleep Med. 2008;4(5):487–504.
41. Stepanski EJ, Wyatt JK. Use of sleep hygiene in the treatment of insomnia. Sleep Med Rev. 2003;7(3):215–25.
42. Shoham-Salomon V, Rosenthal R. Paradoxical interventions: a meta-analysis. J Consult Clin Psychol. 1987;55(1):22–8.
43. Harvey AG, Payne S. The management of unwanted pre-sleep thoughts in insomnia: distraction with imagery versus general distraction. Behav Res Ther. 2002;40(3):267–77.
44. Barlow DH. Behavioral conception and treatment of panic. Psychopharmacol Bull. 1986;22(3):802–6.
45. Barlow DH. Cognitive-behavioral approaches to panic disorder and social phobia. Bull Menninger Clin. 1992;56(2 Suppl A):A14–28.
46. Barlow DH. Cognitive-behavioral therapy for panic disorder: current status. J Clin Psychiatry. 1997;58 Suppl 2:32–6. discussion 36–37.
47. Haynes SN, Moseley D, McGowan WT. Relaxation training and biofeedback in the reduction of frontalis muscle tension. Psychophysiology. 1975;12(5):547–52.
48. Freedman R, Papsdorf JD. Biofeedback and progressive relaxation treatment of sleep-onset insomnia: a controlled, all-night investigation. Biofeedback Self Regul. 1976;1(3):253–71.
49. Borkovec TD, Fowles DC. Controlled investigation of the effects of progressive and hypnotic relaxation on insomnia. J Abnorm Psychol. 1973;82(1):153–8.
50. Afonso RF, Hachul H, Kozasa EH, et al. Yoga decreases insomnia in postmenopausal women: a randomized clinical trial. Menopause. 2012;19(2):186–93.
51. Khalsa SB. Treatment of chronic insomnia with yoga: a preliminary study with sleep-wake diaries. Appl Psychophysiol Biofeedback. 2004;29(4):269–78.
52. Irwin MR, Olmstead R, Carrillo C, et al. Cognitive behavioral therapy vs. Tai Chi for late life insomnia and inflammatory risk: a randomized controlled comparative efficacy trial. Sleep. 2014;37(9):1543–52.
53. Ong JC, Manber R, Segal Z, Xia Y, Shapiro S, Wyatt JK. A randomized controlled trial of mindfulness meditation for chronic insomnia. Sleep. Sep 2014;37(9):1553–63.
54. Lack LC, Wright HR. Treating chronobiological components of chronic insomnia. Sleep Med. 2007;8(6):637–44.
55. Auger RR, Burgess HJ, Emens JS, Deriy LV, Thomas SM, Sharkey KM. Clinical Practice Guideline for the Treatment of Intrinsic Circadian Rhythm Sleep-Wake Disorders: Advanced Sleep-Wake Phase Disorder (ASWPD), Delayed Sleep-Wake Phase Disorder (DSWPD), Non-24-Hour Sleep-Wake Rhythm Disorder (N24SWD), and Irregular Sleep-Wake Rhythm Disorder (ISWRD). An Update for 2015: An American Academy of Sleep Medicine Clinical Practice Guideline. J Clin Sleep Med. 2015;11(10):1199–236.
56. Friedman L, Zeitzer JM, Kushida C, et al. Scheduled bright light for treatment of insomnia in older adults. J Am Geriatr Soc. 2009;57(3):441–52.
57. Suhner AG, Murphy PJ, Campbell SS. Failure of timed bright light exposure to alleviate age-related sleep maintenance insomnia. J Am Geriatr Soc. 2002;50(4):617–23.
58. Kyle SD, Morgan K, Spiegelhalder K, Espie CA. No pain, no gain: an exploratory within-subjects mixed-methods evaluation of the patient experience of sleep restriction therapy (SRT) for insomnia. Sleep Med. 2011;12(8):735–47.

59. Riedel BW, Lichstein KL. Strategies for evaluating adherence to sleep restriction treatment for insomnia. Behav Res Ther. 2001;39(2):201–12.
60. Patel SR, Malhotra A, White DP, Gottlieb DJ, Hu FB. Association between reduced sleep and weight gain in women. Am J Epidemiol. 2006;164(10):947–54.
61. Spiegel K, Tasali E, Leproult R, Van Cauter E. Effects of poor and short sleep on glucose metabolism and obesity risk. Nat Rev Endocrinol. 2009;5(5):253–61.
62. Ye YY, Zhang YF, Chen J, et al. Internet-based cognitive behavioral therapy for insomnia (ICBT-i) improves comorbid anxiety and depression-A meta-analysis of randomized controlled trials. PLoS One. 2015;10(11):e0142258.
63. Blom K, Jernelov S, Kraepelien M, et al. Internet treatment addressing either insomnia or depression, for patients with both diagnoses: a randomized trial. Sleep. 2015;38(2):267–77.
64. Manber R, Edinger JD, Gress JL, San Pedro-Salcedo MG, Kuo TF, Kalista T. Cognitive behavioral therapy for insomnia enhances depression outcome in patients with comorbid major depressive disorder and insomnia. Sleep. 2008;31(4):489–95.
65. Morin CM, Bastien C, Guay B, Radouco-Thomas M, Leblanc J, Vallieres A. Randomized clinical trial of supervised tapering and cognitive behavior therapy to facilitate benzodiazepine discontinuation in older adults with chronic insomnia. Am J Psychiatry. 2004;161(2):332–42.
66. Lichstein KL, Nau SD, Wilson NM, et al. Psychological treatment of hypnotic-dependent insomnia in a primarily older adult sample. Behav Res Ther. 2013;51(12):787–96.
67. Hauri PJ. Can we mix behavioral therapy with hypnotics when treating insomniacs? Sleep. 1997;20(12):1111–8.
68. Milby JB, Williams V, Hall JN, Khuder S, McGill T, Wooten V. Effectiveness of combined triazolam-behavioral therapy for primary insomnia. Am J Psychiatry. 1993;150(8):1259–60.
69. Morin CM, Colecchi C, Stone J, Sood R, Brink D. Behavioral and pharmacological therapies for late-life insomnia: a randomized controlled trial. JAMA. 1999;281(11):991–9 [see comment].
70. Morin CM, Vallieres A, Guay B, et al. Cognitive behavioral therapy, singly and combined with medication, for persistent insomnia: a randomized controlled trial. JAMA. 2009;301(19):2005–15.
71. Jacobs GD, Pace-Schott EF, Stickgold R, Otto MW. Cognitive behavior therapy and pharmacotherapy for insomnia: a randomized controlled trial and direct comparison. Arch Intern Med. 2004;164(17):1888–96.
72. Zavesicka L, Brunovsky M, Horacek J, et al. Trazodone improves the results of cognitive behaviour therapy of primary insomnia in non-depressed patients. Neuro Endocrinol Lett. 2008;29(6):895–901.
73. Morin CM, Hauri PJ, Espie CA, Spielman AJ, Buysse DJ, Bootzin RR. Nonpharmacologic treatment of chronic insomnia. An American Academy of Sleep Medicine review. Sleep. 1999;22(8):1134–56.
74. Murtagh DR, Greenwood KM. Identifying effective psychological treatments for insomnia: a meta-analysis. J Consult Clin Psychol. 1995;63(1):79–89.
75. Smith MT, Perlis ML, Park A, et al. Comparative meta-analysis of pharmacotherapy and behavior therapy for persistent insomnia. Am J Psychiatry. 2002;159(1):5–11.
76. Morin CM, Bootzin RR, Buysse DJ, Edinger JD, Espie CA, Lichstein KL. Psychological and behavioral treatment of insomnia: update of the recent evidence (1998–2004). Sleep. 2006;29(11):1398–414.
77. Johnson JA, Rash JA, Campbell TS, et al. A systematic review and meta-analysis of randomized controlled trials of cognitive behavior therapy for insomnia (CBT-I) in cancer survivors. Sleep Med Rev. 2015;27:20–8.
78. Trauer JM, Qian MY, Doyle JS, Rajaratnam SM, Cunnington D. Cognitive behavioral therapy for chronic insomnia: a systematic review and meta-analysis. Ann Intern Med. 2015;163(3):191–204.
79. Koffel EA, Koffel JB, Gehrman PR. A meta-analysis of group cognitive behavioral therapy for insomnia. Sleep Med Rev. 2015;19:6–16.

80. Wu JQ, Appleman ER, Salazar RD, Ong JC. Cognitive behavioral therapy for insomnia comorbid with psychiatric and medical conditions: a meta-analysis. JAMA Intern Med. 2015;175(9):1461–72.
81. Geiger-Brown JM, Rogers VE, Liu W, Ludeman EM, Downton KD, Diaz-Abad M. Cognitive behavioral therapy in persons with comorbid insomnia: a meta-analysis. Sleep Med Rev. 2015;23:54–67.
82. Smith MT, Finan PH, Buenaver LF, et al. Cognitive-behavioral therapy for insomnia in knee osteoarthritis: a randomized, double-blind, active placebo-controlled clinical trial. Arthritis Rheumatol. 2015;67(5):1221–33.
83. Savard J, Simard S, Ivers H, Morin CM. Randomized study on the efficacy of cognitive-behavioral therapy for insomnia secondary to breast cancer, part II: immunologic effects. J Clin Oncol. 2005;23(25):6097–106.
84. Rybarczyk B, Stepanski E, Fogg L, Lopez M, Barry P, Davis A. A placebo-controlled test of cognitive-behavioral therapy for comorbid insomnia in older adults. J Consult Clin Psychol. 2005;73(6):1164–74.
85. Clarke G, McGlinchey EL, Hein K, et al. Cognitive-behavioral treatment of insomnia and depression in adolescents: a pilot randomized trial. Behav Res Ther. 2015;69:111–8.
86. Trockel M, Karlin BE, Taylor CB, Manber R. Cognitive Behavioral Therapy for insomnia with Veterans: evaluation of effectiveness and correlates of treatment outcomes. Behav Res Ther. 2014;53:41–6.
87. Manber R, Carney C, Edinger J, et al. Dissemination of CBTI to the non-sleep specialist: protocol development and training issues. J Clin Sleep Med. 2012;8(2):209–18.
88. Karlin BE, Trockel M, Taylor CB, Gimeno J, Manber R. National dissemination of cognitive behavioral therapy for insomnia in veterans: therapist- and patient-level outcomes. J Consult Clin Psychol. 2013;81(5):912–7.
89. Edinger JD, Sampson WS. A primary care "friendly" cognitive behavioral insomnia therapy. Sleep. 2003;26(2):177–82.
90. Germain A, Moul DE, Franzen PL, et al. Effects of a brief behavioral treatment for late-life insomnia: preliminary findings. J Clin Sleep Med. 2006;2(4):403–6.
91. Buysse DJ, Germain A, Moul DE, et al. Efficacy of brief behavioral treatment for chronic insomnia in older adults. Arch Intern Med. 2011;171(10):887–95.
92. Troxel WM, Germain A, Buysse DJ. Clinical management of insomnia with brief behavioral treatment (BBTI). Behav Sleep Med. Oct 2012;10(4):266–79.
93. Ellis JG, Cushing T, Germain A. Treating acute insomnia: a randomized controlled trial of a "single-shot" of cognitive behavioral therapy for insomnia. Sleep. 2015;38(6):971–8.
94. Mohr DC, Schueller SM, Montague E, Burns MN, Rashidi P. The behavioral intervention technology model: an integrated conceptual and technological framework for eHealth and mHealth interventions. J Med Internet Res. 2014;16(6):e146.
95. Holmqvist M, Vincent N, Walsh K. Web- vs. telehealth-based delivery of cognitive behavioral therapy for insomnia: a randomized controlled trial. Sleep Med. 2014;15(2):187–95.
96. Ritterband LM, Thorndike FP, Gonder-Frederick LA, et al. Efficacy of an Internet-based behavioral intervention for adults with insomnia. Arch Gen Psychiatry. 2009;66(7):692–8.
97. Ritterband LM, Bailey ET, Thorndike FP, Lord HR, Farrell-Carnahan L, Baum LD. Initial evaluation of an Internet intervention to improve the sleep of cancer survivors with insomnia. Psychooncology. 2012;21(7):695–705.
98. Espie CA, Kyle SD, Williams C, et al. A randomized, placebo-controlled trial of online cognitive behavioral therapy for chronic insomnia disorder delivered via an automated media-rich web application. Sleep. 2012;35(6):769–81.
99. Cheng SK, Dizon J. Computerised cognitive behavioural therapy for insomnia: a systematic review and meta-analysis. Psychother Psychosom. 2012;81(4):206–16.

Chapter 7
Pharmacological Treatment of Insomnia

Paula K. Schweitzer and Stephen D. Feren

Abstract Medications used for the treatment of insomnia include prescription and non-prescription drugs approved by the US Food and Drug Administration (FDA) for the treatment of insomnia, prescription drugs approved by the FDA for treatment of another condition but used "off-label" for the treatment of insomnia, and unregulated substances such as herbal preparations and dietary supplements. These drugs differ in their pharmacological properties and in their efficacy and safety in the treatment of insomnia. This chapter reviews the key pharmacological characteristics of these medications, their mechanisms of action, and the available efficacy and safety data in the treatment of primary and comorbid insomnia. This review is followed by a discussion of the implementation and optimization of pharmacological treatment of insomnia for specific subtypes of insomnia.

Keywords Insomnia • Pharmacotherapy • Hypnotics • Benzodiazepine receptor agonists • Melatonin receptor agonists • Orexin antagonist • Antidepressants • Antipsychotics • Melatonin • Pharmacologic treatment of insomnia

Introduction

Medications used for the treatment of insomnia include prescription and non-prescription drugs approved by the US Food and Drug Administration (FDA) for the treatment of insomnia, prescription drugs approved by the FDA for treatment of another condition but used "off-label" for the treatment of insomnia, and unregulated substances such as herbal preparations and dietary supplements. Off-label use of prescription medications for insomnia is extremely common [1]. In 2007 the antidepressant trazodone and the antipsychotic quetiapine were prescribed for

P.K. Schweitzer, Ph.D. (✉)
Sleep Medicine and Research Center, St. Luke's Hospital,
232 S. Woods Mill Road, Chesterfield, MO 63017, USA
e-mail: paula.schweitzer@stlukes-stl.com

S.D. Feren, M.D.
Department of Neurology and Sleep Medicine, Kaiser Permanente,
Atlanta, GA, USA

© Springer International Publishing Switzerland 2017
H.P. Attarian (ed.), *Clinical Handbook of Insomnia*, Current Clinical Neurology,
DOI 10.1007/978-3-319-41400-3_7

insomnia as frequently as the zolpidem and eszopiclone, hypnotics with FDA indication for insomnia [2]. Both the complexity of the neurochemical regulation of sleep-wake behavior and the complexity of insomnia itself have driven the development of and use of drugs to treat insomnia. Choice of medication to optimize treatment of insomnia requires awareness of the pharmacologic properties of the available medications, knowledge of the research literature on efficacy and safety of these drugs in different insomnia subtypes, and knowledge of individual patient characteristics, including timing and frequency of the sleep complaint as well as the presence of comorbidities such as medical and psychiatric disorders, pain, or substance abuse. The drugs available for treatment of insomnia differ in their pharmacologic properties, in their efficacy and safety among subtypes of insomnia, and in the breadth of research data available in different insomnia subtypes. This chapter reviews current knowledge about medications used to promote sleep and discusses implementation and optimization of pharmacological treatment for insomnia. With the exception of melatonin, unregulated substances are not discussed. Tables 7.1 and 7.2 list medications used to treat insomnia and their key pharmacologic properties.

Key Pharmacologic Issues

Important factors relevant to the effects of a drug on sleep-wake behavior include (1) pharmacokinetic properties, particularly time to peak concentration (t_{max}) and half-life; (2) receptor-binding profile, which determines both mechanism of action and adverse effects; and (3) route of metabolism.

t_{max} determines how rapidly the clinical effect occurs. A t_{max} greater than 2 h is likely to be ineffective in promoting rapid sleep onset. Half-life, coupled with dose, determines the duration of the clinical effect. Drugs with short half-life are likely to be ineffective in maintaining sleep throughout the night, while drugs with very long half-life are more likely to promote sleep toward the end of the night but are also more likely to cause residual sedation. Higher doses increase both the likelihood of, and duration of, a clinical effect. In addition, pharmacological effects may differ with drug dose. For example, doxepin at low doses is predominantly a histamine antagonist, but at higher doses, it also inhibits reuptake of serotonin and norepinephrine, and exhibits anticholinergic and anti-adrenergic effects [3].

The receptor-binding profiles of most drugs approved by the FDA for treatment of insomnia have high pharmacologic specificity. That is, their effects are produced by activity at a single receptor type, without significant action at other receptors. For example, benzodiazepine receptor agonists bind to the benzodiazepine receptor-binding site, Ramelteon binds to melatonin 1 and 2 (MT_1, MT_2) receptors, low-dose doxepin (Silenor) blocks histamine 1 (H_1) receptors, and suvorexant blocks orexin receptors 1 and 2 (OX_1, OX_2). In contrast, most prescription drugs used "off-label" to treat insomnia (primarily sedating antidepressants and antipsychotics) affect multiple receptors, and thus may have multiple side effects [4].

Table 7.1 Pharmacology of drugs with FDA indication for insomnia

Generic name	Trade name	FDA indication	Receptor-binding profile					t_{max} (h)	$t_{1/2}$ (h)	Metabolism[a]	Dose range for insomnia (mg)
			GABA$_A$ specificity	MT$_1$–MT$_2$	Anti-OX$_1$–OX$_2$	Anti-H$_1$	Anti-mACh				
Benzodiazepine receptor agonists											
Estazolam	Prosom	Insomnia	Nonspecific					1.5–2	10–24	3A4	1–2
Flurazepam	Dalmane	Insomnia	Nonspecific					0.5–1.5	48–120[b]	3A4	15–30
Quazepam	Doral	Insomnia	Nonspecific					2	39–73[b]	2C19, 3A4	7.5–15
Temazepam	Restoril	Insomnia	Nonspecific					1–3	8–20	3A4, UGT	15–30
Triazolam	Halcion	Insomnia	Nonspecific					1–3	2–6	3A4, 3A5	0.125–0.25
Eszopiclone	Lunesta	Insomnia	Nonspecific					1.3–1.6	6–7	3A4, 2E1	1–3
Zaleplon	Sonata	Insomnia	$\alpha_1 > \alpha_{2,3,5}$					1.1	1	AO, 3A4	5–20
Zolpidem	Ambien	Insomnia	$\alpha_1 \gg \alpha_{2,3,5}$						1.5–2.4	3A4, 2C9	5–10
Zolpidem modified release	Ambien CR	Insomnia	$\alpha_1 \gg \alpha_{2,3}$ no α_5					1.7–2.5	1.6–4.5	3A4, 2C9	6.25–12.5
Zolpidem sublingual	Intermezzo	Insomnia	$\alpha_1 \gg \alpha_{2,3}$ no α_5					0.3–1.3	1.5–2.4	3A4, 2C9	1.75–3.5
Zolpidem sublingual	Edluar	Insomnia	$\alpha_1 \gg \alpha_{2,3}$ no α_5					0.5–3	2.6–2.8	3A4, 2C9	5–10
Zolpidem oral spray	Zolpimist	Insomnia	$\alpha_1 \gg \alpha_{2,3}$ no α_5					0.9	2.7–2.8	3A4, 2C9	5–10
Melatonin receptor agonist											
Ramelteon	Rozerem	Insomnia		+++				0.7–0.9	0.8–2	1A2, 2PC, 3A4	8
Orexin receptor antagonist											

(continued)

Table 7.1 (continued)

Generic name	Trade name	FDA indication	Receptor-binding profile					t_{max} (h)	$t_{1/2}$ (h)	Metabolism[a]	Dose range for insomnia (mg)
			GABA$_A$ specificity	MT$_1$–MT$_2$	Anti-OX$_1$–OX$_2$	Anti-H$_1$	Anti-mACh				
Suvorexant	Belsomra	Insomnia			+++			0.5–6	12	3A, 2C19	5–20
Histamine receptor antagonists											
Doxepin	Silenor	Insomnia				+++		3.5	15.3–31[b]	2C10, 2D6, 1A2, 2C9	3–6
Diphenhydramine	Benadryl	Allergy, sleep aid				+++	+++	2–3	5–11	2D6, 1A2, 2CP, 2C19	25–50
Doxylamine	Unisom	Allergy, sleep aid				+++	+++	1.5–2.5	10–12	2D6, 1A2, 2CP	25

GABA$_A$ γ[gamma]-aminobutyric acid type A receptor agonist, *MT$_1$–MT$_2$* melatonin 1 and 2 receptor agonist, *anti-OX$_1$–OX$_2$* orexin 1 and 2 receptor antagonist, *anti-H$_1$* histamine 1 receptor antagonist, *anti-mACh* muscarinic anticholinergic receptor antagonist, *t$_{max}$* time to peak concentration, *t$_{1/2}$* elimination half-life, *AO* aldehyde oxidase

[a]All entries beginning with numbers refer to specific CYP enzymes in the cytochrome P-450 system

Table 7.2 Pharmacology of drugs used "off-label" for insomnia

Generic name	Trade name	FDA indication	Receptor-binding profile							t_{max} (h)	$t_{1/2}$ (h)	Metabolism[a]	Dose range for insomnia (mg)
			GABA$_A$ specificity	MT$_1$–MT$_2$	Anti-H$_1$	Anti-5HT$_2$	Anti-alpha$_1$	Anti-dopa-mine	Anti-mACh				
Benzodiazepines													
Alprazolam	Xanax	Anxiety	Nonspecific							1–3	12–14	3A4, 3A55, 2C19	0.25–1.0
Alprazolam extended release	Xanax XR	Anxiety	Nonspecific							1–2	6.3–27	3A4, 3A55, 2C19	0.5–3
Chlordiazepoxide	Librium	Anxiety, alcohol withdrawal	Nonspecific							0.5–4	5–100	2B, 2C19, 3A4	5–10
Clonazepam	Klonopin	Anxiety, seizures	Nonspecific							1–2	35–40	2B, 3A4	0.25–2.0
Diazepam	Valium	Anxiety, muscle spasm, seizures	Nonspecific							0.5–2	20–50	2B, C19, CYP3A4	2–10
Lorazepam	Ativan	Anxiety	Nonspecific							1–3	12–15	UGT	0.25–2
Antidepressants													
Amitriptyline	Elavil	Depression			++	+	+++		+++	2–8	5–45	2D6, 2C19, 1A2, 3A4	25–150
Doxepin	Sinequan	Depression, anxiety			+++	+	+++		++	2–8	10–30	2D6, 2C19, 1A2, 3A4	10–150
Trimipramine	Surmontil	Depression			+++	+	+++		++	2–8	15–40	2D6, 2C19, 1A2, 3A4	25–150
Mirtazapine	Remeron	Depression			+++	+++	++			0.25–2	20–40	2D6, 3A4	7.5–30

(continued)

Table 7.2 (continued)

Generic name	Trade name	FDA indication	Receptor-binding profile							t_{max} (h)	$t_{1/2}$ (h)	Metabolism[a]	Dose range for insomnia (mg)
			GABA$_A$ specificity	MT$_1$–MT$_2$	Anti-H$_1$	Anti-5HT$_2$	Anti-alpha$_1$	Anti-dopa-mine	Anti-mACh				
Trazodone	Desyrel	Depression			+	+++	+++			1–2	7–15	3A4, 2D6, 1A2	25–150
Antipsychotics													
Olanzapine	Zyprexa	Schizophrenia bipolar disorder			+++	+++	++	++	+++	4–6	30	1A2	2.5–20
Quetiapine	Seroquel	Schizophrenia			++	+	+++	+		1–2	7	2D6, 3A4	25–250
Anticonvulsants													
Gabapentin	Neurontin	Seizures, neuropathic pain								2–3.5	5–7		300
Pregabalin	Lyrica	Seizures, neuropathic pain								1.5	6.3		100
Tiagabine	Gabitril	Seizures	GAT$_1$ inhibition							0.75	2–9	3A	2–12
Other													
Melatonin	Melatonin	None		+++							1–3	1A2, 2C19	0.1–75
Prazosin	Minipress	Hypertension					+++			3	2–3		2–20

GABA$_A$ γ[gamma]-aminobutyric acid type A receptor agonist, *MT$_1$–MT$_2$* melatonin 1 and 2 receptor agonist, *anti-H1* histamine 1 receptor antagonist, *anti-5HT$_2$* serotonin type 2 receptor antagonist, *anti-dopamine* dopamine receptor antagonist, *anti-mACh* muscarinic anticholinergic receptor antagonist, *t$_{max}$* time to peak concentration, *t$_{1/2}$* elimination half-life, *UGT* uridine 5′-diphospho-glucuronosyltransferase, *AO* aldehyde oxidase, *GAT$_1$* GABA transporter 1

[a]All entries beginning with numbers refer to specific CYP enzymes in the cytochrome P-450 system

The receptor-binding profile affects the adverse event profile, usually in a dose-dependent manner. Effects associated with drugs that bind to the benzodiazepine receptor site (e.g., benzodiazepine receptor agonists) include sedation, dizziness, ataxia, memory effects, and abuse potential. Drugs with anticholinergic effects (e.g., amitriptyline, diphenhydramine, olanzapine) may produce dizziness, dry mouth, blurred vision, constipation, and urinary retention. Drugs with alpha$_1$-adrenergic blocking properties (e.g., amitriptyline, doxepin, trazodone, quetiapine, olanzapine) have an increased risk for orthostatic hypotension. Drugs which block dopamine receptors carry the potential for extrapyramidal movement disorders, but these are rare with the drugs typically used to treat insomnia (quetiapine, olanzapine, risperidone) [5].

Finally, the route of metabolism is important for predicting interactions with other drugs.

Prescription and Non-prescription Agents Approved by FDA for Treatment of Insomnia

Benzodiazepine Receptor Agonists

Mechanism of Action

BzRA hypnotics promote sleep by enhancing the effect of GABA, the primary inhibitory neurotransmitter in the central nervous system, at the GABA$_A$ receptor complex [6]. GABA$_A$ receptors are a family of ligand-gated chloride channel inhibitory receptors. Each receptor consists of subunits that form a pentamer [7], with the most common expressions consisting of two α[alpha], two β[beta], and one γ[gamma] subunit [8, 9]. BzRAs bind to a site between the α[alpha] and γ[gamma] subunits, increasing the frequency of the chloride channel opening in the presence of GABA. The net result is an increase in inhibitory activity in wake-promoting regions of the brain, resulting in decreased arousal, thereby facilitating sleep. Experimental evidence generally associates the sedative effect of BzRAs with receptors containing α[alpha]$_1$ subunits, anxiolysis with α[alpha]$_{2-3}$ subunits, and memory function with α[alpha]$_5$ subunits [10]. However, receptor subtype function has not been established in humans. Barbiturates, alcohol, anesthetics, neurosteroids, and anticonvulsants also similarly influence the GABA$_A$ channel, but they bind at other unique locations on the receptor complex [11].

BzRA hypnotics are typically classified by chemical structure as either benzodiazepines (drugs with a benzodiazepine chemical structure, consisting of a fused benzene and diazepam ring) or non-benzodiazepines (drugs with different chemical structures). However, both classes bind to the benzodiazepine-receptor site located at the interface between the α[alpha] and the γ[gamma] subunits. BzRAs with a benzodiazepine chemical structure (temazepam, triazolam, estazolam, flurazepam, and quazepam) bind with equal affinity to four alpha subunits (1, 2, 3, 5) [12]. Non-benzodiazepine BzRAs bind more selectively. Zolpidem and zaleplon have a relatively higher affinity for the α[alpha]$_1$ subunit, although zaleplon additionally retains some affinity for α[alpha]$_5$ [13]. While eszopiclone has greatest affinity for α[alpha]$_1$, it has intermediate affinities for α[alpha]$_2$ and α[alpha]$_3$, suggesting possible anxiolytic properties. The significance of these differences among the BzRAs in relative affinity for the various GABA$_A$ α[alpha] subunits has not been demonstrated in clinical trials, however, and should be considered an unreliable basis for speculation in the clinic, given the complexity of the GABA$_A$ receptor family.

Pharmacokinetics

BzRA hypnotics differ primarily in their pharmacokinetic properties, primarily half-life (see Table 7.1). Drugs with very short elimination half-lives, such as zaleplon and the sub-lingual form of zolpidem (Intermezzo), may be taken in the middle of the night without risk for carryover sedation. Drugs with slightly longer half-lives, such as zolpidem and triazolam, may be useful for sleep-onset difficulties, but may be less effective in treating sleep maintenance problems. Drugs with intermediate half-lives, such as eszopiclone, temazepam, estazolam, and the controlled-release formulation of zolpidem (Ambien CR), may be more effective with sleep maintenance complaints but may also have increased risk for morning sedation. Drugs with very long half-lives, or with active metabolites, such as flurazepam and quazepam, can accumulate with daily dosing. Because half-life affects duration of action of a drug, different formulations of drugs such as zolpidem have been developed to target specific sleep complaints, including difficulties with sleep onset only, sleep maintenance only, or the combination.

BzRAs have quick onset of action, as nearly all are rapidly absorbed, reaching a peak concentration within 1–1.5 h. The zolpidem spray and sub-lingual tablet formulations have quicker rates of absorption [14, 15] and partially avoid first-pass metabolism in the liver by directly entering the systemic circulation through the oral mucosa, translating into a faster onset of clinical effect [16]. Because food reduces the absorption of zolpidem [17] (including the fast-dissolving sub-lingual tablet) and eszopiclone, thereby delaying the time to peak concentration, these drugs should not be taken with food.

All BzRAs are metabolized in the liver, but the specific enzymatic path varies (see Table 7.1). The clearance of BzRAs metabolized through the P450 pathway can be increased by concurrent use of a CYP3A4 enzyme inducers (e.g., rifampicin, modafinil, carbamazepine, phenytoin) and can be decreased by CYP3A4 inhibitors (e.g., diltiazem, erythromycin, azole antifungals, saquinavir, verapamil) [18]. This enzyme induction/inhibition effect is most pronounced for triazolam, which is metabolized primarily through the CYP3A family, but it is also relevant for zolpidem [19]. Individuals with gene polymorphisms that decrease or increase activity of CYP3A4, 2C9, 2C19 [20], or 2E1 may similarly demonstrate increased or decreased plasma drug concentrations. Gender differences in metabolism may occur. Drug clearance is reduced in women [21], especially among elderly women, leading to lower recommended therapeutic dose ranges. Temazepam can undergo oxidation through CYP3A4, but the primary path for excretion of temazepam is conjugation of the unaltered parent molecule to glucuronic acid [22], suggesting that it may be preferred in cases complicated by concurrent use of a CYP inducer/inhibitor. Zaleplon is unique among the hypnotics in that it appears to undergo metabolism primarily through aldehyde oxidase [23]. Aldehyde oxidase inhibition by cimetidine has been demonstrated to reduce clearance of zaleplon, however, requiring a reduction in dose to at least 5 mg [24]. Lower doses should similarly be used in individuals with even mild-moderate liver disease, because of substantial first-pass metabolism of zaleplon in the liver before entering the systemic circulation.

Efficacy

The efficacy of BzRA hypnotics, measured by polysomnography as well as subjective report, is well established for treatment of primary insomnia in adults 18–65 and in adults older than 65 for periods of several nights up to 4 weeks [5]. Evidence of sustained efficacy with longer term use (3–12 months), without evidence for tolerance or rebound insomnia, has been demonstrated for eszopiclone [25–27] and extended-release zolpidem [28]. In an open-label 6–12-month extension trial in older adults, zaleplon 5–10 mg persistently improved latency to persistent sleep, total sleep, and number of awakenings, without evidence for rebound insomnia upon discontinuation [29]. Efficacy of non-nightly administration of zolpidem 10 mg for a period of 12 weeks has also been shown, without evidence of rebound insomnia [30].

Most BzRAs decrease sleep latency and increase total sleep time. The exception is zaleplon, which, consistent with its very short half-life, did not improve total sleep time or wake after sleep onset when taken nightly for 5 weeks [31]. However, when taken in the middle of the night, zaleplon 10 mg reliably improved both ability to return to sleep and increased total amount of sleep, without increased residual sedation even 4–5 h after dosing [32].

A number of BzRA efficacy trials have been carried out for insomnia comorbid with other medical or psychiatric conditions, documenting very similar improvements in sleep measures. The majority of studies have been done with zolpidem and eszopiclone, but one of the earliest studies showed improved sleep with triazolam in patients with rheumatoid arthritis [33]. Zolpidem 10 mg increased total sleep time and improved sleep quality in a 4-week placebo-controlled study in depressed patients with refractory insomnia despite adequate control of depressive symptoms with selective serotonin reuptake inhibitor (SSRI) medication [34]. Zolpidem extended-release coadministered with escitalopram improved subjective insomnia symptoms in patients with comorbid anxiety [35] and depression [36], without changes in symptoms of anxiety or depression. In contrast, eszopiclone coadministered with either escitalopram (in patients with generalized anxiety disorder) or fluoxetine (in patients with major depression) not only improved sleep but also further reduced symptoms of anxiety or depression [37, 38].

Both zolpidem and eszopiclone improved sleep- and menopause-related symptoms in menopausal women [39, 40]. Eszopiclone has also been shown to be effective in treating insomnia comorbid with chronic low back pain [41], rheumatoid arthritis [42], PTSD [43], and schizophrenia [44].

In the past, the study of the effect of hypnotics on daytime function has been limited to the assessment of residual sedation. More recently, there have been studies evaluating whether improvement in sleep by hypnotic medication is accompanied by improvement in daytime function. The few studies that have assessed daytime measures report improvements in daytime alertness, ability to function, and physical well-being with eszopiclone treatment of insomnia [25, 26].

Safety

Residual Effects

Sedation

The side effects typically associated with BzRA use, including residual sedation, impaired psychomotor function, and amnesia, are related to their primary hypnotic effect at inopportune times, and to the potentiation of GABA-mediated inactivation of neuronal circuits not involved in sleep-wake systems. Residual sedation, a prolongation of the sedating effect of the drug into the waking period, can result in sleepiness as well as impaired psychomotor performance, including driving impairment. The potential for a BzRA to cause residual sedation the following day is determined by the drug's duration of action, which is determined by half-life, drug dose, and rate of drug metabolism, which may be slower in women and in the elderly. Long-acting medications like flurazepam and quazepam are particularly associated with increased daytime sleepiness [45]. Shorter-acting agents like zolpidem and triazolam cause little residual sleepiness 6–8 h after administration [46] unless taken at higher than typical doses [47]. Short-acting drugs like zaleplon and the sublingual formulation of zolpidem cause no substantial sedation even 4 h after dose administration [48, 49].

Driving Performance

Epidemiological data indicate that risk of motor vehicle accidents in individuals taking hypnotics increases with increasing half-life [50]. Studies in healthy normals show no impairment in on-the-road driving performance assessed 4 h post-dose with zaleplon 10 and 20 mg [51], or sublingual zolpidem 2.5 mg [52]. However, small deviations were seen in lateral car position 4 and 6 h after administration of zolpidem 10 mg but not at later time points [53].

While the majority of studies assessing driving performance following hypnotic use have been done in healthy normals, there are a few studies in patients with insomnia. The magnitude of driving impairment following a single night of zopiclone (a BzRA typically used as a positive control in on-the-road driving studies, not available in the USA) was less in a group of middle-aged chronic BzRA users compared to healthy controls, suggesting that studies in healthy volunteers may slightly overestimate the effect in insomnia patients with chronic hypnotic use [54]. Zolpidem 10 mg over 1 week did not impair driving simulator performance of primary insomnia patients assessed 9 h post-dose, in contrast to zopiclone 7.5 mg and lormetazepam 1 mg [55]. In a driving simulator study of female primary insomnia patients, zolpidem 10 mg and temazepam 20 mg did not differ from placebo on mean time to collision 5.5 h post-dose, but 2 of the 18 patients had multiple collisions, and zolpidem produced greater lane position deviation [56]. These results underlie the importance of allowing sufficient time following hypnotic ingestion prior to performing certain tasks as well as the importance of individual responses to drug effects.

Fall Risk

Increased risk of falling is another psychomotor side effect commonly attributed to BzRA treatment. The inability to balance against gravity, represented prosaically as a fall, is the failure of a complex integration of central and peripheral motor, sensory, and vestibular functions, some known to be sensitive to the effects of GABA activation. This is of most concern in the elderly. Evidence suggests that insomnia itself may be a substantial contributing factor to fall risk in the elderly [57, 58], particularly elderly women with untreated insomnia [59]. Nursing home residents with untreated insomnia, similar to the elderly at large, are at increased risk of falling [60].

Benzodiazepines as a class, but not BzRA medications specifically for sleep, are associated with a greater risk of falls in the elderly [61], whether short- or long-acting [62]. In another study, injurious falls were associated with benzodiazepines but only in the setting of polypharmacy [63]. When comorbid medical conditions were controlled, antidepressants, opiates, and anticonvulsants, but not sedatives, predicted injurious falls, but sedatives did not [64]. In elderly males with insomnia, both non-benzodiazepine and benzodiazepine use were associated with a modest increase in risk for falls [65]. A study of nursing home residents reported increased risk of hip fracture in new users of non-benzodiazepines, with the risk greatest for individuals who required limited assistance to transfer [66].

Amnesia

BzRAs impair the ability to form new memories, as do most sedative medications, and the effect is proportionally related to plasma drug concentration, maximal at peak drug levels [67, 68]. The anterograde amnesia resolves with clearance of the drug [69]. Only studies of acute memory effects have been carried out in primary insomniacs, but no tolerance to the amnestic effect is evident over 3–4 weeks of nightly hypnotic use in healthy non-insomniac males taking extended-release zolpidem 12.5 mg [70]. Memory effects may not be significant for zaleplon. Healthy young adults administered 10 and 20 mg doses did not differ from placebo with respect to immediate and delayed word recall when assessed 1.25 and 8.25 h after dose administration [71]. Sleep also has an independent amnestic effect that should be considered separately from the direct BzRA effect, as maintaining wakefulness despite the hypnotic effect attenuates the BzRA-associated amnesia [72].

Complex Behaviors During Sleep

Talking, walking [73, 74], and other complex behaviors while in a sleep-like state have been reported to occur in association with use of some BzRAs, typically zolpidem and zopiclone but also zaleplon [75]. Zopiclone is a racemic mixture of eszopiclone and its inactive stereoisomer is available in Europe but not in the USA. The range of reported behaviors is wide, including driving, eating, emailing, taking additional hypnotic, sex, and shopping [76, 77]. Cases have been reported complicated by death [78] or injury. Hypnotic doses have been therapeutic to supratherapeutic, and other substances such as alcohol, antidepressants, and benzodiazepines have been co-implicated in some situations. The reports in the scientific literature almost exclusively take the form of a case or short case series. No controlled, prospective studies exist. The incidence of these events and predictive factors is not known, although higher hypnotic dose is associated in some analyses, especially when administered above the typical therapeutic range [79]. Unfortunately, the quality of evidence with respect to these events is low, and even basic information characterizing state of wakefulness/sleep is not known.

Mortality Risk

There is controversy over whether sedative hypnotic use, particularly BzRA use, is associated with increased mortality [80]. Kripke et al. [81], in a large retrospective study, reported a 3.5–5.5 increased hazard for death in patients prescribed hypnotics for insomnia compared to a matched cohort of non-hypnotic users. This study, however, did not control for psychiatric comorbidities, nor were the groups matched for underlying sleep disorders [82]. Kriegsbaum et al. [83], in a similarly large study, documented that the association of hypnotic use with increased mortality was markedly reduced when psychiatric comorbidities and socioeconomic class were taken into account, with hazard ratios of 1.22–1.43. A large prospective study of the French population showed similar results [84]. Moreover, when baseline sleep complaints were also controlled in that study, the risk of mortality over the next 12 years was not significantly associated with hypnotic use. Neutel and Johansen [85] present data suggesting that the association between hypnotic use and increased mortality may be confounded by the increased use of hypnotics in the months proximal to death for palliative management of terminal illness. In a study of 8862 deaths compared to almost 900,000 controls in a single year, increasingly larger proportions of the prospective deaths received prescriptions for BzRAs as death approached, approximating almost 45 % of that group during the last 2 months prior to death. Moreover, the frequency of BzRA use was similar at all ages in the prospective-death cohort, but increased with increasing age in the controls. In summary, the available evidence suggests that BzRA use may be associated with a modestly increased mortality risk, but comorbid medical and psychiatric disease, sleep problems, and other classes of medications have larger to much larger effects on mortality risk. Clarifying the role of potential mediators of this relationship (e.g., cancer incidence, falls, substance abuse) may better define the true nature and magnitude of the mortality risk associated with BzRA use.

Tolerance, Dependence, Abuse Potential

In most BzRA efficacy trials, there is no evidence for tolerance (loss of effect over time). Recent studies of eszopiclone [25–27], zolpidem [86], and zolpidem extended-release [28] in adults and zaleplon in older adults [29] found no evidence of tolerance or withdrawal for 6–12 months. In the study by Roehrs et al. [86], designed specifically to assess the potential for primary insomniacs to develop tolerance, there was no increase in self-administration over a 1-year period. Studies of intermittent dosing of zolpidem and zolpidem extended-release for periods of 2–6 months show no increases in dose frequency over time [87], which is consistent with epidemiologic studies of medication use by chronic insomniacs over longer periods of treatment [88].

Studies of the reinforcing effects of these drugs indicate that they have a low-to-moderate behavioral dependence liability, which may be higher in individuals with a history of alcohol/drug abuse or comorbid anxiety/depression [89–92]. Risk for dependence likely depends on the specific drug, dosage, comorbid disease, and individual differences [5].

Data on the incidence of abuse of hypnotic medications, independent of other sedatives, is not available. However, a population-based study indicated that 2.3 % of the US population reported nonmedical use of sedatives and tranquilizers, with approximately 0.002 % of the population meeting the criteria for substance abuse [93].

Discontinuation Effects

Insomnia can transiently worsen when BzRAs are stopped, exceeding baseline severity for 1–2 nights in most cases. This rebound of insomnia is not uncommon when discontinuing short and intermediate half-life agents [94], especially at higher doses; but it is uncommon when discontinuing very-long-half-life medications, such as flurazepam or quazepam, that effectively "self-taper."

Rebound insomnia should be distinguished from recrudescence, or return of symptoms to pretreatment levels. Because primary insomnia is conceptualized as a lifelong disorder, some risk of recurrence following treatment discontinuation is expected. Rebound insomnia should also be differentiated from withdrawal, which is characterized by the appearance of additional symptoms that were not present before treatment, and which typically last for a longer period of time. Rebound is not a sign of tolerance or dependence. Rebound insomnia does not increase the likelihood of hypnotic self-administration [95]. Patient education about the temporary nature of the rebound can help patients understand that this is not a sign of dependence.

Melatonin Receptor Agonists

Ramelteon

Ramelteon is a melatonin receptor agonist which binds with high affinity to MT_1 and MT_2 receptors [96]. Compared to melatonin, ramelteon has a greater affinity (3–16 times) and selectivity (1000-fold greater) for MT_1/MT_2. Ramelteon likely promotes sleep via the MT_1 receptor by attenuating wake-promoting signals from the suprachiasmatic nucleus and may affect the timing of sleep via the MT_2 receptor [97].

Polysomnographic and subjective data indicate that ramelteon decreases sleep latency in adults with primary insomnia [98] with efficacy maintained for up to 6 months [99]. Similar improvements in sleep latency have been reported in elderly primary insomniacs treated with ramelteon [100]. Effects on total sleep time are less consistent, with improvement in polysomnographically recorded TST only for short-term use, and no consistent improvement in subjective TST during short- or long-term use [101].

Ramelteon has no abuse potential. The most common adverse effects are somnolence, dizziness, fatigue, and nausea, with safety demonstrated over 6 months of nightly use [99].

Melatonin

Melatonin is considered a dietary supplement and, therefore, not regulated by the FDA. It is discussed in later in this chapter.

Orexin Antagonists

Suvorexant, the first drug of this class to be approved for treatment of insomnia, promotes sleep by blocking orexin receptors [102]. Suvorexant is a dual-orexin receptor antagonist (DORA) with similar potency at both orexin receptors, OX_1 and OX_2. Orexin is a peptide produced by neurons in the lateral hypothalamus that are essential for maintenance of wakefulness. Decrease in orexinergic tone is essential for initiation and maintenance of sleep [103]. Antagonism of orexin appears to improve sleep in insomnia patients by reduction in hyperarousal [104]. Following oral administration, suvorexant is rapidly absorbed, has an average t_{max} of 1.5–4 h, and has a half-life of about 12 h [105].

Randomized placebo-controlled clinical trials indicate that suvorexant improves polysomnographic measures of sleep (SL, sleep maintenance) in both younger and older (≥65) adults for up to 3 months [106]. Improvement in subjective measures

(SL, TST, sleep maintenance, sleep quality) has been demonstrated for up to 1 year of treatment in the same age groups [107]. Increases in TST were mainly attributable to an increase in REM sleep, and to a lesser extent stage 2 sleep [108]. In an exploratory study [109], the power spectral density profile during sleep after 1 month of suvorexant treatment was unchanged compared to placebo in both healthy and insomnia subjects, in contrast to other drugs commonly used to treat insomnia. For example, zolpidem, which acts on the GABA system, decreased power in the theta band, and both zolpidem and the antidepressant, trazodone, increased power in the sigma band. This suggests that orexin antagonism might lead to improvement in sleep without major neurophysiologic changes to the EEG.

The most common side effect noted with suvorexant is somnolence; fatigue and dry mouth are less common but more frequent than placebo [107]. Abrupt discontinuation after 1 year of treatment was not associated with rebound insomnia or withdrawal [107]. Suvorexant was not associated with any clinically significant respiratory effects during sleep in adults (40 mg dose) with mild-to-moderate obstructive sleep apnea or COPD, or in older adults (≥ 65; 30 mg dose) with COPD [110, 111]. In addition, suvorexant does not appear to impair next-day driving in healthy (non-insomnia) volunteers less than 65 years old [112]. However, there were some individuals who displayed impairment.

Histamine (H₁) Antagonists

Selective H₁ Antagonist: Doxepin 3–6 mg

Doxepin in low doses (3–6 mg) is a more potent and selective H_1 antagonist than drugs generally classified as antihistamines [113]. At these doses, doxepin has little effect on serotonergic, adrenergic, or muscarinic cholinergic receptors, unlike the doses (75–150 mg) typically used for treatment of depression. The selective blockade of histamine results in sleep promotion during the middle and end of the night when other wake-promoting systems (norepinephrine, orexin, serotonin, acetylcholine) are minimally active [114].

Doxepin, in clinical trials with primary insomnia patients, improved objective and subjective measures of sleep maintenance in adults (3–6 mg) for 5 weeks and in older adults (1–3 mg) for 12 weeks [115, 116]. Similar to suvorexant, doxepin 1–6 mg improved sleep during the last quarter of the night without residual daytime effects. Most notably, the largest effect size for doxepin 1–6 mg was during the last hour (hour 8) of the night.

Despite therapeutic efficacy during the last hour of the night there was no evidence of residual sedation during clinical trials. Nor was there any indication of rebound insomnia or symptoms of withdrawal upon drug discontinuation. The most frequent adverse effects in clinical trials were sedation and headache.

Nonselective H₁ Antagonists: Diphenhydramine, Doxylamine

Diphenhydramine or doxylamine is the principal ingredient in most over-the-counter medications with FDA indication for use as a sleep aid. These drugs are nonselective H1 antagonists, as they also exhibit muscarinic cholinergic antagonism, which contributes to their effects on sleep as well as to their side effects.

Although sedation is a common side effect of the first-generation antihistamines, evidence for efficacy in treating insomnia is limited. Among the few randomized, placebo-controlled studies of diphenhydramine, there is weak evidence for improvement in subjective sleep measures and mixed evidence for improvement in polysomnographic measures [117, 118]. There are no placebo-controlled trials of doxylamine.

The most commonly reported adverse effects of over-the-counter antihistamines are anticholinergic effects such as dry mouth, blurred vision, urinary retention, and confusion. Other adverse effects include sedation, dizziness, and weight gain. Agitation and insomnia have occasionally been reported. Daytime sedation may be a problem given the relatively long elimination half-life of these drugs. Indeed, plasma concentration of diphenhydramine 12 h post-dose correlates with the degree of H_1 receptor occupancy [119]. Tolerance to the sedating effects of daily daytime (tid) administration of diphenhydramine develops within 3–4 days [120, 121]. Tolerance to intermittent use and to nighttime administration has not been studied.

Prescription Agents Used Off-Label for Treatment of Insomnia

Other BzRAS

Other benzodiazepines not approved as hypnotics by the FDA but frequently used to treat insomnia include lorazepam, clonazepam, and alprazolam [122]. These drugs are indicated for treatment of anxiety or panic disorders. Clonazepam is also indicated in treatment of seizures and is used off-label to treat REM behavior disorder [123]. The pharmacologic properties of these drugs are similar to benzodiazepine hypnotics; thus, while efficacy in insomnia has not been extensively studied with these drugs, they appear to have similar effects on sleep and similar side effects. Their half-lives are relatively long (11–40 h).

Antidepressants

Sedating antidepressants are commonly used for the treatment of insomnia despite relatively little data on safety and efficacy for this treatment purpose. Not only is trazodone the most frequently used antidepressant for insomnia, it has been among the most frequently prescribed of all drug treatments for insomnia over the past 20 years [1, 2]. Mirtazapine and amitriptyline are also commonly used. These drugs are typically prescribed for insomnia in doses lower than those clinically indicated for treatment of depression.

Trazodone

Trazodone, FDA approved for the treatment of major depression (200–600 mg), is typically used for insomnia at doses of 25–150 mg. Trazodone promotes sleep primarily by antagonism of serotonin $5HT_{2A}$, alpha$_1$-adrenergic, and histamine H_1 receptors [6]. At the higher doses used for treatment of depression, trazodone also blocks the serotonin transporter. The effects of trazodone can vary significantly because of its active metabolite mCPP and its metabolism by CYP3A4 and CPY2D6 pathways.

There have been two placebo-controlled trials of trazodone in patients with primary insomnia. In the first study, trazodone 50 mg improved subjective measures of sleep latency and duration during the first week of treatment, but these results were not sustained during the second week [124]. In a polysomnographic study, trazodone 50 mg, given for seven consecutive nights, decreased number of awakenings and stage 1 sleep but had no effect on sleep latency or sleep efficiency [125].

There are four placebo-controlled studies of trazodone treatment of insomnia with comorbid illness. Following alcohol detoxification, trazodone improved sleep efficiency [126] and sleep quality [127]. However, in a study of patients on methadone maintenance, trazodone failed to improve either subjective or objective sleep measures [128]. In patients with persistent insomnia following treatment of depression with fluoxetine or bupropion, trazodone improved indices of insomnia [129]. There were no direct measures of sleep in that study.

Common side effects of trazodone include sedation, dizziness, orthostatic hypotension, headache, dry mouth, and blurred vision [5]. Priapism is a rare occurrence. In a study of primary insomnia patients given trazodone for 1 week, there were small but significant impairments in short-term memory, verbal learning, and equilibrium [125]. There is no evidence of abuse.

Mirtazapine

Mirtazapine promotes sleep via antagonism of serotonin $5HT_2$, $5HT_3$, histamine H_1, and alpha$_1$-adrenergic receptors. Its half-life is very long (20–40 h). Metabolic clearance is reduced in women and in older adults.

There have been no placebo-controlled trials of mirtazapine for the treatment of primary insomnia or comorbid insomnia. However, three studies on esmirtazapine (the S(+) enantiomer of mirtazapine) documented improvement in polysomnographic measures of sleep in patients with primary insomnia [130]. Esmirtazapine has a shorter half-life (10 h) than mirtazapine. It is no longer being developed as a hypnotic.

Studies of mirtazapine in major depressive disorder indicate that the most common side effects are sedation, increased appetite, weight gain, dry mouth, and constipation [131]. It has no potential for abuse.

Tricyclic Antidepressants

Tricyclic antidepressants frequently used to treat insomnia include amitriptyline, doxepin, and trimipramine, typically in doses lower than those used for treatment of depression. Tricyclics promote sleep primarily by antagonism of norepinephrine, histamine, and acetylcholine. Amitriptyline and doxepin also inhibit serotonin and norepinephrine reuptake transporters. Amitriptyline is the most anticholinergic of the tricyclics, while doxepin is a more potent H1 antagonist than most drugs classified as antihistamines. In very low doses, doxepin is a relatively selective histamine antagonist, with minimal effects on norepinephrine, acetylcholine, or serotonin. Its low-dose formulation (trade name Silenor) is approved for treatment of insomnia and discussed in Sect. 3.4.1. Tricyclic antidepressants antagonize peripheral alpha-adrenergic receptors, which accounts for their cardiovascular effects.

In the treatment of primary insomnia, doxepin 25–50 mg and trimipramine 50–200 mg improved sleep efficiency and subjective sleep quality when used for up to 4 weeks [132–136]. Amitriptyline, doxepin, and trimipramine, in antidepressant doses, improved sleep in patients treated for depression [137–139]. Sleep indices were improved with doxepin 10 mg in patients with Parkinson's disease [140].

Dose-dependent side effects [141] include sedation and weight gain (related to histamine antagonism), orthostatic hypotension (related to $alpha_1$ antagonism), and dry mouth, blurred vision, constipation, and urinary retention (related to muscarinic cholinergic antagonism). A less common but serious side effect is impairment of cardiac conduction, which can lead to heart block or seizures. These drugs can be lethal in overdose. There is no abuse potential.

Antipsychotics

The antipsychotic drug most commonly used off-label to treat insomnia is quetiapine, but olanzapine has also been used with greater frequency than other antipsychotics. These drugs are more likely to be used to treat insomnia in patients with comorbid psychiatric disease. Their sedating effects come from antagonism of multiple receptors, including H_1, $alpha_1$-adrenergic, serotonin $5HT_2$, and dopamine. Olanzapine, in addition, antagonizes muscarinic receptors. Olanzapine's t_{max} of 4–6 h and half-life of 20–54 h make it unlikely to be efficacious for sleep-onset difficulties and likely to have residual sedation.

There has been a single randomized control trial of quetiapine 25 mg for primary insomnia and none for olanzapine [142]. There was a trend for improvement in subjective SL and TST; the lack of a significant effect may have been the result of insufficient power ($n = 6$–7 per group). The only other study of quetiapine in primary insomnia was an uncontrolled open-label study which reported improvements in polysomnographic measures of TST and sleep efficiency with doses of 25–75 mg [143]. Both quetiapine and olanzapine have been studied in patients with insomnia and comorbid disorders [4, 144], but most studies lack placebo control and are compromised by small sample size, short duration of treatment, and lack of objective measures of sleep. However, the few placebo-controlled studies indicate that quetiapine improves subjective measures of sleep in patients with major depressive disorder [145], bipolar depression [146], generalized anxiety disorder [147], and fibromyalgia [148].

Common side effects are sedation, dizziness, dry mouth, blurred vision, urinary retention, increased appetite, and weight gain [149–151]. There is also increased risk for impaired cognition and cardiac-related mortality in older adults, particularly those with dementia [152].

Anticonvulsants

Anticonvulsant drugs used to treat insomnia include gabapentin, pregabalin, and, less frequently, tiagabine. Gabapentin and pregabalin, while structural analogues of GABA, do not appear to interact with $GABA_A$ receptors or inhibit reuptake of GABA. They promote sleep by decreasing the wake-promoting glutamate and norepinephrine systems via selective binding to the $alpha_2$ delta subunit of N-type voltage-gated calcium channels [153, 154]. Tiagabine promotes sleep by inhibiting GABA reuptake. Given the long t_{max} (2–3.5 h), gabapentin is unlikely to improve sleep-onset difficulty.

Gabapentin, in adults reporting occasional disturbed sleep and undergoing transient insomnia via phase advance, demonstrated improvement in TST and wake after sleep onset [155, 156]. The only study of gabapentin in the treatment of primary insomnia was an open-label study which reported improvement in sleep efficiency, primarily via decrease in wake time, and an increase in slow-wave sleep [157]. Improvements in polysomnographic and subjective measures of sleep have been reported with gabapentin and pregabalin in patients with restless leg syndrome [158, 159], fibromyalgia [160, 161], neuropathic pain [162, 163], hot flashes [164], and epilepsy [165]. One author suggested that pregabalin has a direct effect on sleep that is separate from its analgesic, anxiolytic, and anticonvulsant effects [166]. Placebo-controlled studies of tiagabine in primary insomnia patients show an increase in slow-wave sleep, but inconsistent results on polysomnographic measures of sleep [167, 168].

Principal side effects are ataxia and diplopia with gabapentin; dry mouth, cognitive impairment, peripheral edema, and weight gain with pregabalin; and nausea with tiagabine.

Alpha₁-Adrenergic Antagonists

Prazosin is an antihypertensive agent used in the treatment of nightmares and sleep disturbance in post-traumatic stress disorder (PTSD). The mechanism for treatment of nightmares is unknown, but sleep is promoted by preventing arousal that occurs when norepinephrine binds to alpha₁-adrenergic receptors [169]. There are no studies of prazosin in the treatment of primary insomnia. However, there is evidence that patients with insomnia have elevated levels of norepinephrine [170]. In patients with PTSD, prazosin decreased nightmares and improved sleep quality in four placebo-controlled trials [171–174]. In a fifth study, prazosin increased polysomnographic total sleep time and REM, along with improving clinical symptoms [175]. Orthostatic hypotension and dizziness are possible side effects.

Melatonin

Melatonin is widely used by consumers to treat insomnia. Melatonin, an endogenous hormone secreted by the pineal gland and primarily involved in the synchronization of circadian rhythms, is available as a supplement that is not regulated by the FDA. As with ramelteon, melatonin likely promotes sleep via the MT_1 receptor and circadian synchronization via the MT_2 receptor. However melatonin has much less affinity and selectivity for these receptors compared to ramelteon. The half-life of melatonin is short (35–60 min) [176]; thus it is unlikely to be useful for sleep maintenance. However, a prolonged-release formula is available by prescription for adults ≥55 in Europe and other countries. Because melatonin is unregulated in the USA, it is available in a wide range of doses.

Interpretation of studies on melatonin is complicated by the large range of doses used, formulation (immediate vs. prolonged-release), timing of administration (a few minutes to many hours before bedtime), heterogeneity of the study population (age, presence of comorbid disorders, different types of sleep disorders), and small sample size. Overall, the available data suggests that melatonin has a therapeutic but weak effect on SL (both subjective and objective), but little effect on sleep duration (subjective, actigraphic, polysomnographic) [177, 178]. Studies of prolonged-release melatonin produce somewhat more consistent results than those of exogenous melatonin in adults 55 and older [179]. Exogenous melatonin may be more useful in delayed sleep-phase disorder, as it advances the sleep-wake rhythm when given at the appropriate time [180].

There are few reports of adverse events in controlled trials with melatonin [181]. A National Academy of Sciences report states that short-term use of 10 mg or less appears to be safe in healthy adults but recommended caution in children/adolescents and during pregnancy [182]. Headache, somnolence, nausea, hypotension, and hypertension have been reported in higher doses [183].

Pharmacologic Management of Insomnia

Indications for Pharmacological Treatment

Insomnia patients not only perceive daytime dysfunction and exhibit neurobehavioral impairment [184], but they also have reduced quality of life [185], increased risk for psychiatric disorders [186], higher health care use and cost [187], increased accidents and errors at work [188], and increased absenteeism from work [189]. When the clinician and patient decide that, without treatment, these consequences are sufficiently significant, pharmacotherapy can be considered as a treatment option.

Pharmacotherapy is an acceptable treatment for short-term insomnia, particularly situational forms of insomnia such as may occur while traveling or during periods of predictable and transiently increased stress. There is no basis to believe that cognitive behavioral therapy (CBT) would substantially less beneficial for acute insomnia than for chronic insomnia, but rapidly implementing CBT shortly after insomnia onset may be difficult.

Treatment options for chronic insomnia include CBT, pharmacotherapy, or their combination [190]. There are no practice parameters on pharmacotherapy for chronic insomnia nor is there a consensus regarding long-term pharmacologic treatment for chronic insomnia. General guidelines indicate the use of the lowest effective dose, with tapering of medication when feasible. However chronic use of hypnotics medication may be indicated for severe or refractory insomnia or comorbid insomnia. Published studies of eszopiclone, zaleplon, and zolpidem extended-release indicate maintenance of efficacy without tolerance for up to 12 months. Relying on pharmacotherapy alone, however, is not ideal. CBT should be considered, comorbid conditions addressed, psychosocial stressors managed, and healthy lifestyles promoted.

Contraindications to Pharmacological Treatment

The safety of hypnotic medications has not been demonstrated in pregnancy. All BzRAs, ramelteon, doxepin, and suvorexant are considered Class C when assessing potential for fetal harm. The risk for dependence and tolerance to BzRAs is very likely increased for those with a personal or family history of substance abuse. Prescription hypnotics should be avoided if the patient is concurrently using alcohol or other sedating medications. Individuals with substantial liver disease may ineffectively metabolize and consequently accumulate increased concentrations of BzRAs, suvorexant, doxepin, and trazodone.

Since BzRAs are respiratory suppressants and have myorelaxation effects, their use in pulmonary disorders should be carefully considered. Older BzRAs have been demonstrated to worsen sleep apnea [191], but this effect is less clear for newer non-benzodiazepine BzRAs. Eszopiclone 3 mg had no effect on the apnea-hypopnea index (AHI) in mild-to-moderate sleep apnea [192] and even reduced the AHI in moderate-severe obstructive sleep apnea in a subject group selected for increased arousal threshold [193]. Zolpidem reduced AHI in central sleep apnea [194]. Triazolam 0.125–0.25 mg and zolpidem 5–10 mg did not exacerbate nocturnal desaturations in a small study of subjects with mild-to-moderate COPD [195] and in mild-to-severe but stable COPD without pre-existing severe daytime desaturations or CO_2 retention [196]. Eszopiclone, taken during the first 2 weeks of continuous positive airway pressure (CPAP) treatment for sleep apnea, improved CPAP compliance over the first 6 months of therapy [197].

The most common contraindication to pharmacotherapy is the amount of time available to sleep. For most hypnotic medications, there should be a period of 7–8 h immediately following dosing that is dedicated solely to sleep. Shorter windows of time, 4–5 h, are appropriate for agents designed for middle-of-the-night dosing. Extensions in the length of this period of protected time should be considered based on factors likely to prolong duration of action—higher than typical dose, other sedating medications, advanced age, or female gender.

Finally, pharmacotherapy may be contraindicated for caregivers with insomnia who must be able to rise easily during the night and navigate without risk of falling.

Implementing Pharmacological Treatment

Starting Treatment

Optimizing pharmacological treatment requires knowledge of the patient's temporal pattern of sleep difficulty; past history of hypnotic medication use, including effectiveness and side effects; and comorbidities. Patient education is essential before beginning pharmacotherapy. This includes discussion of the pathophysiology of insomnia and potential aggravating factors; treatment options, including CBT and pharmacotherapy or their combination; a good baseline assessment of sleep pattern prior to initiating treatment in order to monitor response to therapy; and instructions regarding medication use, particularly time allotted for sleep after dosing; potential adverse effects. Dose and treatment regimen should be individualized, agreed to by the patient, and monitored by the physician. Starting dose should be the lowest clinically indicated dose. Dose adjustment should be made by the physician, with effectiveness and side effects monitored within 3–7 days of starting medication.

Stopping Treatment

Discontinuing treatment, even if only temporarily, is useful as a strategy to reduce long-term risk of tolerance, to determine retrospectively if treatment was helpful, and to assess whether the insomnia has improved to the point that pharmacotherapy is no longer needed. There is no evidence basis for how and when to taper hypnotic medications. Some practitioners follow a schedule, with medication tapers every 3–6 months. Others taper during periods characterized by reduced daytime demand, improvements in level of psychosocial stress, vacations, or holidays. Patients should be warned in advance about the potential for rebound insomnia for 1–2 nights once the medication is completely discontinued. Tapers can take the form of a regular decrease in dose size at the same dosing frequency, or a decrease in the number of doses by 1–2 per week. CBT can facilitate medication tapering and discontinuation.

Reasonable strategies for managing rebound include patient education, non-nightly hypnotic use, lower doses, and slow tapering [198]. Patient expectations and anxieties about discontinuing treatment can be a significant factor. A reliable placebo effect occurs with insomnia treatment [199, 200], and rebound occurs even when discontinuing a placebo.

Treatment Considerations Based on Temporal Pattern of Insomnia

Specific medications are more appropriate for insomnia at the beginning of the night, the middle of the night, or near the end of the night, based on the pharmacokinetic profile and efficacy data.

Difficulty with Sleep Onset Only

For difficulty with insomnia only at the beginning of the night, zaleplon, zolpidem, and ramelteon are effective and less likely than alternative medications to cause residual morning sedation. If there are factors preventing the use of these medications (e.g., prior history of ineffectiveness, side effects, cost), eszopiclone, temazepam, or sustained-release zolpidem can be considered.

For individuals who have intermittent problems falling asleep and can predict when they are likely to have a bad night, taking medication only on the nights they expect to have sleep difficulty is optimal. If prediction is not possible, taking medication only after a specified period of time without falling asleep is typically a poor option. CBT should be considered in these circumstances.

For individuals with nightly problems falling asleep, an intermittent medication taper and drug-holiday are reasonable. However, it should be noted that zaleplon, zolpidem, and ramelteon have demonstrated effectiveness of at least 6 months of nightly treatment without evidence of tolerance.

Difficulty with Sleep Maintenance Only

Difficulty maintaining sleep is the most common sleep complaint [201]. Two options for treatment exist: administer either a short-acting medication at the time of awakening or take a medication with demonstrated effectiveness for sleep maintenance at the beginning of the night. Zaleplon and sublingual zolpidem (Intermezzo) can be taken as needed during middle-of-the-night awakenings, assuming at least 4 h of time in bed remain. If sleep-maintenance insomnia is occurring on a nightly basis, taking a PRN medication in the middle of every night can become a burden. Regular bedtime dosing of doxepin 3–6 mg, sustained-release zolpidem, or suvorexant would be reasonable. For individuals with sleep difficulties specifically during the last 2 h of the night, the best options are bedtime dosing of doxepin 3–6 mg or suvorexant, as both drugs have demonstrated efficacy during the last third of the night without next-day impairment. In particular, doxepin 3–6 mg is efficacious during hour 8 of the night. With nightly administration, an intermittent medication taper and drug-holiday are recommended.

Difficulty with Both Sleep Onset and Sleep Maintenance

Drugs with demonstrated efficacy for sleep onset and sleep maintenance include eszopiclone, temazepam, sustained-release zolpidem, and suvorexant. For individuals with sleep maintenance difficulties encompassing the last 2 h of the night, consideration can be given to bedtime administration of both a short-acting drug such as ramelteon, zaleplon, or zolpidem with doxepin 3–6 mg, although this is not ideal. If there is nightly administration, an intermittent taper and drug-holiday are recommended.

Treatment Considerations Based on Comorbid Conditions

Insomnia is common in patients with chronic pain, depression, anxiety, and substance abuse [201]. The guidelines described above, based on time of night of insomnia symptoms, can be applied to treatment of insomnia in these situations. However, as we learn more about sleep-wake regulation, which should guide the development of alternate therapies, we should be able to tailor drug treatment of insomnia more specifically than merely by time of night. There is currently limited data on pharmacologic treatment of comorbid insomnia. However, the available data suggests that options for treatment of insomnia comorbid with some chronic pain conditions include gabapentin and pregabalin. Benzodiazepines can also be considered because of their anxiolytic and myorelaxant properties. For insomnia comorbid with major depression or general anxiety disorder, there is evidence that eszopiclone is efficacious, particularly in patients treated with SSRI medication. Zolpidem and clonazepam have shown efficacy in treating insomnia in patients with depression as well. While quetiapine has been studied in patients with depression, anxiety, and bipolar disorder, its side effect profile may limit its usefulness. Theoretically, an orexin antagonist, such as suvorexant, could be useful in anxious patients, as anxiety-related increases in arousal are believed to be mediated by inputs to orexin neurons in brain areas linked to anxiety [114, 202]. Similarly, suvorexant could be considered in patients with a history of, or increased risk for, substance abuse, as arousal associated with loss of reward is believed to be mediated by inputs from reward areas of the brain to orexin [114]. Prazosin is the drug of choice for treatment of nightmares and insomnia associated with PTSD.

Because of the paucity of placebo-controlled trials with sedating antidepressants, their use cannot be recommended for treatment of insomnia except in individuals who fail other treatments or for whom other treatments are contraindicated. While antipsychotic medications cannot be routinely recommended for insomnia, both because of the lack of data and the side effect profile, these drugs may be useful in individuals with psychotic or mood disorders, and could be considered for use in individuals in whom substance abuse is a concern.

Conclusion

Substantial advances have occurred over the last few decades in our ability to safely and effectively treat insomnia, such that pharmacotherapy can now be increasingly tailored to many different clinical situations. Improved knowledge about treatment of insomnia comorbid with various medical and psychiatric conditions, and the growing diversity of accessible receptor targets, contributes to more reliable and more appropriate pharmacotherapy. Variations in pharmacokinetics inform drug selection for insomnia at the beginning, middle, or end of the night. Safety is a perennial concern in drug therapy, and predictable differences in metabolism among certain patient groups, the aged and females for example, improve clinician ability to manage risk. Despite these advances, our knowledge of insomnia pharmacotherapy cannot be described as robust; and there are many unresolved clinically relevant questions: How is pharmacotherapy best combined with CBT, how best can we improve daytime symptoms, and how effective are currently available drugs in the typical clinic patient?

Acknowledgement The authors gratefully acknowledge the assistance of Angela C. Randazzo, Ph.D., in the preparation of this chapter.

References

1. Walsh JK. Drugs used to treat insomnia in 2002: regulatory-based rather than evidence-based medicine. Sleep. 2004;27(8):1441–2.
2. Schweitzer PK, Curry DT, Eisenstein RD. Pharmacological treatment of insomnia. In: Attarian H, Schuman C, editors. Clinical handbook of insomnia. 2nd ed. New York: Humana Press; 2010.
3. Roth T, Rogowski R, Hull S, Schwartz H, Koshorek G, Corser B, Seiden D, Lankford A. Efficacy and safety of doxepin 1, 3 and 6 mg in adults with primary insomnia. Sleep. 2007;30:1555–61.
4. Buysse D. Clinical pharmacology of other drugs used as hypnotics. In: Kryger MH, Roth T, Dement WC, editors. Principles and practice of sleep medicine. 5th ed. St. Louis: Elsevier; 2011.

5. Krystal AD. A compendium of placebo-controlled trials of the risks/benefits of pharmacological treatments for insomnia: the empirical basis for U.S. clinical practice. Sleep Med Rev. 2009;13(4):265–74.

6. Stahl S. Stahl's essential psychopharmacology: neuroscientific basis and practical applications. 4th ed. New York: Cambridge University Press; 2013.

7. Miller PS, Aricescu AR. Crystal structure of a human GABA$_A$ receptor. Nature. 2014;512(7514):270–5.

8. Sieghart W, Sperk G. Subunit composition, distribution and function of GABA$_A$ receptor subtypes. Curr Topics Med Chem. 2002;2:795–816.

9. Olsen RW, Sieghert W. Subtypes of the γ[gamma]-aminobutyric acidA receptors: classification on the basis of subunit composition, pharmacology, and function. Pharmacol Rev. 2008;60(3):243–60.

10. Rudolph U, Crestani F, Benke D, Brünig I, Benson JA, Fritschy JM, Martin JR, Bluethmann H, Möhler H. Benzodiazepine actions mediated by specific gamma-aminobutyric acid(A) receptor subtypes. Nature. 1999;401(6755):796–800.

11. Li P, Akk G. Synaptic-type α1β2γ2L GABA$_A$ receptors produce large persistent currents in the presence of ambient GABA and anesthetic drugs. Mol Pharmacol. 2015;87(5):776–81.

12. Sieghart W, Sperk G. Subunit composition, distribution and function of GABA(A) receptor subtypes. Curr Top Med Chem. 2002;2:795–816.

13. Sanna E, Busonero F, Talani G, Carta M, Massa F, Peis M, Maciocco E, Biggio G. Comparison of the effects of zaleplon, zolpidem, and triazolam at various GABAA receptor subtypes. Eur J Pharmacol. 2002;451:103–10.

14. Greenblatt DJ, Harmatz JS, Roth T, Singh NN, Moline ML, Harris SC, Kapil RP. Comparison of pharmacokinetic profiles of zolpidem buffered sublingual tablet and zolpidem oral immediate-release tablet: results from a single-center, single-dose, randomized, open-label crossover study in healthy adults. Clin Ther. 2013;35(5):604–11.

15. Neubauer DN. ZolpiMist™: a new formulation of zolpidem tartrate for the short-term treatment of insomnia in the US. Nat Sci Sleep. 2010;2:79–84.

16. Yang LP, Deeks ED. Sublingual zolpidem (Edluar™; Sublinox™). CNS Drugs. 2012;26(11):1003–10.

17. Greenblatt DJ, Harmatz JS, Singh NN, Roth T, Harris SC, Kapil RP. Influence of food on pharmacokinetics of zolpidem from fast dissolving sublingual zolpidem tartrate tablets. J Clin Pharmacol. 2013;53(11):1194–8.

18. Wang JS, DeVane CL. Pharmacokinetics and drug interactions of the sedative hypnotics. Psychopharmacol Bull. 2003;37(1):10–29.

19. Von Moltke LL, Greenblatt DJ, Granda BW, Duan SX, Grassi JM, Venkatakrishnan K, Harmatz JS, Shader RI. Zolpidem metabolism in vitro: responsible cytochromes, chemical inhibitors, and in vivo correlations. Br J Clin Pharmacol. 1999;48:89–97.

20. Fukasawa T, Yasui-Furukori N, Aoshima T, Suzuki A, Tateishi T, Otani K. Single oral dose pharmacokinetics of quazepam is influenced by CYP2C19 activity. Ther Drug Monit. 2004;26(5):529–33.

21. Greenblatt DJ, Harmatz JS, Singh NN, Steinberg F, Roth T, Moline ML, Harris SC, Kapil RP. Gender differences in pharmacokinetics and pharmacodynamics of zolpidem following sublingual administration. J Clin Pharmacol. 2014;54(3):282–90.

22. Schwarz HJ. Pharmacokinetics and metabolism of temazepam in man and several animal species. Br J Clin Pharmacol. 1979;8:23S–9.

23. Lake BG, Ball SE, Kao J, Renwick AB, Price RJ, Scatina JA. Metabolism of zaleplon by human liver: evidence for involvement of aldehyde oxidase. Xenobiotica. 2002;32(10):835–47.

24. Renwick AB, Ball SE, Tredger JM, Price RJ, Walters DG, Kao J, Scatina JA, Lake BG. Inhibition of zaleplon metabolism by cimetidine in the human liver: in vitro studies with subcellular fractions and precision-cut liver slices. Xenobiotica. 2002;32(10):849–62.

25. Krystal AD, Walsh JK, Laska E, Caron J, Amato DA, Wessel TC, et al. Sustained efficacy of eszopiclone over 6 months of nightly treatment: results of a randomized, double-blind, placebo-controlled study in adults with chronic insomnia. Sleep. 2003;26:793–9.

26. Walsh JK, Krystal AD, Amato DA, et al. Nightly treatment of primary insomnia with eszopiclone for six months: effect on sleep, quality of life and work limitations. Sleep. 2007;30:959–68.
27. Roth T, Walsh J, Krystal A, et al. An evaluation of the efficacy and safety of eszopiclone over 12 months in patients with chronic primary insomnia. Sleep Med. 2005;6:487–95.
28. Krystal AD, Erman M, Zammit GK, et al. ZOLONG Study Group. Long-term efficacy and safety of zolpidem extended-release 12.5 mg, administered 3 to 7 nights per week for 24 weeks, in patients with chronic primary insomnia: a 6-month, randomized, double-blind, placebo-controlled, parallel-group, multicenter study. Sleep. 2008; 31:79–90.
29. Ancoli-Israel S, Richardson GS, Mangano RM, Jenkins L, Hall P, Jones WS. Long-term use of sedative hypnotics in older patients with insomnia. Sleep Med. 2005;6(2):107–13.
30. Perlis M, McCall WV, Krystal A, et al. Long-term, non-nightly administration of zolpidem in the treatment of patients with primary insomnia. J Clin Psychiatry. 2004;65:1128–37.
31. Walsh JK, Vogel GW, Scharf M, Erman M, William Erwin C, Schweitzer PK, Mangano RM, Roth T. A five week, polysomnographic assessment of zaleplon 10 mg for the treatment of primary insomnia. Sleep Med. 2000;1(1):41–9.
32. Zammit GK, Corser B, Doghramji K, Fry JM, James S, Krystal A, Mangano RM. Sleep and residual sedation after administration of zaleplon, zolpidem, and placebo during experimental middle-of-the-night awakening. J Clin Sleep Med. 2006;2(4):417–23.
33. Walsh JK, Muehlbach MJ, Lauter SA, Hilliker NA, Schweitzer PK. Effects of triazolam on sleep, daytime sleepiness, and morning stiffness in patients with rheumatoid arthritis. J Rheumatol. 1996;23(2):245–52.
34. Asnis GM, Chakraburtty A, DuBoff EA, Krystal A, Londborg PD, Rosenberg R, Roth-Schechter B, Scharf MB, Walsh JK. Zolpidem for persistent insomnia in SSRI-treated depressed patients. J Clin Psychiatry. 1999;60(10):668–76.
35. Fava M, Asnis GM, Shrivastava R, Lydiard B, Bastani B, Sheehan D, Roth T. Zolpidem extended-release improves sleep and next-day symptoms in comorbid insomnia and generalized anxiety disorder. J Clin Psychopharmacol. 2009;29(3):222–30.
36. Fava M, Asnis GM, Shrivastava RK, Lydiard B, Bastani B, Sheehan DV, Roth T. Improved insomnia symptoms and sleep-related next day functioning in patients with comorbid major depressive disorder and insomnia following concomitant zolpidem extended-release 12.5 mg and escitalopram treatment: a randomized controlled trial. J Clin Psychiatry. 2011;72(7):914–28.
37. Pollack M, Kinrys G, Krystal A, McCall WV, Roth T, Schaefer K, Rubens R, Roach J, Huang H, Krishnan R. Eszopiclone coadministered with escitalopram in patients with insomnia and comorbid generalized anxiety disorder. Arch Gen Psychiatry. 2008;65(5):551–62.
38. Fava M, McCall WV, Krystal A, Rubens R, Caron J, Wessel T, Amato T, Roth T. Eszopiclone coadministered with fluoxetine in patients with insomnia co-existing with major depressive disorder. Biol Psychiatry. 2006;59(11):1052–60.
39. Dorsey CM, Lee KA, Scharf MB. Effect of zolpidem on sleep in women with perimenopausal and postmenopausal insomnia: a 4-week, randomized, multicenter, double-blind, placebo-controlled study. Clin Ther. 2004;26(10):1578–86.
40. Soares CN, Joffe H, Rubens R, Caron J, Roth T, Cohen L. Eszopiclone in patients with insomnia during perimenopause and early postmenopause: a randomized controlled trial. Obstet Gynecol. 2006;108(6):1402–10.
41. Goforth HW, Preud'homme XA, Krystal AD. A randomized, double-blind, placebo-controlled trial of eszopiclone for the treatment of insomnia in patients with chronic low back pain. Sleep. 2014;37(6):1053–60.
42. Roth T, Price JM, Amato DA, Rubens RP, Roach JM, Schnitzer TJ. The effect of eszopiclone in patients with insomnia and coexisting rheumatoid arthritis: a pilot study. Prim Care Companion J Clin Psychiatry. 2009;11(6):292.
43. Pollack MH, Hoge EA, Worthington JJ, Moshier SJ, Wechsler RS, Brandes M, Simon NM. Eszopiclone for the treatment of posttraumatic stress disorder and associated insomnia: a randomized, double-blind, placebo-controlled trial. J Clin Psychiatry. 2011;72(7):892–7.

44. Tek C, Palmese LB, Krystal AD, Srihari VH, DeGeorge PC, Reutenauer EL, Guloksuz S. The impact of eszopiclone on sleep and cognition in patients with schizophrenia and insomnia: a double-blind, randomized, placebo-controlled trial. Schizophr Res. 2014;160(1–3):180–5.
45. Bliwise D, Seidel W, Karacan I, Mitler M, Roth T, Zorick F, Dement W. Daytime sleepiness as a criterion in hypnotic medication trials: comparison of triazolam and flurazepam. Sleep. 1983;6(2):156–63.
46. Roehrs TA, Roth T. Gender differences in the efficacy and safety of chronic nightly zolpidem. J Clin Sleep Med. 2016;12(3):319–25.
47. Walsh JK, Schweitzer PK, Sugerman JL, Muehlbach MJ. Transient insomnia associated with a 3-hour phase advance of sleep time and treatment with zolpidem. J Clin Psychopharmacol. 1990;10(3):184–9.
48. Walsh JK, Pollak CP, Scharf MB, Schweitzer PK, Vogel GW. Lack of residual sedation following middle-of-the-night zaleplon administration in sleep maintenance insomnia. Clin Neuropharmacol. 2000;23(1):17–21.
49. Roth T, Hull SG, Lankford DA, Rosenberg R, Scharf MB, Intermezzo Study Group. Low-dose sublingual zolpidem tartrate is associated with dose-related improvement in sleep onset and duration in insomnia characterized by middle-of-the-night (MOTN) awakenings. Sleep. 2008;31(9):1277–84.
50. Vermeeren A. Residual effects of hypnotics: epidemiology and clinical implications. CNS Drugs. 2004;18(5):297–328.
51. Verster JC, Volkerts ER, Schreuder AH, Eijken EJ, van Heuckelum JH, Veldhuijzen DS, Verbaten MN, Paty I, Darwish M, Danjou P, Patat A. Residual effects of middle-of-the-night administration of zaleplon and zolpidem on driving ability, memory functions, and psychomotor performance. J Clin Psychopharmacol. 2002;22(6):576–83.
52. Vermeeren A, Vuurman EF, Leufkens TR, Van Leeuwen CJ, Van Oers AC, Laska E, Rico S, Steinberg F, Roth T. Residual effects of low-dose sublingual zolpidem on highway driving performance the morning after middle-of-the-night use. Sleep. 2014;37(3):489–96.
53. Leufkens TR, Lund JS, Vermeeren A. Highway driving performance and cognitive functioning the morning after bedtime and middle-of-the-night use of gaboxadol, zopiclone and zolpidem. J Sleep Res. 2009;18(4):387–96.
54. Leufkens TR, Ramaekers JG, de Weerd AW, Riedel WJ, Vermeeren A. Residual effects of zopiclone 7.5mg on highway driving performance in insomnia patients and healthy controls: a placebo controlled crossover study. Psychopharmacology. 2014;231:2785–98.
55. Staner L, Ertlé S, Boeijinga P, Rinaudo G, Arnal MA, Muzet A, Luthringer R. Next-day residual effects of hypnotics in DSM-IV primary insomnia: a driving simulator study with simultaneous electroencephalogram monitoring. Psychopharmacology (Berl). 2005;181(4):790–8.
56. Partinen M, Hirvonen K, Hublin C, Halavaara M, Hiltunen H. Effects of after-midnight intake of zolpidem and temazepam on driving ability in women with non-organic insomnia. Sleep Med. 2003;4(6):553–61.
57. Brassington GS, King AC, Bliwise DL. Sleep problems as a risk factor for falls in a sample of community-dwelling adults aged 64–99 years. J Am Geriatr Soc. 2000;48(10):1234–40.
58. Helbig AK, Döring A, Heier M, Emeny RT, Zimmermann AK, Autenrieth CS, Ladwig KH, Grill E, Meisinger C. Association between sleep disturbances and falls among the elderly: results from the German Cooperative Health Research in the Region of Augsburg-Age study. Sleep Med. 2013;14(12):1356–63.
59. Kuo HK, Yang CC, Yu YH, Tsai KT, Chen CY. Gender-specific association between self-reported sleep duration and falls in high-functioning older adults. J Gerontol A Biol Sci Med Sci. 2010;65(2):190–6.
60. Avidan AY, Fries BE, James ML, Szafara KL, Wright GT, Chervin RD. Insomnia and hypnotic use, recorded in the minimum data set, as predictors of falls and hip fractures in Michigan nursing homes. J Am Geriatr Soc. 2005;53(6):955–62.
61. Ham AC, Swart KM, Enneman AW, van Dijk SC, Oliai Araghi S, van Wijngaarden JP, van der Zwaluw NL, Brouwer-Brolsma EM, Dhonukshe-Rutten RA, van Schoor NM, van der

Cammen TJ, Lips P, de Groot LC, Uitterlinden AG, Witkamp RF, Stricker BH, van der Velde N. Medication-related fall incidents in an older, ambulant population: the B-PROOF study. Drugs Aging. 2014;31(12):917–27.

62. Ensrud KE, Blackwell TL, Mangione CM, Bowman PJ, Whooley MA, Bauer DC, Schwartz AV, Hanlon JT, Nevitt MC, Study of Osteoporotic Fractures Research Group. Central nervous system-active medications and risk for falls in older women. J Am Geriatr Soc. 2002;50(10):1629–37.

63. Richardson K, Bennett K, Kenny RA. Polypharmacy including falls risk-increasing medications and subsequent falls in community-dwelling middle-aged and older adults. Age Ageing. 2015;44(1):90–6.

64. Kelly KD, Pickett W, Yiannakoulias N, Rowe BH, Schopflocher DP, Svenson L, Voaklander DC. Medication use and falls in community-dwelling older persons. Age Ageing. 2003;32(5):503–9.

65. Diem SJ, Ewing SK, Stone KL, Ancoli-Israel S, Redline S, Ensrud KE. The Osteoporotic Fractures in Men (MrOS) Study Group. Use of non-benzodiazepine sedative hypnotics and risk of falls in older men. J Gerontol Geriatr Res. 2014;3(3):158.

66. Berry SD, Lee Y, Cai S, Dore DD. Nonbenzodiazepine sleep medication use and hip fractures in nursing home residents. JAMA Intern Med. 2013;173(9):754–61.

67. Greenblatt DJ, Harmatz JS, Shapiro L, Engelhardt N, Gouthro TA, Shader RI. Sensitivity to triazolam in the elderly. N Engl J Med. 1991;324(24):1691–8.

68. Roth T, Roehrs TA, Stepanski EJ, Rosenthal LD. Hypnotics and behavior. Am J Med. 1990;88(3A):43S–6.

69. Uemura SI, Kanbayashi T, Wakasa M, Satake M, Ito W, Shimizu K, Shioya T, Shimizu T, Nishino S. Residual effects of zolpidem, triazolam, rilmazafone and placebo in healthy elderly subjects: a randomized double-blind study. Sleep Med. 2015;16(11):1395–402.

70. Kleykamp BA, Griffiths RR, McCann UD, Smith MT, Mintzer MZ. Acute effects of zolpidem extended-release on cognitive performance and sleep in healthy males after repeated nightly use. Exp Clin Psychopharmacol. 2012;20(1):28–39.

71. Troy SM, Lucki I, Unruh MA, Cevallos WH, Leister CA, Martin PT, Furlan PM, Mangano R. Comparison of the effects of zaleplon, zolpidem, and triazolam on memory, learning, and psychomotor performance. J Clin Psychopharmacol. 2000;20(3):328–37.

72. Roehrs T, Zorick FJ, Sicklesteel JM, Wittig RM, Hartse KM, Roth T. Effects of hypnotics on memory. J Clin Psychopharmacol. 1983;3(5):310–3.

73. Yang W, Dollear M, Muthukrishnan SR. One rare side effect of zolpidem—sleepwalking: a case report. Arch Phys Med Rehabil. 2005;86(6):1265–6.

74. Harazin J, Berigan TR. Zolpidem tartrate and somnambulism. Mil Med. 1999;164(9):669–70.

75. Chen YW, Tseng PT, Wu CK, Chen CC. Zaleplon-induced anemsic somnambulism with eating behaviors under once dose. Acta Neurol Taiwan. 2014;23(4):143–5.

76. Poceta JS. Zolpidem ingestion, automatisms, and sleep driving: a clinical and legal case series. J Clin Sleep Med. 2011;7(6):632–8.

77. Dolder CR, Nelson MH. Hypnosedative-induced complex behaviours: incidence, mechanisms and management. CNS Drugs. 2008;22(12):1021–36.

78. Usumoto Y, Kudo K, Sameshima N, Sato K, Tsuji A, Ikeda N. An autopsy case of abnormal behaviour induced by zolpidem. Fukuoka Igaku Zasshi. 2015;106(6):202–5.

79. Chen CS, Huang MF, Hwang TJ, Chen ST, Ko CH, Yen CN, Chen TT, Su PW, Yeh YC, Lin JJ, Yen CF. Clinical correlates of zolpidem-associated complex sleep-related behaviors: age effect. J Clin Psychiatry. 2014;75(11):e1314–8.

80. Kay-Stacey M, Attarian H. Advances in the management of chronic insomnia. Br Med J. 2016 (In Press).

81. Kripke DF, Langer RD, Kline LE. Hypnotics' association with mortality or cancer: a matched cohort study. BMJ Open. 2012;2(1):e000850.

82. Lallukka T, Podlipskyte A, Sivertsen B, et al. Insomnia symptoms and mortality: a register-linked study among women and men from Finland, Norway and Lithuania. J Sleep Res. 2015. doi:10.1111/jsr.12343.

83. Kriegbaum M, Hendriksen C, Vass M, et al. Hypnotics and mortality—partial confounding by disease, substance abuse and socioeconomic factors? Pharmacoepidemiol Drug Saf. 2015;24(7):779–83.
84. Jaussent I, Ancelin ML, Berr C, et al. Hypnotics and mortality in an elderly general population: a 12-year prospective study. BMC Med. 2013;11:212.
85. Neutel CI, Johansen HL. Association between hypnotics use and increased mortality: causation or confounding? Eur J Clin Pharmacol. 2015;71:637–42.
86. Roehrs TA, Randall S, Harris E, Maan R, Roth T. Twelve months of nightly zolpidem does not lead to dose escalation: a prospective placebo-controlled study. Sleep. 2011;34(2):207–12.
87. Walsh JK, Roth T, Randazzo A, Erman M, Jamieson A, Scharf M, Schweitzer PK, Ware JC. Eight weeks of non-nightly use of zolpidem for primary insomnia. Sleep. 2000;23(8):1087–96.
88. Balter MB, Uhlenhuth EH. New epidemiologic findings about insomnia and its treatment. J Clin Psychiatry. 1992;53(Suppl):34–9. discussion 40–42.
89. Licata SC, Penetar DM, Dunlap S, Lukas SE. A therapeutic dose of zolpidem has limited abuse-like effects in drug-naïve females: a pilot study. Eur J Pharmacol. 2008;598(1–3):64–7.
90. Evans SM, Funderburk FR, Griffiths RR. Zolpidem and triazolam in humans: behavioral and subjective effects and abuse liability. J Pharmacol Exp Ther. 1990;255(3):1246–55.
91. Rush CR, Baker RW, Wright K. Acute behavioral effects and abuse potential of trazodone, zolpidem and triazolam in humans. Psychopharmacology (Berl). 1999;144(3):220–33.
92. Griffiths RR, Johnson MW. Relative abuse liability of hypnotic drugs: a conceptual framework and algorithm for differentiating among compounds. J Clin Psychiatry. 2005;66 Suppl 9:31–41.
93. Becker WC, Fiellin DA, Desai RA. Non-medical use, abuse and dependence on sedatives and tranquilizers among U.S. adults: psychiatric and socio-demographic correlates. Drug Alcohol Depend. 2007;90:280–7.
94. Monti JM, Attali P, Monti D, Zipfel A, de la Giclais B, Morselli PL. Zolpidem and rebound insomnia—a double-blind, controlled polysomnographic study in chronic insomniac patients. Pharmacopsychiatry. 1994;27(4):166–75.
95. Roehrs T, Merlotti L, Zorick F, et al. Rebound insomnia and hypnotic self administration. Psychopharmacology. 1992;107:480–4.
96. Kato K, Hirai K, Nishiyama K, Uchikawa O, Fukatsu K, Ohkawa S, et al. Neurochemical properties of ramelteon (TAK-375), a selective MT1/MT2 receptor agonist. Neuropharmacology. 2005;48(2):301–10.
97. Miayamoto M. Pharmacology of ramelteon, a selective MT1/MT2 receptor agonist: a novel drug for sleep disorders. CNS Neurosci Ther. 2009;15:32–51.
98. Erman M, Seiden D, Zammit G, Sainati S, Zheng J. An efficacy, safety and dose-response study of Ramelteon in patients with chronic primary insomnia. Sleep Med. 2006;7:17–24.
99. Mayer G, Wang-Wiegand S, Roth-Schechter B, Lehmann R, Staner C, Partinen M. Efficacy and safety of 6-month nightly ramnelteon administration in adults with primary insomnia. Sleep. 2009;32(3):351–60.
100. Roth T, Seiden D, Sainati S, Wang-Weigand S, Zhang J, Zee P. Effects of ramelteon on patient-reported sleep latency in older adults with chronic insomnia. Sleep Med. 2006;7:312–8.
101. Kuriyama A, Honda M, Hayashino Y. Ramelteon for the treatment of insomnia in adults: a systematic review and meta-analysis. Sleep Med. 2014;15:385–92.
102. Winrow CJ. Promotion of sleep by suvorexant-a novel dual orexin receptor antagonist. J Neurogenet. 2011;25:52–61.
103. de Lecea L, Huerta R. Hypocretin (orexin) regulation of sleep-to-wake transitions. Front Pharmacol. 2014;5:16.
104. Riemann D, Spiegelhalder K, Feige B, et al. The hyperarousal model of insomnia: a review of the concept and its evidence. Sleep Med Rev. 2010;14:19–31.

105. Sun H, Kennedy WP, Wilbraham D, et al. Effects of suvorexant, an orexin receptor antagonist, on sleep parameters as measured by polysomnography in healthy men. Sleep.
2013;36:259–67.
106. Herring W, Connor K, Ivgy-May N, Snyder E, Liu K, Snavely D, Krystal A, Walsh J, Benca
R, Rosenberg R, Sangal R, Budd K, Hutzelmann J, Liebensperger H, Froman S, Lines C,
Roth T, Michelson D. Suvorexant in patients with insomnia: results from two 3-month randomized clinical trials. Biol Psychiatry. http://dx.doi.org/10.1016/j.biopsych.2014.10.003
107. Michelson D, Snyder E, Paradis E, Chengan-Liu M, Hutzelman J, Walsh J, Krystal A, Benca
R, Cohn M, Lines C, Roth T, Herring W. Safety and efficacy of suvorexant during 1-year
treatment of insomnia with subsequent abrupt treatment discontinuation: a phase 3 randomised, double-blind, placebo-controlled trial. Lancet Neurol. 2014;13:461–71.
108. Herring W, Snyder E, Budd K, Hutzelmann J, Snavely D, Liu K, Lines C, Roth T, Michelson
D. Orexin receptor antagonism for treatment of insomnia: a randomized clinical trial of
suvorexant. Neurology. 2012;79:2265–74.
109. Ma J, Svetnik V, Snyder E, Lines C, Roth T, Herring WJ. Electroencephalographic power
spectral density profile of the orexin receptor antagonist suvorexant in patients with primary
insomnia and healthy subjects. Sleep. 2014;37(10):1609–19.
110. Sun H, Palcza J, Card D, Gipson A, Rosenberg R, Kryger M, Lines C, Wagner J, Troyer
M. Effects of suvorexant, an orexin receptor antagonist, on respiration during sleep in patients
with obstructive sleep apnea. J Clin Sleep Med. 2016;12(1):9–17.
111. Sun H, Palcza J, Rosenberg R, Kryger M, Siringhaus T, Rose J, Lines C, Wagner J, Troyer
M. Effects of suvorexant, an orexin receptor antagonist, on breathing during sleep in patients
with chronic obstructive pulmonary disease. Respir Med. 2015;109(3):416–26. doi:10.1016/j.
rmed.2014.12.010. Epub 2015 Jan 5.
112. Vermeeren A, Sun H, Vuurman E, Jongen S, Van Leeuwen C, Van Oers A, Palcza J, Li X,
Laethem T, Heirman I, Bautmans A, Troyer M, Wrishko R, McCrea J. On-the-road driving
performance the morning after bedtime use of suvorexant 20 and 40 mg: a study in non-
elderly healthy volunteers. Sleep. 2015;38(11):1803–13.
113. Weber J, Siddiqui M, Wagstaff A. Low-dose doxepin: in the treatment of insomnia. CNS
Drugs. 2010;24:713–20.
114. Krystal AD, Richelson E, Roth T. Review of the histamine system and the clinical effects of
H1 antagonists: basis for a new model for understanding the effects of insomnia medications.
Sleep Med Rev. 2013;17(4):263–72.
115. Krystal AD, Lankford A, Durrence HH, Ludington E, Jochelson P, Rogowski R, et al.
Efficacy and safety of doxepin 3 and 6 mg in a 35-day sleep laboratory trial in adults with
chronic primary insomnia. Sleep. 2011;34:1433–42.
116. Krystal AD, Durrence HH, Scharf M, Jochelson P, Rogowski R, Ludington E, et al. Efficacy
and safety of doxepin 1 mg and 3 mg in a 12-week sleep laboratory and outpatient trial of
elderly subjects with chronic primary insomnia. Sleep. 2010;33:1553–61.
117. Rickels K, Morris RJ, Newman H, Rosenfeld H, Schiller H, Weinstock R. Diphenhydramine
in insomniac family practice patients: a double-blind study. J Clin Pharmacol.
1983;23(5–6):234–42.
118. Morin C, Koetter U, Bastien C, Ware JC, Wooten V. Valerian-hops combination and diphenhydramine for treating insomnia: a randomized placebo-controlled clinical trial. Sleep.
2005;28(11):1465–71.
119. Zhang D, Tashiro M, Shibuya K, Okamura N, Funake Y, Yoshikawa T, Kato M, Yanai K. Next
day residual sedative effect after nighttime administration of an over-the-counter antihista-
mine sleep aid, diphenhydramine, measured by positron emission tomography. J Clin
Psychopharm. 2010;30(6):694–701.
120. Schweitzer PK, Muehlbach MJ, Walsh JK. Sleepiness and performance during three-day
administration of cetirizine or diphenhydramine. J Allergy Clin Immunol. 1994;94:716–24.
121. Richardson GS, Roehrs TA, Rosenthal L, Koshorek G, Roth T. Tolerance to daytime sedative
effects of H1 antihistamines. J Clin Psychopharmacol. 2002;22:511–5.

122. Roehrs T, Roth T. 'Hypnotic' prescription patterns in a large managed-care population. Sleep Med. 2004;5(5):463–6.
123. Ferri R, Zucconi M, Marelli S, Plazzi G, Schenck CH, Ferini-Strambi L. Effects of long-term use of clonazepam on nonrapid eye movement sleep patterns in rapid eye movement sleep behavior disorder. Sleep Med. 2013;14(5):399–406.
124. Walsh J, Erman M, Erwin C, et al. Subjective hypnotic efficacy of trazodone and zolpidem in DSMIII-R primary insomnia. Hum Psychopharmacol. 1998;13:191–8.
125. Roth A, McCall W, Liguori A. Cognitive, psychomotor and polysomnographic effects of trazodone in primary insomniacs. J Sleep Res. 2011;20:552–8.
126. Le Bon O, Murphy JR, Staner L, Hoffmann G, Kormoss N, Kentos M, Dupont P, Lion K, Pelc I, Verbanck P. Double-blind, placebo-controlled study of the efficacy of trazodone in alcohol post-withdrawal syndrome: polysomnographic and clinical evaluations. J Clin Psychopharmacol. 2003;23(4):377–83.
127. Friedmann PD, Rose JS, Swift R, Stout RL, Millman RP, Stein MD. Trazodone for sleep disturbance after alcohol detoxification: a double-blind, placebo-controlled trial. Alcohol Clin Exp Res. 2008;32(9):1652–60.
128. Stein MD, Kurth ME, Sharkey KM, Anderson BJ, Corso RP, Millman RP. Trazodone for sleep disturbance during methadone maintenance: a double-blind, placebo-controlled trial. Drug Alcohol Depend. 2012;120(1–3):65–73.
129. Nierenberg A, Adler L, Peselow E, Zornberg G, Rosenthal M. Trazodone for antidepressant-associated insomnia. Am J Psychiatry. 1994;151:1069–72.
130. Ivgy-May N, Ruwe F, Krystal A, Roth T. Esmirtazapine in non-elderly adult patients with primary insomnia: efficacy and safety form a randomized, 6-week sleep laboratory trial. Sleep Med. 2015;16:838–44.
131. Fawcett J, Barkin RL. Review of the results from clinical studies on the efficacy, safety and tolerability of mirtazapine for the treatment of patients with major depression. J Affect Disord. 1998;51(3):267–85.
132. Rodenbeck A, Cohrs S, Jordan W, Huether G, Ruther E, Hajak G. The sleep-improving effects of doxepin are paralleled by a normalized plasma cortisol secretion in primary insomnia. Psychopharmacology (Berl). 2003;170:423–8.
133. Hajak G, Rodenbeck A, Adler L, Huether G, Bandelow B, Herrendorf G, Staedt J, Rüther E. Nocturnal melatonin secretion and sleep after doxepin administration in chronic primary insomnia. Pharmacopsychiatry. 1996;29(5):187–92.
134. Hajak G, Rodenbeck A, Voderholzer U, Riemann D, Cohrs S, Hohagen F, Berger M, Rüther E. Doxepin in the treatment of primary insomnia: a placebo-controlled, double-blind, polysomnographic study. J Clin Psychiatry. 2001;62(6):453–63.
135. Riemann D, Voderholzer U, Cohrs S, Rodenbeck A, Hajak G, Ruther E, Wiegand M, Laakmann G, Baghai T, Fischer W, Hoffmann M, Hohagen F, Mayer G, Berger M. Trimipramine in primary insomnia: results of a polysomographic double-blind controlled study. Pharmacopsychiatry. 2002;35(5):165–74.
136. Hohagen F, Montero RF, Weiss E. Treatment of primary insomnia with trimipramine: an alternative to benzodiazepine hypnotics? Eur Arch Psychiatry Clin Neurosci. 1994;244(2):65–72.
137. Kupfer DJ, Spiker DG, Coble P, et al. Amitriptyline and EEG sleep in depressed patients: I. Drug effect. Sleep. 1978;1:149–59.
138. Roth T, Zorick F, Wittig R, McLenaghan A, Roehrs T. The effects of doxepin HCl on sleep and depression. J Clin Psychiatry. 1982;43(9):366–8.
139. Ware JC, Brown FW, Moorad Jr PJ, Pittard JT, Cobert B. Effects on sleep: a double-blind study comparing trimipramine to imipramine in depressed insomniac patients. Sleep. 1989;12(6):537–49.
140. Rios Romenets S, Creti L, Fichten C, Bailes S, Libman E, Pelletier A, Postuma RB. Doxepin and cognitive behavioural therapy for insomnia in patients with Parkinson's disease—a randomized study. Parkinsonism Relat Disord. 2013;19(7):670–5.

141. Nelson JC. Tricyclic and tetracyclic drugs. In: Schatzberg Am Nemeroff C, editor. The American Psychiatric Publishing textbook of psychopharmacology. Washington, DC: American Psychiatric Publishing; 2004. p. 207–20.
142. Tassniyom K, Paholpak S, Tassniyom S, Kiewyoo J. Quetiapine for primary insomnia: a double blind, randomized controlled trial. J Med Assoc Thai. 2010;93(6):729–34.
143. Wiegand M, Landry T, Bruckner T, Pohl C, Zdenko V, Jahn T. Quetiapine in primary insomnia: a pilot study. Psychopharmacology. 2008;196:337–8.
144. Anderson S, Vande GJ. Quetiapine for insomnia: a review of the literature. Am J Health Syst Pharm. 2014;71:394–402.
145. Trivedi M, Bandelow B, Demyttenaere K, Papakosts G, Szamosi J, Earley W, Eriksson H. Evaluation of the effects of extended release quetiapine fumarate monotherapy on sleep disturbance in patients with major depressive disorder: a pooled analysis of four randomized acute studies. Int J Neuropsychopharmacol. 2013;16:1733–44.
146. Endicott J, Paulsson B, Gustafsson U, et al. Quetiapine monothcrapy in the treatment of depressive episodes of bipolar I and II disorder: improvements in quality of life and quality of sleep. J Affect Disord. 2008;111:306–19.
147. Stein D, Bandelow B, Merideth C, et al. Efficacy and tolerability of extended release quetiapine fumarate (quetiapine XR) monotherapy in patients with generalized anxiety disorder: an analysis of pooled data from 3 8-week placebo-controlled studies. Hum Psychopharmacol. 2011;26:614–28.
148. Potvin S, Morin M, Cloutier C, Gendron A, Bissonnette A, Marchand D. Add-on treatment of quetiapine for fibromyalgia. A pilot, randomized, double-blind, placebo-controlled 12-week trial. J Clin Psychopharmacol. 2012;32:684–7.
149. Cates ME, Jackson CW, Feldman JM, et al. Metabolic consequences of using low dose quetiapine for insomnia in psychiatric patients. Community Ment Health J. 2009;45:251–4.
150. Gugger JJ, Cassagnol M. Low-dose quetiapine is not a benign sedative-hypnotic agent. Am J Addict. 2008;17:454–5.
151. Coe HV, Hong IS. Safety of low doses of quetiapine when used for insomnia. Ann Pharmacother. 2012;46:718–22.
152. Kirshner H. Controversies in behavioral neurology: the use of atypical antipsychotic drugs to treat neurobehavioral symptoms in dementia. Curr Neurol Neurosci Rep. 2008;8(6):471–4.
153. Rose M, Kam CA. Gabapentin: pharmacology and it's use in pain management. Anaesthesia. 2002;57:451–62.
154. Gajraj N. Pregabalin: its pharmacology and use in pain management. Anesth Analg. 2007;105(6):1805–15.
155. Rosenberg R, Hull S, Lankford D, Mayleben D, Seiden D, Furey S, Jayawardena S, Roth T. A randomized, double-blind, single-dose, placebo-controlled, multicenter, polysomnographic study of gabapentin in transient insomnia induced by sleep phase advance. J Clin Sleep Med. 2014;10(10):1093–100.
156. Furey S, Hull S, Leibowitz MT, Jayawardena S, Roth T. A randomized, double-blind, placebo-controlled, multicenter, 28-day, polysomnographic study of gabapentin in transient insomnia induced by sleep phase advance. J Clin Sleep Med. 2014;10(10):1101–9.
157. Lo H-S, Yang C-M, Lo H, Lee C-Y, Ting H, Tzang B-S. Treatment effects of gabapentin for primary insomnia. Clin Neuropharmacol. 2010;22:84–90.
158. Winkelman J, Bogan R, Schmidt M, Hudson J, DeRossett S, Hill-Zabala C. Randomized polysomnography study of gabapentin enacarbil in subjects with restless legs syndrome. Mov Disord. 2011;26(11):2065–72.
159. Garcia-Borreguero D, Patrick J, DuBrava S, Becker P, Lankford A, Chen C, Miceli J, Knapp L, Allen R. Pregabalin versus pramipexole: effects on sleep disturbance in restless legs syndrome. Sleep. 2014;37(4):635–43.
160. Arnold LM, Goldenberg DL, Stanford SB, Lalonde JK, Sandhu HS, Keck Jr PE, Welge JA, Bishop F, Stanford KE, Hess EV, Hudson JI. Gabapentin in the treatment of fibromyalgia: a randomized, double-blind, placebo-controlled, multicenter trial. Arthritis Rheum. 2007;56(4):1336–44.

161. Roth T, Lankford D, Bhadra P, Whalen E, Resnick E. Effect of pregabalin on sleep in patients with fibromyalgia and sleep maintenance disturbance: a randomized, placebo-controlled, 2-way crossover Polysomnography study. Arthritis Care Res (Hoboken). 2012;64(4):597–606.

162. Sabatowski R, Gálvez R, Cherry DA, Jacquot F, Vincent E, Maisonobe P, Versavel M, 1008–045 Study Group. Pregabalin reduces pain and improves sleep and mood disturbances in patients with post-herpetic neuralgia: results of a randomised, placebo-controlled clinical trial. Pain. 2004;109(1–2):26–35.

163. Boyle J, Eriksson ME, Gribble L, Gouni R, Johnsen S, Coppini DV, Kerr D. Randomized, placebo-controlled comparison of amitriptyline, duloxetine, and pregabalin in patients with chronic diabetic peripheral neuropathic pain: impact on pain, polysomnographic sleep, daytime functioning, and quality of life. Diabetes Care. 2012;35(12):2451–8.

164. Yurcheshen ME, Guttuso Jr T, McDermott M, Holloway RG, Perlis M. Effects of gabapentin on sleep in menopausal women with hot flashes as measured by a Pittsburgh Sleep Quality Index factor scoring model. J Womens Health (Larchmt). 2009;18(9):1355–60.

165. De Haas S, Otte A, de Weerd A, van Erp G, Cohen A, van Gerven J. Exploratory polysomnographic evaluation of pregabalin on sleep disturbance in patients with epilepsy. J Clin Sleep Med. 2007;3(5):473–8.

166. Roth T, Arnold L, Garcia-Borreguero D, Resnick M, Clair A. A review of the effects of pregabalin on sleep disturbance across multiple clinical conditions. Sleep Med Rev. 2014;18(3):261–71.

167. Walsh JK, Perlis M, Rosenthal M, Krystal A, Jiang J, Roth T. Tiagabine increases slow-wave sleep in a dose-dependent fashion without affecting traditional efficacy measures in adults with primary insomnia. J Clin Sleep Med. 2006;2(1):35–41.

168. Walsh JK, Randazzo AC, Frankowski S, Shannon K, Schweitzer PK, Roth T. Dose-response effects of tiagabine on the sleep of older adults. Sleep. 2005;28(6):673–6.

169. Krystal AD. New developments in insomnia medications of relevance to mental health disorders. Psychiatr Clin N Am. 2015;38:843–60.

170. Irwin M, Clark C, Kennedy B, et al. Nocturnal catecholamines and immune function in insomniacs, depressed patients, and control subjects. Brain Behav Immun. 2003;17(5):365–72.

171. Germain A, Richardson R, Moul DE, Mammen O, Haas G, Forman SD, Rode N, Begley A, Nofzinger EA. Placebo-controlled comparison of prazosin and cognitive-behavioral treatments for sleep disturbances in US Military Veterans. J Psychosom Res. 2012;72(2):89–96.

172. Raskind MA, Peskind ER, Hoff DJ, et al. A parallel group placebo controlled study of prazosin for trauma nightmares and sleep disturbance in combat veterans with post-traumatic stress disorder. Biol Psychiatry. 2007;61(8):928–34.

173. Raskind MA, Peskind ER, Kanter ED, Petrie EC, Radant A, Thompson CE, Dobie DJ, Hoff D, Rein RJ, Straits-Tröster K, Thomas RG, McFall MM. Reduction of nightmares and other PTSD symptoms in combat veterans by prazosin: a placebo-controlled study. Am J Psychiatry. 2003;160(2):371–3.

174. Raskind MA, Peterson K, Williams T, et al. A trial of prazosin for combat trauma PTSD with nightmares in active-duty soldiers returned from Iraq and Afghanistan. Am J Psychiatry. 2013;170(9):1003–10.

175. Taylor FB, Martin P, Thompson C, et al. Prazosin effects on objective sleep measures and clinical symptoms in civilian trauma posttraumatic stress disorder: a placebo-controlled study. Biol Psychiatry. 2008;63(6):629–32.

176. DeMuro RL, Nafziger AN, Blask DE, Menhinick AM, Bertino Jr JS. The absolute bioavailability of oral melatonin. J Clin Pharmacol. 2000;40:781–4.

177. Ferracioli-Oda E, Qawasmi A, Bloch M. Meta-analysis: melatonin for the treatment of primary sleep disorders. PLoS One. 2013;8(5), e63773. doi:10.1371/journal.pone.0063773.

178. Wilson S, Nutt D, Alford C, Argyropoulos S, Baldwin D, Bateson A, Britton T, Crowe C, Dijk D-J, Espie C, Gringras P, Hajak G, Idzikowski C, Krystal A, Nash J, Selsick H, Sharpley A, Wade A. British Association for Psychopharmacology consensus statement on evidence-based treatment of insomnia, parasomnias and circadian rhythm disorders. J Psychopharmacol. 2010;23(11):1577–600.

179. Wade AG, Ford I, Crawford G, McConnachie A, Nir T, Laudon M, Zisapel N. Nightly treatment of primary insomnia with prolonged release melatonin for 6 months: a randomized placebo controlled trial on age and endogenous melatonin as predictors of efficacy and safety. BMC Med. 2010;8:51. doi:10.1186/1741-7015-8-51.

180. Van Geijlswijk IM, Korzilius HP, Smits MG. The use of exogenous melatonin in delayed sleep phase disorder: a meta-analysis. Sleep. 2010;33(12):1605–14.

181. Buscemi N, Vandermeer B, Hooton N, et al. The efficacy and safety of exogenous melatonin for primary sleep disorders. A meta-analysis. J Gen Intern Med. 2005;20:1151–8.

182. Committee on the Framework for Evaluating the Safety of the Dietary Supplements FaNB, Board on Life Sciences, Institute of Medicine and National Research Council of the National Academies. Dietary supplements: a framework for evaluating safety. Washington, DC: The National Academies Press; 2005.

183. Auger RRA, Burgess HJ, Emens JS, Deriy L, Thomas SM, Sharkey K. Clinical practice guideline for the treatment of intrinsic circadian rhythm sleep-wake disorders: advanced sleep-wake phase disorder (ASWPD), delayed sleep-wake phase disorder (DSWPD), non-24-hour sleep-wake rhythm disorder (N24SWD), and irregular sleep-wake rhythm disorder (ISWRD). An update for 2015. An American Academy of Sleep Medicine Clinical Practice Guideline. J Clin Sleep Med. 2015;11(10):1199–236.

184. Shekleton JA, Flynn-Evans EE, Miller B, Epstein LJ, Kirsch D, Brogna LA, Burke LM, Bremer E, Murray JM, Gehrman P, Lockley SW, Rajaratnam SM. Neurobehavioral performance impairment in insomnia: relationships with self-reported sleep and daytime functioning. Sleep. 2014;37(1):107–16.

185. Zammit GK, Weiner J, Damata N, et al. Quality of life in people with insomnia. Sleep. 1999;22 Suppl 2:S379–85.

186. Breslau N, Roth T, Rosenthal L, et al. Sleep disturbance and psychiatric disorders: a longitudinal epidemiological study of young adults. Biol Psychiatry. 1996;39:411–8.

187. Ozminkowski RJ, Wang S, Walsh JK. The direct and indirect costs of untreated insomnia in adults in the United States. Sleep. 2007;30:263–73.

188. Shahly V, Berglund PA, Coulouvrat C, Fitzgerald T, Hajak G, Roth T, Shillington AC, Stephenson JJ, Walsh JK, Kessler RC. The associations of insomnia with costly workplace accidents and errors: results from the America Insomnia Survey. Arch Gen Psychiatry. 2012;69(10):1054–63.

189. Kucharczyk ER, Morgan K, Hall AP. The occupational impact of sleep quality and insomnia symptoms. Sleep Med Rev. 2012;16(6):547–59.

190. Schutte-Rodin S, Broch L, Buysse D, Dorsey C, Sateia M. Clinical guideline for the evaluation and management of chronic insomnia in adults. J Clin Sleep Med. 2008;4(5):487–504.

191. Dolly FR, Block AJ. Effect of flurazepam on sleep-disordered breathing and nocturnal oxygen desaturation in asymptomatic subjects. Am J Med. 1982;73(2):239–43.

192. Rosenberg R, Roach JM, Scharf M, Amato DA. A pilot study evaluating acute use of eszopiclone in patients with mild to moderate obstructive sleep apnea syndrome. Sleep Med. 2007;8(5):464–70.

193. Eckert DJ, Owens RL, Kehlmann GB, Wellman A, Rahangdale S, Yim-Yeh S, White DP, Malhotra A. Eszopiclone increases the respiratory arousal threshold and lowers the apnoea/hypopnoea index in obstructive sleep apnoea patients with a low arousal threshold. Clin Sci (Lond). 2011;120(12):505–14.

194. Quadri S, Drake C, Hudgel DW. Improvement of idiopathic central sleep apnea with zolpidem. J Clin Sleep Med. 2009;5(2):122–9.

195. Steens RD, Pouliot Z, Millar TW, Kryger MH, George CF. Effects of zolpidem and triazolam on sleep and respiration in mild to moderate chronic obstructive pulmonary disease. Sleep. 1993;16(4):318–26.

196. Timms RM, Dawson A, Hajdukovic RM, Mitler MM. Effect of triazolam on sleep and arterial oxygen saturation in patients with chronic obstructive pulmonary disease. Arch Intern Med. 1988;148(10):2159–63.

197. Lettieri CJ, Shah AA, Holley AB, Kelly WF, Chang AS, Roop SA, CPAP Promotion and Prognosis-The Army Sleep Apnea Program Trial. Effects of a short course of eszopiclone on continuous positive airway pressure adherence: a randomized trial. Ann Intern Med. 2009;151(10):696–702.
198. Roehrs T, Merlotti L, Zorick F, Roth T. Rebound insomnia in normals and patients with insomnia after abrupt and tapered discontinuation. Psychopharmacology (Berl). 1992;108(1–2):67–71.
199. Bélanger L, Vallières A, Ivers H, Moreau V, Lavigne G, Morin CM. Meta-analysis of sleep changes in control groups of insomnia treatment trials. J Sleep Res. 2007;16(1):77–84.
200. Winkler A, Rief W. Effect of placebo conditions on polysomnographic parameters in primary insomnia: a meta-analysis. Sleep. 2015;38(6):925–31.
201. Walsh JK, Coulouvrat C, Hajak G, Lakoma MD, Petukhova M, Roth T, Sampson NA, Shahly V, Shillington A, Stephenson JJ, Kessler RC. Nighttime insomnia symptoms and perceived health in the America Insomnia Survey (AIS). Sleep. 2011;34(8):997–1011.
202. Krystal AD, Benca R, Kilduff T. Understanding the sleep-wake cycle: sleep, insomnia, and the orexin system. J Clin Psychiatry. 2013;74 Suppl 1:3–20.

Part II
Insomnia in Special Populations

Chapter 8
Insomnias of Childhood: Assessment and Treatment

Daniel S. Lewin and Edward Huntley

Abstract Insomnia in childhood includes difficulty initiating and maintaining sleep and bedtime resistance. These sleep problems are common in childhood and largely result from interactions between the caregivers or parents and their children. However that are other causes and origins of insomnia that can include child temperament, psychopathology, or variation in sleep need that can include decreased need for sleep and atypical circadian regulation. Chronic insomnia symptoms often precipitate a range of functional daytime impairments (e.g., academic impairment, hyperactivity, inattention, irritability, tiredness) which may further undermine subsequent parent–child interactions including the transition to sleep. Evidence-based interventions for childhood insomnia can address these sleep difficulties and family stress. However, dissemination of evidence-based interventions is limited by the dearth of clinicians trained to deliver these interventions, access to sleep disorder centers, and cost. This chapter provides an overview of approaches to diagnosis and management of childhood insomnia.

Keywords Cognitive-behavioral therapy (CBT) • Insomnia • Evidence-based practice • Child • Parent–child relations • Sleep initiation • Maintenance

D.S. Lewin, Ph.D. (✉)
Department of Pulmonary and Sleep Medicine, Children's National Medical Center, George Washington University School of Medicine,
111 Michigan Avenue, N.W, Washington, DC 20010, USA
e-mail: DLewin@cnmc.org

E. Huntley, Ph.D.
Survey Research Center, Institute for Social Research, University of Michigan,
426 Thompson St., Ann Arbor, MI 48106-1248, USA
e-mail: huntleye@umich.edu

© Springer International Publishing Switzerland 2017
H.P. Attarian (ed.), *Clinical Handbook of Insomnia*, Current Clinical Neurology,
DOI 10.1007/978-3-319-41400-3_8

Introduction

The insomnias of childhood include bedtime resistance, sleep initiation sleep, and maintenance problems. These bedtime and sleep problems can place a significant burden on caregivers and parents who may be required to spend significant time attending to a child at the beginning or middle of the night and sometimes early in the morning. The resulting sleep loss can impact parents' and children's daytime functioning and increase bedtime-related conflict and influence family dynamics [1]. Even when sleep problems do not meet criteria for a disorder, they are a common cause of stress in parent–child relationships. Childhood sleep problems can be an indicator of poor regulatory capacity in the infant or child, and there is evidence that sleep problems presenting in the first few years of life can be a marker of a diathesis for psychopathology and health problems [2–5]. Even though sleep problems in early childhood are quite common and there are well-established interventions for these problems, little is understood about the etiology pathophysiology of childhood sleep disorders. This chapter reviews common causes of insomnia from infancy through the school-age years that can persist into middle childhood and adolescence. The discussion of pathophysiology will be followed by a detailed practical approach to evaluating and treating insomnias in this age group.

Definitions

While most children have at least minor or transient problems initiating and maintaining sleep, between 15 and 20 % of children have persistent insomnia [6, 7]. The International Classification of Sleep Disorders (ICSD) Third Edition has harmonized with the DSM-5 [8] by consolidating insomnia into chronic and short-term categories, and eliminating prior subtypes. Insomnia may be diagnosed after the age of 6 months at which time the nocturnal sleep of typically developing children has become more consolidated and nighttime feedings are minimal to none. All insomnia subtypes including the behavioral insomnias of childhood (BIC) are no longer independent diagnostic categories but are discussed as descriptors that may have some clinical utility as they suggest etiology. The BIC will be the primary focus of this chapter and treated as a sub-category of insomnia as there is a large evidence-based literature demonstrating the efficacy of insomnia interventions.

The BIC are divided into three diagnostic categories: sleep-onset association type and limit-setting type and a mixed type with features of both sleep-onset association and bedtime resistance difficulties. The specific features of BIC subtypes, as defined in the second edition of the ICSD, are presented in Table 8.1. It is important to note that the criteria for the BIC do not include specific time periods for sleep-onset latency (SOL) and wake time after sleep onset (WASO). However duration criteria differentiate chronic insomnia (3 months or greater with symptoms present three or more times a week) and short-term insomnia (<3 months and may be

Table 8.1 Definition of behavioral insomnias of childhood, ICSD-2 [9]

Behavioral insomnias of childhood	
Sleep Onset Association Disorder	Limit Setting Sleep Disorder

• Prevalence: 10–30 %
 • Age: 6–36 months
 • Clinical features:
   (a) Delayed sleep onset and nighttime awakenings
   (b) Sleep onset becomes associated with exogenous cues
   (c) Sleep onset at bedtime or middle of night will not occur without cue
	• Prevalence: 25–30 %
	 • Age: 18–60 months
	 • Clinical features:
	   (a) Delayed bedtime
	   (b) Caregivers reinforce undesirable behavior at bedtime
	   (c) Inconsistent limit setting
	   (d) Otherwise normal nocturnal sleep

episodic and occur <3 times a week) [9, 10]. While the primary focus of this chapter is on the BIC subtypes that occur primarily in children 6 years of age and younger, there will also be some discussion of chronic and short-term insomnia. In part because the age range of insomnia has been extended down to 6 months of age, there is a dearth of research on prevalence and treatment. The chapter also focuses on recent advances in the evaluation of cognitive behavior therapy for insomnia (CBTI) in school-age children (6–12 years).

The primary features of BIC subtypes include parent reports of bedtime resistance, involvement of the parent in wake-to-sleep transitions at the beginning and the middle of the night, and sleep/wake schedule conflicts with environmental demands. In children younger than 6 years, it is a parent who typically identifies the sleep problem and brings it to the attention of a pediatrician, mental health provider, or sleep specialist. On occasion, an educator or childcare provider will report changes in daytime functioning including academic impairment, hyperactivity, inattention, and tiredness and has an atypical need for sleep during the day. While even very young children can describe sleep problems, their sleep complaints seldom lead to a referral.

Pathophysiology of BIC

For both children and adults, and perhaps all species of animals, the transition from wake to sleep is a vulnerable period as it requires the letting down of vigilance. While most people currently live in relatively safe and secure environments and have the luxuries of strong locks, lights, and secure homes, this was not the case for most of human history. Bedtime routines and repetitive and familiar behavior sequences facilitate the letting down of vigilance and help to assure that the sleep environment is safe and free of threats. From an evolutionary perspective, these routines allay fears and worries. Across all species, routinized behavior prior to the wake-to-sleep transition is common and typically involves checking the immediate environment for threats and seeking out indicators of safety such as a being in close proximity to one's clan or pack. Human infants and young children are dependent on their parents for the implementation of routines and maintenance of a safe environment. When individual or environmental factors interfere with routines or cause chronic psychophysiological arousal or hypervigilance at bedtime, wake-to-sleep transitions can be negatively affected.

The origins of BIC and insomnia are often heterogeneous. In some cases it is important to understand the cause as it can maintain the sleep problem. In other cases, the causes are remote and less relevant to intervention. These initial causes, which may occur alone but often co-occur and can sometimes be compounding, can be divided into several categories. The most common cause is *parental reinforcement* of a child's attention-seeking behavior, or dependence on the parent's involvement in wake-to-sleep transitions. Included in this category are feeding problems and poor sleep hygiene. Children who have medical problems (e.g., gastroesophageal reflux or colic) may have an increased risk of developing sleep problems. A sentinel event such as a separation from parents, the birth of a sibling, or an accident can precipitate a subsequent sleep disturbance that then persists. Children with a diathesis for psychopathology, temperamental hyperarousal, or hyperactivity often have increased anxiety and hypervigilance at bedtime. Conflict between environmental demands (e.g., child care or parent work schedules) and the child's intrinsic circadian phase may result in delayed sleep onset and insufficient sleep during the day. Finally, sleep disorders such as obstructive sleep apnea syndrome and restless leg syndrome can cause insomnia. Further explanation of these categories is warranted as their contributions to the sleep problems may inform the treatment approach.

Parental Reinforcement

Parental reinforcement refers to routines established at wake-to-sleep transitions that involve a child's bid for attention and a response from the parents that increases the likelihood that the child will repeat their behavior. Over the course of development the wake-to-sleep transition is the first significant period of separation for the child–parent dyad and can lead to heightened arousal and ambivalence on the part of the parent and child. Therefore, an assessment of the child and parent attachment and interactions is critical to understanding the nature of sleep disturbances in young children. Parents' contributions to the child's problematic sleep-to-wake transitions and bedtime resistance may occur for a variety of reasons. For example, parents may simply prefer to be present when the child is falling asleep or may learn that their presence results in a faster and easier transition to sleep. When the bedtime routines and the wake-to-sleep transition involve parental presence (e.g., feeding the child, rocking the child, bed sharing, or parental presence in the child's bedroom), the child may become dependent on this very powerful indicator of safety and security. When the child protests being left alone and the parent repeatedly returns to the child's room, the parent's repeated visits reward the child for calling out and reinforce the child's dependence on the parent. The parent is in turn reinforced by the child's rapid calming and relatively rapid return to sleep. Ambivalence may be amplified if the child has a history of medical problems and/or if parents who work long hours or more than one job and have limited time with their child due to conflicts in their work schedule.

It is a widely accepted assumption that by teaching the child to transition to sleep independently at the beginning of the night, the child generalizes this learning to middle of the night awakenings. If the parent attempts to leave the room when the child is awake, or is not present for any or all of the multiple awakenings that occur during a normal night of sleep, the child may have difficulty returning to sleep if the child has not learned to initiate sleep independently.

Parental reinforcement is the most important root cause of behavioral insomnias of childhood and perhaps an initiating cause of insomnia that then follows an independent course and persists from childhood into adolescence. Parents may quickly modify routines and their children will generally adapt quite quickly. When chronic and more severe bedtime and nighttime conflict between the parent and child is present, these interactions can become part of the learned bedtime ritual and may carry over to parent–child interactions during the day. Over time, the child may become labeled by a caregiver or self-identify as a "poor" or "bad sleeper." One of the goals of treatment is to break this cycle of conflict and to replace impressions that the child is inherently a poor sleeper with the knowledge that the child can learn to be a "good sleeper."

Feeding Behavior

An infant and young child's feeding patterns can contribute to irregular sleep/wake patterns. It is common for a mother to nurse or feed her infant during the wake-to-sleep transition. This association between feeding and sleep onset is quite powerful as it involves both physical closeness and sustenance. In older infants the association between feeding and sleep onset can become problematic when the infant becomes dependent on parental presence. If the infant cannot re-initiate sleep independently when natural awakenings occur throughout the night, sleep is then disrupted for the parent and 24-h feeding patterns become irregular for the infant, causing further problems in biological cycling for both. After 6 months of age most typically developing infants do not need to feed at the beginning or middle of the sleep period. Modifying the feeding pattern prior to a sleep intervention is an important first—and in some cases the only necessary—step in establishing an independent wake-to-sleep transition.

Medical Problems

Various medical problems can contribute to a child's sleep problems and can shape parents' patterns of response that can in turn complicate the wake-to-sleep transition. Medical problems associated with pain and physical discomfort, as well as medications and procedures, can result in a child developing negative associations with the crib or bed. Parents' responses to their child's illnesses can be quite complex. Parental worry that arises from ongoing illness or that is conditioned based on a prior illness can result in some parents having ambivalent feelings about separating from their child at bedtime. Parental guilt, a common and normal response to a child's illness, can also result in parents having ambivalent or conflicting feelings about separating from their child at bedtime. For example, a child who has gastroesophageal reflux or colic, and consequently has long bouts of screaming and crying at bedtime that cannot be soothed, can cause both the parents and child to develop a negative association with bedtime. While the well-established behavioral treatments for BIC are effective for children with medical illnesses, it is usually optimal to aggressively treat the underlying illness before implementing a behavioral sleep intervention and to help parents understand their child's and their own negative associations and aversions.

Sentinel Events

A sentinel event in the child's or family's life may cause insomnia symptoms and lead to chronic insomnia. The event may cause increased vigilance and worry or a short-term change in routine could lead to dependence on parental presence, and short- or long-term sleep problems at the wake-to-sleep transition. A short-term positive adaptation in a family that has suffered a trauma might involve the parents taking the child into their own bed during the acute response phase. Once the trauma becomes more remote and the parents attempt to shift the child back to his or her bed, the separation at bedtime may reignite fear in the child, parental guilt, and/or parental ambivalence about co-sleeping or being present when the child transitions to sleep. In these cases, treatment may focus on fears that are related to a past event, parental ambivalence, and a behavioral intervention involving a gradual approach to establishing an independent wake-to-sleep transition. If the trauma is severe, or is associated with sleep or bedtime (e.g., sexual abuse or a home fire), a referral to a pediatric mental health specialist for assessment and treatment of post-traumatic stress disorders would be warranted.

Psychopathology and Temperament

There are now well-established links between child sleep disturbances and anxiety disorders [11] as well as the later emergence of mental health problems [12]. There are also significantly increased rates of sleep problems among children with developmental disorders (e.g., autism) [13–15], attention-deficit hyperactivity disorder (ADHD) [6, 16], and other psychiatric disorders [17]. Therefore, a psychiatric history and assessment of mental status are of particular importance. If a comorbid sleep and psychiatric disorder is suspected, a referral for treatment is in order. However, there is some evidence that an intervention for the child's sleep problems may improve the psychiatric symptoms [18].

The wake-to-sleep transition is one of the first significant separations that a child experiences in his or her development. The ability of the child to self-sooth in order to regulate his or her internal states during these separations may be mediated by the attachment between child and parent. Attachment, as conceptualized by Bowlby [19], is a biologically based bond between the child and parent that ensures safety and survival of the child and over the course of development has components of both physiological and psychological bonds [20]. Attachment patterns develop through a series of separations and reunions with the child and parent and, over time, lead to a stable and predictable relationship that the child internalizes. This internal model of the parent facilitates increasing self-regulatory capacity and independence over time. During infancy the sleep/wake cycle involves multiple separations and reunions. Thus, the wake-to-sleep transitions represent a critically important phenomenon in the emerging patterns of parent–child interactions [21]. A transactional model of sleep/wake development proposed by Anders [22] illustrates how intrinsic (e.g., biomedical factors, infant temperament) and external contexts (e.g., cultural and social norms, family stress, parental psychopathology, SES) interact bidirectionally. When problems arise in the attachment relationship, they may appear first as BIC symptoms of the child but in some instances may also be understood as a function of problems of the child–parent dyad. For example, over-identification with the child and/or guilt over neglect and abandonment may trigger parental separation anxiety, which subsequently becomes generalized by the child as bedtime resistance from and/or difficulty initiating sleep onset. Therefore the child–parent dyad plays an essential role for establishing and maintaining healthy sleep behaviors early in life, and assessment of the child–parent relationship is essential for understating the complex transactions that occur within the context of a family system.

Some children with stable personality characteristics involving avoidance, hyper-arousal, and hyper-reactivity to environmental stimuli may have increased rates of sleep problems [22]. These children may be overly attentive to cues in their environment that threaten their sense of safety and may have difficulty letting down vigilance. Attachment disorders may also increase the risk for sleep problems in children [23]. For example, children who have been adopted from other countries and have been raised in nurseries may be overly attached to parents or may be unable to accept nurturance and calming offered by parents. Criteria for diagnosing these types of problems can be found in the Zero to Three Diagnostic Manual [24]. In addition, there is some evidence that suggests that children adopted from overseas may experience increased rates of sleep problems [25].

There are also some established links between postpartum depression and mother-infant sleep problems. Specifically, maternal depression may be worsened by inadequate sleep which is common during the infant's first 6 months of life, and maternal depression may result in irritability, withdrawal, and/or impairment in mother–child bonding [26, 27]. Treatment of postpartum depression and behavioral–educational interventions designed to promote maternal and infant sleep resulted in increased maternal nighttime sleep time and longer infant nighttime sleep periods with fewer infant nighttime awakenings [28].

Co-sleeping can also be linked to marital and family relational problems. In a marriage in which there is conflict, sexual, or emotional abuse, or avoidance of sexual relations, a child in the parental bed or a parent co-sleeping in a child's bed may facilitate avoidance or serve as a buffer against further conflict. These parental psychiatric problems and marital problems can contribute significantly to the maintenance of a child's sleep problems, and referral to an adult psychiatrist or a family therapist may be a necessary adjunctive approach.

Environmental and Circadian Factors

There are a variety of environmental demands that may have a negative impact on the child's sleep period. Based on preference, and economic or career demands, some parents enforce a sleep schedule on the infant. For example, parents who have to return to work soon after the birth of their child and initiate childcare when the child is 6 weeks of age may be required to wake their child early or put them to bed late. There is currently no consensus on the impact of sleep training or scheduling. Some infants may take easily to an enforced day and nighttime sleep schedule as a result of their being adaptable and having flexibility in mechanisms regulating their circadian phase. Other infants may have difficulty adapting. If the scheduled sleep periods are in direct conflict with the infant's homeostatic and circadian drive, then sleep problems may immerge; either the infant has difficulty falling asleep at the required time or extended periods of wakefulness lead to poor regulatory capacity and the infant has difficulty settling. While there is no scientific evidence that children who are overtired and who have had insufficient sleep have more difficulty settling and do not sleep as well, this is accepted in clinical practice as a relatively robust phenomena [29–31].

The timing of sleep and nap periods can be difficult to navigate as there are vast individual differences in children's sleep needs: the timing of their day and nighttime periods of highest sleep propensity, their intrinsic flexibility to tolerate sleeping at different time periods, and their ability to tolerate varying durations of wakefulness between sleep periods during the day. There is a good deal of variability in published normative trends regarding the timing and sleep needs in infants and children (refer to Table 8.2) and no validated or clinically feasible approaches for

Table 8.2 Estimated normative values for total sleep time from birth to 18 years

Age group	National Institutes of Health [83][a]	Population Study Switzerland [84]
Infants [84–86]	16–18 h	13.9–14.2 h
Toddlers and pre-school (1–5 years)	11–12 h	11.4–13.5 h
School age (6–10 years)	≥10 h	9.9–11 h
Teenagers (12–18 years)	8.5–10 h	8.1–9.6 h

[a]https://www.nhlbi.nih.gov/health/health-topics/topics/sdd/howmuch

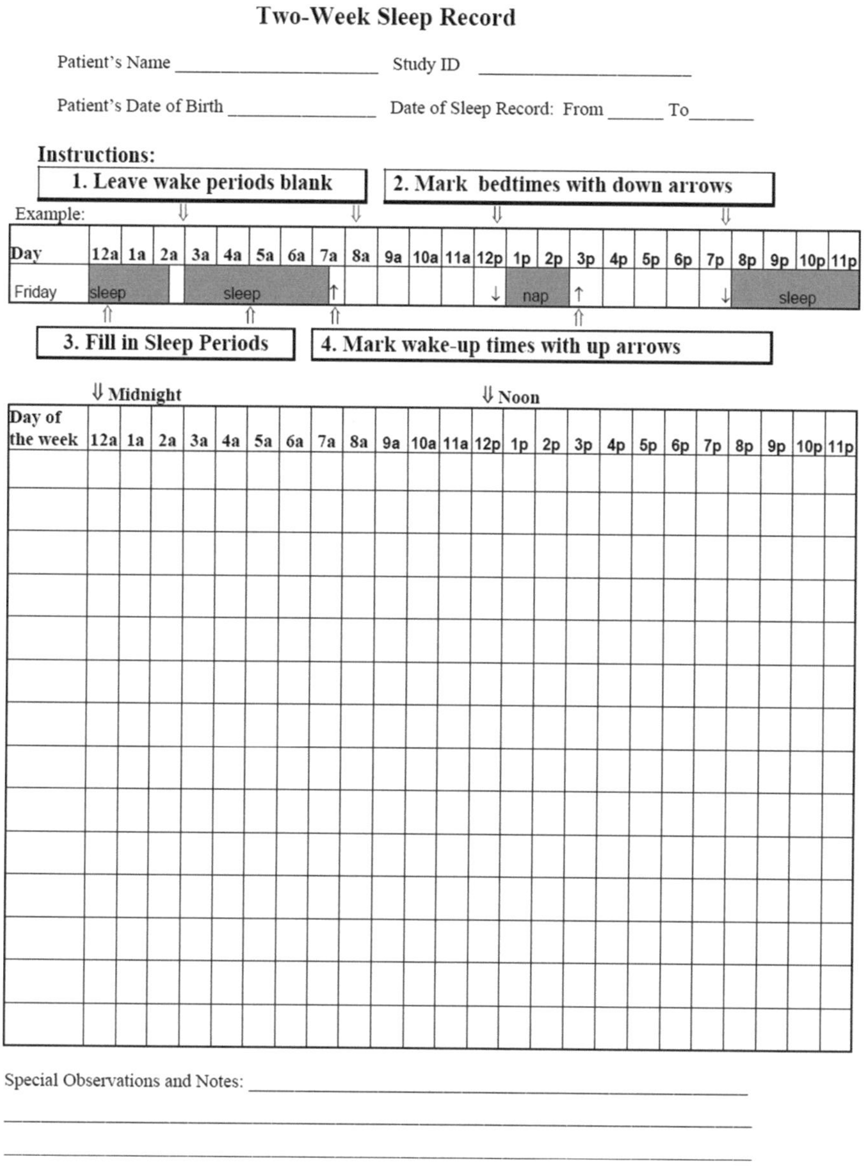

Two-Week Sleep Record

Patient's Name _____   Study ID _____

Patient's Date of Birth _____   Date of Sleep Record: From _____ To _____

Instructions:

| 1. Leave wake periods blank | 2. Mark bedtimes with down arrows |

Example:

Day	12a	1a	2a	3a	4a	5a	6a	7a	8a	9a	10a	11a	12p	1p	2p	3p	4p	5p	6p	7p	8p	9p	10p	11p
Friday	sleep				sleep				↑				↓	nap	↑					↓		sleep		

| 3. Fill in Sleep Periods | 4. Mark wake-up times with up arrows |

⇓ Midnight   ⇓ Noon

Day of the week	12a	1a	2a	3a	4a	5a	6a	7a	8a	9a	10a	11a	12p	1p	2p	3p	4p	5p	6p	7p	8p	9p	10p	11p

Special Observations and Notes: _____

_____

_____

Fig. 8.1 Two-week visual sleep log

their evaluation. Actigraphy and sleep logs (see Fig. 8.1) provide the best approximation of key variables (i.e., number and duration of sleep periods, sleep-onset latency, wake time after sleep onset), but interpretation of these data and the development of a treatment plan require consideration of circadian and homeostatic factors as well as assessment of a child's behavior regulation during the day, and environmental demands.

Sleep Disorders

Several sleep disorders can cause symptoms of insomnia and should be evaluated as part of the assessment. These sleep disorders which cause or are associated with inadequate sleep may account for increased irritability and poor regulatory capacity that can delay sleep onset. For example, obstructive sleep apnea syndrome which has a prevalence of 1 and 4 % in children [32] has been associated with behavioral problems and poor sleep regulation [33, 34]. Restless leg syndrome (RLS) has been estimated to occur in as many as 2–6 % of children [35, 36]. RLS involves limb discomfort that tends to occur in the early evening and can delay sleep onset. In some cases parents are called upon to rub the child's legs to relieve sensations. The child's overactivity at bedtime may relieve RLS sensations, but parents can misinterpret their child's activity as oppositional or hyperactive behavior which can result in parent–child conflict. Parasomnias (e.g., confusional arousals and night terrors), while not a cause of insomnia, can be confused for full awakenings. While it can be difficult to differentiate a full from a partial awakening in a very young child or a child with a developmental disability, educating the parent about partial awakenings is an important consideration in developing a treatment plan.

In summary, behavioral sleep problems in young children can present with varying levels of severity, ranging from transient problems with sleep onset to a diagnosable disorder, and their causes are usually multifactorial. While the vast majority of cases are relatively straightforward and can be evaluated and managed by general practice pediatricians or child mental health or behavioral specialists, persistent problems require a comprehensive evaluation and consideration of sleep/wake mechanisms, child-specific factors, developmental and psychiatric status, family function, and environmental demands.

Insomnia Pathophysiology

The literature on the evaluation and treatment of psychophysiological insomnia in adults and BIC is quite large and there are several excellent review articles that summarize this literature [6, 7, 37, 38]. There are a few recent articles on the pathophysiology of adolescent insomnia [39, 40]. However, there are no published reports that describe insomnia symptoms in children aged 6–12, but this is an important area of focus of future research given that pediatric insomnia is included in the most recent edition of the ICSD and in quality metrics for evaluation and treatment of insomnia recently published by the American Academy of Sleep Medicine [41].

We propose that there are three subgroups of patients between 6 and 18 years of age who meet the criteria for chronic and short-term insomnia in the ICSD (Table 8.3) [42]. The first group is composed of children who will have lifelong difficulty initiating and maintaining sleep that supersedes BIC (Table 8.2) and will eventually be diagnosed with chronic insomnia. The second group is composed of children who have temperamental problems and may meet the criteria for a

Table 8.3 Summary of chronic and short-term insomnia criteria, ICSD-3 [10]

Diagnostic criteria (must meet criteria A–F)
(A) The patient, or the patient's caregiver, observes one or more of the following problems resulting in a general dissatisfaction with sleep:
• Difficulty initiating sleep
• Difficulty maintaining sleep (i.e., waking during the night with difficulty returning to sleep)
• Final awakening occurring earlier than planned or desired
• Resistance to going to bed on a developmentally appropriate schedule
• Difficulty sleeping without caregiver intervention
(B) The patient, or the patient's caregiver, observes one or more of the following related to nighttime sleep difficulty:
• Fatigue or reduced energy
• Cognitive impairment (e.g., reduced attention, concentration, or memory functioning)
• Impaired social, family, occupational, academic performance, or other important areas of functioning
• Mood disturbance/irritability
• Daytime sleepiness
• Behavioral problems (e.g., hyperactivity, impulsivity, aggression)
• Reduced motivation/initiative
• Proneness for errors or accidents
• Concerns or dissatisfaction with sleep
(C) The reported sleep/wake complaints cannot be explained purely by inadequate opportunity (i.e., enough time is allotted for sleep) or inadequate circumstances (i.e., the environment is comfortable, dark, safe, and quiet) for sleep
(D) The sleep disturbance and associated daytime symptoms occur: **Chronic insomnia:** at least three times a week; **short-term insomnia:** may be <3 times per week
(E) The sleep disturbance and associated daytime symptoms have been present for at least: **Chronic insomnia:** 3 months; **short-term insomnia:** <3 months
(F) The sleep/wake difficulty is not explained by another sleep disorder
Other: Insomnia symptoms must be independent of a sentinel event or obvious initiating cause

psychiatric disorder and who also have chronic sleep problems that persist even when psychiatric problems remit. The third group is composed of children who have persistent symptoms of insomnia that may be attributed to an initiating cause (e.g., BIC, a medical illness, sentinel event), but their symptoms persist into childhood or adolescence and they are not responsive to established treatment for BIC.

Assessment

Most sleep problems in young children are relatively straightforward to evaluate and treat, and are often addressed by pediatricians who provide general recommendations. Other problems require a comprehensive evaluation and a nuanced interpretation of data derived from sleep logs, actigraphy, and sleep questionnaires.

Assessment of sleep problems in primary pediatric practices almost exclusively relies on parental report. When children present to a pediatric sleep specialist, they have typically failed other interventions and require more extensive assessment and an individually tailored treatment plan. This thorough assessment typically takes between 60 and 90 min.

The presenting complaint generally involves a conflict at bedtime or bedtime resistance, disrupted child and parental sleep (multiple middle-of-the-night awakenings and/or early morning awakenings), daytime impairment (e.g., irritability, impaired attention), or general concern that the child's sleep quality is poor. The first steps in the assessment are refining the presenting complaint and establishing a consensus treatment goal. The specific domains of assessment are provided in detail in Table 8.4. During the interview, observation of parent–child interactions in the examination room can also be useful in understanding the child's developmental status, regulatory capacity (i.e., their ability to maintain attention or deal with frustration), and their parents' attentiveness to their needs. When taking a history, some assessment of each of the categories discussed above is optimal. The remainder of the evaluation should focus on the five categories of potential causes and facilitators of sleep problems presented in the section above on pathophysiology.

Sleep logs or diaries and sleep questionnaires are well-established assessment tools that have been used in the vast majority of assessment and treatment studies. Sleep logs used over a 2-week period provide more objective data for sleep patterns and can be used to establish a baseline to evaluate clinical interventions [43]. Diaries are typically kept for 1–2 weeks and provide more detailed information that can be tailored to specific insomnia symptoms [44]. They have been shown to have relatively good reliability with actigraphy [45] and are a necessary complement to actigraphs. Optimally, a family should come to their initial assessment session with a completed 2-week sleep log that documents the timing of sleep periods: time in bed, sleep-onset latency (SOL), wake time after sleep onset (WASO), time out of bed,

Table 8.4 Quick review of assessment domains

Assessment domain	Area of focus	Example
Daytime routine	Time out of bed	Variability; parental role; child's mood, and alertness
	Difficulty waking	Frequency; duration; parental role
	Academic difficulties	Poor performance disruptive behavior; inattention; irritability
Sleep routine	Transition to sleep	Child's behavior: bedtime resistance; curtain calls or call outs; parental involvement
	Time to bed	Variability: weekday/weekend; sleep onset latency
	Sleep hygiene	Activity leading up to scheduled bedtime; use of electronic media; caffeine
	Sleep environment	Light; temperature; noise; where and with whom; transitional object
	Nighttime sleep behavior	Full versus partial awakenings; other arousals; restlessness; snoring

and schedule and unplanned naps. It is often helpful to compare sleep periods from school schedules to those obtained on weekends, holidays, or vacations. There are several questionnaires and there are two comprehensive reviews of available questionnaires [46]. Two of the most widely used sleep questionnaires, the Sleep Habits Questionnaire [47] and the Pediatric Sleep Questionnaire [48], can be used to identify potential sleep problems in children and adolescents.

Children's Sleep Habits Questionnaire (CSHQ; [47]). The CSHQ is a comprehensive, parent-report measure for assessing children's sleep with good psychometric properties for both community and sleep-disordered samples for children 4–12 years of age. It yields both a total score and eight subscale scores reflecting key sleep domains that encompass a range of medical and behavioral sleep problems including sleep-disordered breathing, sleep-related anxiety, bedtime refusal, insomnia, parasomnias, and daytime sleepiness. However, it should be noted that the CSHQ does not have established normative values for the total or subscale scores. Items are rated on a three-point scale. The CSHQ has shown adequate internal consistency in both clinical and community samples of children [47]. Two-week test-retest estimates also have been shown to be acceptable (.62 to .79). The CSQH has been primarily used for research to assess sleep at baseline and post-intervention.

The Pediatric Sleep Questionnaire (PSQ; [48]). The PSQ is a validated 74-item questionnaire assessing children's sleeping habits and behaviors in children 2–18 years of age. The PSQ includes a 22-item sleep-related breathing disorder subscale (PSQ-SRBD) that has been shown to predict the risk for PSG-confirmed SDB [49]. In addition, the PSQ includes a four-item Sleepiness Scales (PSQ-SS) that contains items assessing the degree to which sleepiness is a problem rather than perceived sleep propensity in different situations. The PSQ-SS had low-to -moderate validity against an objective measure of sleepiness, the Multiple Sleep Latency Test, which is comparable to what has been observed in the adult literature assessing associations between the Epworth Sleepiness Scale and Multiple Sleep Latency Test [50].

Wrist actigraphy is a cost-effective tool that has a broad array of applications in research and in clinical settings. It estimates sleep by utilizing the difference between reduced activity during a sleep period relative to waking behavior. The actigraph itself is a small battery-operated device (size of a watch) that is worn on the wrist 24 h a day (for up to 2 or more weeks) and records movement sampled several times per second with an accelerometer and stores the sampled data in epochs (typically 1 min). After downloading raw movement data, a computer program applies an algorithm to score sleep/wake periods. Actigraphy has been validated against PSG with agreement rates for minute-by-minute sleep/wake identification of higher than 90 % [51–53]. Actigraphy has been used extensively in clinical and research assessment with children, and there are no risks associated with its use. In addition, actigraphy provides the clinician with the opportunity to collect data from an individual sleeping in her natural sleep environment. Dependent variables derived from actigraphy include total sleep time (TST), sleep efficiency (SE; a ratio of minutes asleep to time in bed), and wake time after sleep onset (WASO). While SOL is also important, actigraphy does not afford reliable measures of this variable.

To aid the assessment of behavioral problems and psychiatric symptoms several of the following validated questionnaires utilizing parent or teacher report may help a clinician characterize behavioral problems and psychiatric symptoms that may be associated with BIC symptoms: (a) general behavioral problems—Child Behavior Checklist (CBCL); (b) depression—Child Depression Inventory (CDI); (c) anxiety—Screen for Child Anxiety-Related Emotional Disorders (SCARED); and (d) ADHD—(Connors). If a co-occurring sleep and psychiatric disorder is suspected, a referral for treatment is in order.

CBCL ([54, 55]). The CBCL is a 113-item parent-report scale assessing a broad range of behavioral problems and social and academic functioning. The CBCL is one of the most extensively tested rating scales available and possesses excellent psychometrics. The measure yields total, internalizing, and externalizing behavior scales, and eight subscale scores. In addition there are a youth self-report version and teacher report form that have been validated and may be considered to supplement the parental report. The measures take about 10 min to complete and 2 min to score.

SCARED ([56, 57]). The SCARED is a 42-item measure of childhood anxiety that includes a child and parent form. Birmaher et al. [57] found that the SCARED was able to differentiate between clinically anxious and non-anxious psychiatrically ill youth. Test-retest reliability coefficients and internal consistency coefficients of the subscales were found to be acceptable.

CDI ([58]). The CDI is the most widely used self-report measure of depressive symptoms in children and is used extensively in pediatric sleep and affective research. The CDI consists of 27 items and yields five factors plus a total score normed according to age and gender. Published reports on the reliability and validity of the CDI are extensive with internal consistency coefficients ranging from .71 to .89 and the test-retest coefficients range from .74 to .83 (time interval 2–3 weeks).

The Connors Rating Scale-Revised (CRS-R; [59]). The CRS-R is an 80-item observer (parent or teacher) or self-report questionnaire used to assess attention-deficit/hyperactivity disorder (ADHD) and evaluate problem behavior in children and adolescents. Short versions of the CRS scales are also available. The CRS-R is comprised of seven factors: cognitive problems, oppositional, hyperactivity-impulsivity, anxious-shy, perfectionism, social problems, and psychosomatic. The CRS-R factors have high internal reliability (alphas = .75–.94) but poor-to-adequate 6-week test-retest reliability (rs = .13—parents and .78).

Treatment

There are several interventions that have established efficacy as treatments of the BIC [7, 37, 60, 61], but only a few studies evaluating the efficacy of cognitive behavior therapy for insomnia in school-age children and adolescents (CBT-I) [62, 63]. The interventions for BIC involve simple and graduated extinction techniques, sleep scheduling, positive routines, sleep hygiene training, and parent education.

The number of sessions and the order in which these interventions are implemented have not been adequately studied, and the demands of the specific case generally dictate priorities. Based on discussions with pediatric sleep specialists, the most common course of treatment involves a thorough in-person assessment and initial treatment recommendations, and then in-person, telephone, or e-mail follow-up.

Treatment for BIC

Initial recommendations should focus on the treatment of medical problems and feeding schedules. Symptoms of untreated gastroesophageal reflux, and recurrent ear infections and other ailments involving pain and discomfort, can undermine usually efficacious interventions. Special attention may need to be given to parents of children who have had medical problems as they may be, with good reason, hypersensitive to their child's condition. Children with illnesses involving pain may have developed an aversion to their crib or bed. When this is suspected, and when possible, a change in the bedroom or the type of bed may break this association. Other behavioral techniques such as systematic desensitization or graduated exposure may be most effective.

Ferber [31] recommends addressing feeding schedules prior to implementing a sleep intervention. Common feeding schedules and issues that interfere with an infant's independent wake-to-sleep transitions can include nursing or bottle feeding the infant. The association between feeding and direct contact with the parents is exceedingly powerful. Middle-of-the-night feedings are equally problematic. While a middle-of-the-night feeding usually results in the infant returning to sleep very rapidly and is rewarding for the overtired parent, it reinforces the child's dependence on the parent and may disrupt daytime feeding schedules. Specifically, after 6 months of age normally developing infants do not need to feed at night. The one caveat is that an infant whose sole nutrition is mother's milk may have difficulty going a whole night without a feeding. In this case the introduction of cereal for infants prior to bedtime can help to sustain the infant throughout the night.

A thorough evaluation establishes the priorities for interventions and specifically the identification of behaviors that are targets for change. An understanding of the behavioral cues that precede it (antecedents) and the responses or consequences that follow the behavior must be understood as critical components of the behavioral plan to eliminate the problematic behavior. Other considerations, which have been discussed in detail above, involve child-, parent-, and environment-specific factors, and the history and course of the sleep problem.

Extinction

Extinction techniques involve removal of reinforcers that maintain or cue an undesirable behavior. *Simple or unmodified extinction* involves the immediate removal of reinforcers [64, 65]. For example, parents ignore the child's bids for attention at bedtime and the middle of the night and over the course of 3–5 days the child learns that crying, call outs, and sometimes more extreme behavior (e.g., throwing toys or other objects and vomiting) do not elicit the desired response from the parent. The child no longer depends on the parents to be present at bedtime because he develops new associations or self-soothing skills, and the attempt to gain the parents' attention ceases. This approach breaks the chain of interactions between parent and child, and the sleep-onset association (i.e., parental presence) is transferred to an object or a self-soothing behavior that decreases or eliminates the child's dependence on the parent. Simple extinction has also been called the "cry-it-out" or cold turkey method. This is generally very effective, although not all parents feel comfortable implementing this plan. The child's crying and call outs can be quite persistent, and it is not uncommon for a child to vomit in their crib as a result of long episodes of crying and upset. If a child vomits during the course of an intervention plan, parents are instructed to clean up immediately, and to provide their child with support but to minimize strong emotional responses (e.g., anger, frustration, physical comforting) that could be reinforcing. Parents who fail to implement simple extinction techniques often inadvertently reinforce longer crying spells and poorer self-regulation.

Graduated extinction (GE) techniques are far easier for parents to tolerate because they involve less crying and more flexibility for parents to regulate the pace of the intervention. The trade-off is that GE can take longer to implement. There are some manualized approaches [65], but most interventions are tailored to the specific needs and preferences of the parent and child. The general principle of a GE intervention is that reinforcement is gradually withdrawn on a set schedule. The variables that are modified over time can include physical contact with the child (e.g., breast feeding, holding, patting), verbal responses, proximity to the child, and frequency and duration of check-ins. Any combination of these variables can be gradually modified. For example, if the parent typically lies in bed with the child until the child falls asleep, the recommendation could involve three nights of sitting next to the child's bed and holding his or her hand until he falls asleep; followed by three nights of sitting further away from the child and using verbalizations to calm the child; followed by three nights sitting in the room and refusing interactions; followed by three nights of check-ins every 5 min as long as the child stays in bed; followed by three nights of check-ins every 10 min.

There are several types of modifications that can be included in a GE intervention. *Fading* refers to a gradual decrease in the intensity or quality of parental reinforcement of the child's behavior. *Shaping* refers to the parents' reinforcement of qualitative changes in the child's behavior. For example, if the child cries for extended periods of time, the parent might only enter the room when there is a pause in the child's crying, thereby reinforcing calming behavior. *Chaining* refers to the parent gradually modifying the child's behavioral response. For example, the parents may tell the child that they will check in with the child as long as the child does not cry, and then the parents may tell the child that they will check in as long as the child does not call out. *Thinning* refers to a gradual decrease in the frequency of parental reinforcement of child-calming behavior.

Positive Routines

Positive routines involve modification of parent–child interactions and behaviors at bedtime to decrease stress and conflict and to establish a relaxed environment that is conducive to a smooth transition to sleep. Positive routines also establish new wake-to-sleep associations. This may be coupled with a shift in the time to bed so that the child has an increased sleep propensity but is not overtired and hyperaroused. In adjusting time to bed, it is also important to consider that there is a naturally occurring increase in arousal level also called the "danger zone." When a regular sequence of activities is established, the child knows what to expect and the sequence should involve increasing calm and relaxing behaviors like reading, close time with parents, and quiet singing. Parental warmth and calm, and positive and supportive statements, reinforce the child's participation in the quiet activities, set the tone, model appropriate behavior, and reinforce and facilitate learning. Once the child learns the routine and transitions to sleep more quickly, the parents can gradually advance the bedtime with the goal of increasing the child's total sleep time. After about 6 months of age, the introduction of a transitional object (a blanket, a plush toy) can become an important part of the bedtime routine and can take the place of the parent or other sleep-onset associations that are problematic. The choice of an object is important because it will sometimes be with the family for years. It should be washable and made of a non-toxic material and parents may want to purchase a duplicate in the event that the object is lost.

Schedule Modification

Schedule modification is sometimes necessary when the child's bedtime is exceedingly early or late or when the timing of naps interferes with bedtime. Schedule problems can arise when a child's optimal sleep time (controlled by their circadian phase) conflicts with parental or other environmental demands. Some young infants have very rigid early morning awakenings that chronically disrupt parents' sleep. While small shifts in the sleep phase can sometimes be achieved, parents may need help in adjusting their schedule or agreeing on an alternating care plan for their child. Helping parents identify the optimal nap times based on the child's age and daytime sleep needs can be complicated. A late-afternoon nap for some children over the age of 3 can erode their ability to fall asleep at night while others need a nap. Eliminating a morning nap between 18 and 24 months of age can extend the duration and improve the quality of the afternoon nap.

Sleep Hygiene Training

Sleep hygiene training involves changes in behaviors, sleep-related activities, or the environment that precede sleep and that interfere with sleep or the process of decreasing arousal. Sleep hygiene education is a common component of behavioral interventions used to address adult sleep problems such as insomnia and is routinely included in behavioral interventions targeted in pediatric populations [66–68]. Sleep hygiene education begins with an assessment of daytime and bedtime routines that delay sleep onset (e.g., exercise, use of electronic media, pets in the bedroom) and degrade sleep quality (e.g., caffeine use, environmental factors like light, noise, and temperature). The clinician works with parents and their child to establish guidelines that are feasible and within reference to developmental norms. During the hour leading up to the child's scheduled bedtime parent and children are instructed to engage in calm and relaxing activities that the child enjoys (e.g., reading). This may require some negotiation between child and parent and activities that have the potential to cause conflict and should be avoided. The timing of bedtime routine activities should be consistent and predictable and the scheduled bedtimes should not deviate significantly (e.g., 30–60 min) from day to day. The bed should only be used for sleeping; therefore, activities other than sleep (e.g., play) should be avoided to strengthen the association between the bed and sleep. Some flexibility can be exercised with calm and focused activities such as reading. It is best practice to keep all electronic devices out of bed and the bedroom. A later bedtime may be warranted especially if a child appears alert and functions well with slightly less sleep. To the extent possible light (e.g., use of a nightlight) and noise should be reduced to promote an optimal sleep environment.

Other Treatment Considerations

Another intervention that can be useful with older children involves the use of a bedtime pass [69, 70]. The child is provided with a token or piece of paper that allows them one opportunity to engage the parent after bedtime. This technique provides the child with more control and helps them to weigh their actual need to see the parent. If passes are not used on successive nights then the child can turn them in for a reward. As part of the intervention, parents should also be informed that following the initial implementation of the intervention, an extinction burst commonly occurs [71]. This phenomenon that occurs in many behavioral interventions involves a temporary return to the undesired behavior. If parents are unaware of the phenomena they may assume that the intervention has failed. They are generally instructed to persist in the treatment plan.

In the interest of managing expectations when discussing interventions for BIC it is important that some caregivers may feel concerned about inducing distress in their child during a critical time in a family transition for infants and their caregivers. These are natural concerns that should be met with empathy and validation. Such concerns provide a clinician with the opportunity that to date there exists no empirical evidence from longitudinal studies indicating long-standing negative behavioral, emotional, psychosocial, or hormonal effects associated with the behavioral strategies to address BIC [72].

CBT-I for School-Age Children

The approach to the assessment of insomnia in school-age children does not differ significantly from that of younger children; however, involving a verbal child in the assessment and treatment plan is likely useful in assuring their understanding and willingness to participate. Cognitive behavioral treatments for insomnia are described elsewhere in this book but a brief overview of the core components of CBT-I with some modifications is provided. CBT-I is a comprehensive, non-pharmacologic, and evidence-based intervention for insomnia that has been developed for adults with well-established short-term and long-term efficacy [73, 74]. CBT-I has been modified to be developmentally appropriate for adolescents [75, 76] and school-age children [63] and includes components intended to promote greater control over sleep, reduce emotional distress, and enhance sleep efficiency.

Following assessment, CBT-I begins with psychoeducation, to provide parents and children with information about the role of sleep, its regulation, and consequences of insufficient sleep framed within a developmentally appropriate context (e.g., school-aged children required 10–11 h of sleep). For some parents it may be helpful to draw on the two-process model of sleep regulation (i.e., homeostatic sleep pressure and circadian rhythm) to provide a framework for sleep regulation [77]. In addition Spielman's 3P model of insomnia may also be a useful heuristic for framing interventions intended to identify and resolve factors perpetuating insomnia [78]. As described above sleep hygiene practices can be included with psychoeducation and used to supplement CBT-I interventions as needed.

The core behavioral components of CBT-I consist of stimulus control therapy and sleep restriction which are well-evaluated interventions used in adults that meet established treatment standards as defined by the American Psychological Association [79] and American Academy of Sleep Medicine [80]. Stimulus control therapy [81] utilizes standardized instructions intended to associate the bed/sleep environment with sleep rather than sleep-incompatible behaviors (e.g., boredom, frustration, or worry at not being able to sleep) and to re-establish a consistent sleep/wake schedule. Sleep restriction therapy aims to increase sleep drive and consolidate sleep by limiting a patient's time in bed to the total sleep time derived from 1 to 2 weeks of sleep diary [82]. Time in bed is subsequently titrated up or down based on response to intervention and minimum time in bed is generally never less than 7.5 h for school-age children and is applied flexibly based on acceptance and adherence to treatment. Prohibits naps at times other than the assigned time in bed.

Although stimulus control and sleep restriction therapy may be adequate behavioral interventions to address insomnia some older school-age children may also benefit from the inclusion of cognitive strategies aimed at reducing cognitive arousal associated with anxious thoughts or identifying and challenging dysfunctional attitudes and beliefs and misconceptions about sleep that contribute to emotional distress and further sleep problems.

The CBT-I interventions described above may be augmented with relaxation training to introduce strategies aimed at reducing somatic tension or intrusive thoughts at bedtime interfering with sleep. Common techniques include diaphragmatic breathing and progressive muscle relaxation.

Conclusion

Behavioral sleep problems during childhood represent a complex group of problems ranging from short-term delays in sleep onset and parental reinforcement of problematic behavior to chronic problems with sleep initiation and maintenance. Thorough assessment is required to define the causes and clinical course of the problems, especially when they are chronic and disrupt the family and/or the child's daytime behavior. There is currently no research on the developmental pathophysiology of behavioral sleep problems in childhood, particularly those that are chronic and persist into later childhood and early adolescence. There is a relatively large literature and several good reviews of behavioral treatment strategies for BIC occurring in infants and children under the age of 7. In most cases, parents can implement these interventions independently or with the assistance of a pediatrician or pediatric nurse. However, persistent problems require the expertise of a sleep specialist.

References

1. Sadeh A, Tikotzky L, Scher A. Parenting and infant sleep. Sleep Med Rev. 2010;14(2):89–96. Epub 2009/07/28.
2. Wong MM, Nigg JT, Zucker RA, Puttler LI, Fitzgerald HE, Jester JM, et al. Behavioral control and resiliency in the onset of alcohol and illicit drug use: a prospective study from preschool to adolescence. Child Dev. 2006;77(4):1016–33.
3. Gregory AM, Caspi A, Eley TC, Moffitt TE, Oconnor TG, Poulton R. Prospective longitudinal associations between persistent sleep problems in childhood and anxiety and depression disorders in adulthood. J Abnorm Child Psychol. 2005;33(2):157–63.
4. Chorney DB, Detweiler MF, Morris TL, Kuhn BR. The interplay of sleep disturbance, anxiety, and depression in children. J Pediatr Psychol. 2008;33(4):339–48. Epub 2007/11/10.
5. Touchette E, Petit D, Tremblay RE, Boivin M, Falissard B, Genolini C, et al. Associations between sleep duration patterns and overweight/obesity at age 6. Sleep. 2008;31(11):1507–14. Epub 2008/11/19.

6. Mindell JA, Kuhn B, Lewin DS, Meltzer LJ, Sadeh A, American Academy of Sleep Medicine. Behavioral treatment of bedtime problems and night wakings in infants and young children. Sleep. 2006;29(10):1263–76 [erratum appears in Sleep. 2006 Nov 1;29(11):1380].
7. Kuhn BR, Elliott AJ. Treatment efficacy in behavioral pediatric sleep medicine. J Psychosom Res. 2003;54:587–97.
8. American Psychiatric Association. Cautionary statement for forensic use of DSM-5. Diagnostic and statistical manual of mental disorders. 5th ed. Arlington, VA: American Psychiatric Publishing; 2013.
9. AASM. The international classification of sleep disorders: diagnostic & coding manual, ICSD-2. 2nd ed. Westchester, IL: American Academy of Sleep Medicine; 2005.
10. American Academy of Sleep Medicine Work Group. International classification of sleep disorders. 3rd ed. Westchester, IL: American Academy of Sleep Medicine; 2014.
11. Alfano CA, Ginsburg GS, Kingery JN. Sleep-related problems among children and adolescents with anxiety disorders. J Am Acad Child Adolesc Psychiatry. 2007;46(2):224–32.
12. Gregory AM, Rijsdijk FV, Dahl RE, McGuffin P, Eley TC. Associations between sleep problems, anxiety, and depression in twins at 8 years of age. Pediatrics. 2006;118(3):1124–32.
13. Dorris L, Scott N, Zuberi S, Gibson N, Espie C. Sleep problems in children with neurological disorders. Dev Neurorehabil. 2008;11(2):95–114.
14. Liu X, Hubbard JA, Fabes RA, Adam JB. Sleep disturbances and correlates of children with autism spectrum disorders. Child Psychiatry Hum Dev. 2006;37(2):179–91.
15. Malow BA, Marzec ML, McGrew SG, Wang L, Henderson LM, Stone WL. Characterizing sleep in children with autism spectrum disorders: a multidimensional approach. Sleep. 2006;29(12):1563–71.
16. Mindell JA, Emslie G, Blumer J, Genel M, Glaze D, Ivanenko A, et al. Pharmacologic management of insomnia in children and adolescents: consensus statement. Pediatrics. 2006;117(6):e1223–32.
17. Ivanenko A, Johnson K. Sleep disturbances in children with psychiatric disorders. Semin Pediatr Neurol. 2008;15(2):70–8.
18. Insomnia therapy may help improve depression treatment. Using cognitive behavioral therapy in insomnia therapy (CBT-I) also may help make depression treatment more effective. Duke Med Health News. 2014;20(2):5. Epub 2014/03/22.
19. Bowlby J. A secure base: parent–child attachment and healthy human development. New York: Basic Books; 1988. p. xii. 205 pp.
20. Gabbard GO. Psychodynamic psychiatry in clinical practice. 4th ed. Washington, DC: American Psychiatric Pub; 2005. p. xiv. 629 pp.
21. Anders TF. Infant sleep, nighttime relationships, and attachment. Psychiatry. 1994;57(1):11–21.
22. Anders TF, Halpern LF, Hua J. Sleeping through the night: a developmental perspective. Pediatrics. 1992;90(4):554–60.
23. Poehlmann J. Representations of attachment relationships in children of incarcerated mothers. Child Dev. 2005;76(3):679–96.
24. Zero to Three. Diagnostic classification: 0–3: diagnostic classification of mental health and developmental disorders of infancy and early childhood. Washington, DC: Zero to Three: National Center for Infants, Toddlers and Families; 1999. 134 p.
25. Rettig MA, McCarthy-Rettig K. A survey of the health, sleep, and development of children adopted from China. Health Soc Work. 2006;31(3):201–7.
26. Dawson G, Hessl D, Frey K. Social influences of early developing biological and behavioral systems related to risk for affective disorder. Dev Psychopathol. 1994;6(4):759–79.
27. Hiscock H, Wake M. Randomised controlled trial of behavioural infant sleep intervention to improve infant sleep and maternal mood. BMJ. 2002;324(7345):1062–5.
28. Stremler R, Hodnett E, Lee K, MacMillan S, Mill C, Ongcangco L, et al. A behavioral-educational intervention to promote maternal and infant sleep: a pilot randomized, controlled trial. Sleep. 2006;29(12):1609–15.
29. Mindell JA, Owens JA. A clinical guide to pediatric sleep: diagnosis and management of sleep problems. New York: Lippincott Williams and Wilkins; 2003.

30. Mindel J. Sleeping through the night. New York: Harper Collins; 1997.
31. Ferber R. Solve your child's sleep problems. New York: Simon & Schuster; 1985.
32. Lumeng JC, Chervin RD. Epidemiology of pediatric obstructive sleep apnea. Proc Am Thorac Soc. 2008;5(2):242–52. Epub 2008/02/06.
33. Owens J, Spirito A, Marcotte A, McGuinn M, Berkelhammer L. Neuropsychological and behavioral correlates of obstructive sleep apnea syndrome in children: a preliminary study. Sleep Breath. 2000;4(2):67–78.
34. Lewin DS, Huntley ED, Eisner M, editors. Neurobehavioral assessment of the effects of sleep restriction on children with obstructive sleep apnea OSA and a healthy comparison group. 18th Annual Meeting of the Associated Professional Sleep Societies (APSS). Philadelphia, PA: American Academy of Sleep Medicine; 2004.
35. Picchietti D, Allen RP, Walters AS, Davidson JE, Myers A, Ferini-Strambi L. Restless legs syndrome: prevalence and impact in children and adolescents—the Peds REST study. Pediatrics. 2007;120(2):253–66. Epub 2007/08/03.
36. Picchietti DL, Bruni O, de Weerd A, Durmer JS, Kotagal S, Owens JA, et al. Pediatric restless legs syndrome diagnostic criteria: an update by the International Restless Legs Syndrome Study Group. Sleep Med. 2013;14(12):1253–9. Epub 2013/11/05.
37. Mindell JA. Empirically supported treatments in pediatric psychology: bedtime refusal and night wakings in young children. J Pediatr Psychol. 1999;24(6):465–81.
38. Harvey AG. A cognitive model of insomnia. Behav Res Ther. 2002;40(8):869–93. Epub 2002/08/21.
39. Dohnt H, Gradisar M, Short MA. Insomnia and its symptoms in adolescents: comparing DSM-IV and ICSD-II diagnostic criteria. J Clin Sleep Med. 2012;8(3):295–9. Epub 2012/06/16.
40. Richardson CE, Gradisar M, Barbero SC. Are cognitive "insomnia" processes involved in the development and maintenance of delayed sleep wake phase disorder? Sleep Med Rev. 2015;26:1–8. Epub 2015/07/05.
41. Edinger JD, Buysse DJ, Deriy L, Germain A, Lewin DS, Ong JC, et al. Quality measures for the care of patients with insomnia. J Clin Sleep Med. 2015;11(3):311–34. Epub 2015/02/24.
42. Medicine AAoS. International classification of sleep disorders. Sateia M, editor. 3rd ed. Darien, IL: American Academy of Sleep Medicine; 2014.
43. Owens JA, Babcook D, Blumer J, Chervin RD, Ferber R, Goetting M, et al. The use of pharmacotherapy in the treatment of pediatric insomnia in primary care: rational approaches. A consensus meeting summary. J Clin Sleep Med. 2005;1(1):49–59.
44. Carney CE, Buysse DJ, Ancoli-Israel S, Edinger JD, Krystal AD, Lichstein KL, et al. The consensus sleep diary: standardizing prospective sleep self-monitoring. Sleep. 2012;35(2):287–302. Epub 2012/02/02.
45. Werner H, Molinari L, Guyer C, Jenni OG. Agreement rates between actigraphy, diary, and questionnaire for children's sleep patterns. Arch Pediatr Adolesc Med. 2008;162(4):350–8.
46. Spruyt K, Gozal D. Development of pediatric sleep questionnaires as diagnostic or epidemiological tools: a brief review of dos and don'ts. Sleep Med Rev. 2011;15(1):7–17. Epub 2010/10/19.
47. Owens JA, Spirito A, McGuinn M. The Children's Sleep Habits Questionnaire (CSHQ): psychometric properties of a survey instrument for school-aged children. Sleep. 2000;23(8):1043–51.
48. Chervin RD, Hedger K, Dillon JE, Pituch KJ. Pediatric sleep questionnaire (PSQ): validity and reliability of scales for sleep-disordered breathing, snoring, sleepiness, and behavioral problems. Sleep Med. 2000;1(1):21–32.
49. Chervin RD, Weatherly RA, Garetz SL, Ruzicka DL, Giordani BJ, Hodges EK, et al. Pediatric sleep questionnaire: prediction of sleep apnea and outcomes. Arch Otolaryngol Head Neck Surg. 2007;133(3):216–22.
50. Chervin RD, Ruzicka DL, Giordani BJ, Weatherly RA, Dillon JE, Hodges EK, et al. Sleep-disordered breathing, behavior, and cognition in children before and after adenotonsillectomy. Pediatrics. 2006;117(4):e769–78.

51. Ancoli-Isreal S. Actigraphy. In: Kryger MH, Roth T, Dement WC, editors. Principles and practice of sleep medicine. Philadelphia, PA: Elsevier/Saunders; 2005. p. xxxiii. 1517 p.
52. Sadeh A, Acebo C. The role of actigraphy in sleep medicine. Sleep Med Rev. 2002;6(2):113–24.
53. Sadeh A, Alster J, Urbach P. Actigraphically based sleep-wake scoring. J Ambulat Monit. 1989;2:209–16.
54. Achenbach TM. Manual for the child behavior checklist/4–18. Burlington, VT: Department of Psychiatry, University of Vermont; 1991.
55. Achenbach TM. Manual for the child behavior checklist/2–3 and 1992 profile. Burlington, VT: Department of Psychiatry, University of Vermont; 1992. p. xi. 210 pp.
56. Birmaher B, Brent DA, Chiappetta L, Bridge J, Monga S, Baugher M. Psychometric properties of the Screen for Child Anxiety Related Emotional Disorders (SCARED): a replication study. J Am Acad Child Adolesc Psychiatry. 1999;38(10):1230–6.
57. Birmaher B, Khetarpal S, Brent D, Cully M, Balach L, Kaufman J, et al. The Screen for Child Anxiety Related Emotional Disorders (SCARED): scale construction and psychometric characteristics. J Am Acad Child Adolesc Psychiatry. 1997;36(4):545–53.
58. Kovacs M. The children's depression, inventory (CDI). Psychopharmacol Bull. 1985;21(4):995–8.
59. Conners CK, Sitarenios G, Parker JD, Epstein JN. The revised Conners' Parent Rating Scale (CPRS-R): factor structure, reliability, and criterion validity. J Abnorm Child Psychol. 1998;26(4):257–68.
60. Minde K, Faucon A, Falkner S. Sleep problems in toddlers: effects of treatment on their daytime behavior. J Am Acad Child Adolesc Psychiatry. 1994;33(8):1114–21.
61. Mindell J, Kuhn B, Lewin D, Meltzer L, Sadeh A. Behavioral treatment of bedtime problems and night wakings in infants and young children. Sleep. 2006;29(10):1263–76.
62. Clarke G, McGlinchey EL, Hein K, Gullion CM, Dickerson JF, Leo MC, et al. Cognitive-behavioral treatment of insomnia and depression in adolescents: a pilot randomized trial. Behav Res Ther. 2015;69:111–8. Epub 2015/04/29.
63. Paine S, Gradisar M. A randomised controlled trial of cognitive-behaviour therapy for behavioural insomnia of childhood in school-aged children. Behav Res Ther. 2011;49(6–7):379–88. Epub 2011/05/10.
64. France KG. Behavior characteristics and security in sleep-disturbed infants treated with extinction. J Pediatr Psychol. 1992;17(4):467–75.
65. Adams LA, Rickert VI. Reducing bedtime tantrums: comparison between positive routines and graduated extinction. Pediatrics. 1989;84(5):756–61.
66. Bootzin RR, Stevens SJ. Adolescents, substance abuse, and the treatment of insomnia and daytime sleepiness. Clin Psychol Rev. 2005;25(5):629–44.
67. Degotardi PJ, Klass ES, Rosenberg BS, Fox DG, Gallelli KA, Gottlieb BS. Development and evaluation of a cognitive-behavioral intervention for juvenile fibromyalgia. J Pediatr Psychol. 2006;31(7):714–23.
68. Weiss MD, Wasdell MB, Bomben MM, Rea KJ, Freeman RD. Sleep hygiene and melatonin treatment for children and adolescents with ADHD and initial insomnia. J Am Acad Child Adolesc Psychiatry. 2006;45(5):512–9.
69. Moore BA, Friman PC, Fruzzetti AE, MacAleese K. Brief report: evaluating the Bedtime Pass Program for child resistance to bedtime—a randomized, controlled trial. J Pediatr Psychol. 2007;32(3):283–7.
70. Freeman KA. Treating bed time resistance with the bed time pass: a systematic replication and component analysis with 3-year-olds. J Appl Behav Anal. 2006;39(4):423–8.
71. France KG, Blampied NM, Wilkinson P. Treatment of infant sleep disturbance by trimeprazine in combination with extinction. J Dev Behav Pediatr. 1991;12(5):308–14.
72. Price AM, Wake M, Ukoumunne OC, Hiscock H. Five-year follow-up of harms and benefits of behavioral infant sleep intervention: randomized trial. Pediatrics. 2012;130(4):643–51. Epub 2012/09/12.

73. Irwin MR, Cole JC, Nicassio PM. Comparative meta-analysis of behavioral interventions for insomnia and their efficacy in middle-aged adults and in older adults 55+ years of age. Health Psychol. 2006;25(1):3–14. Epub 2006/02/02.

74. Morin CM, Bootzin RR, Buysse DJ, Edinger JD, Espie CA, Lichstein KL. Psychological and behavioral treatment of insomnia: update of the recent evidence (1998–2004). Sleep. 2006;29(11):1398–414. Epub 2006/12/14.

75. de Bruin EJ, Bogels SM, Oort FJ, Meijer AM. Efficacy of cognitive behavioral therapy for insomnia in adolescents: a randomized controlled trial with internet therapy, group therapy and a waiting list condition. Sleep. 2015;38:1913–26. Epub 2015/07/15.

76. de Bruin EJ, Oort FJ, Bogels SM, Meijer AM. Efficacy of internet and group-administered cognitive behavioral therapy for insomnia in adolescents: a pilot study. Behav Sleep Med. 2014;12(3):235–54. Epub 2013/06/19.

77. Borbély AA, Achermann P. Sleep homeostasis and models of sleep regulation. In: Kryger MH, Roth T, Dement WC, editors. Principles and practices of sleep medicine. Philadelphia: Elsevier Saunders; 2005. p. 405–17.

78. Spielman AJ. Assessment of insomnia. Clin Psychol Rev. 1986;6(1):11–25.

79. Miller CB, Espie CA, Epstein DR, Friedman L, Morin CM, Pigeon WR, et al. The evidence base of sleep restriction therapy for treating insomnia disorder. Sleep Med Rev. 2014;18(5):415–24. Epub 2014/03/19.

80. Morgenthaler T, Kramer M, Alessi C, Friedman L, Boehlecke B, Brown T, et al. Practice parameters for the psychological and behavioral treatment of insomnia: an update. An American academy of sleep medicine report. Sleep. 2006;29(11):1415–9. Epub 2006/12/14.

81. Bootzin RR, editor. Stimulus control treatment for insomnia. 80th Annual Convention of the American Psychological Association. Washington, DC: American Psychological Association; 1972.

82. Spielman AJ, Saskin P, Thorpy MJ. Treatment of chronic insomnia by restriction of time in bed. Sleep. 1987;10(1):45–56. Epub 1987/02/01.

83. Health NIo. How much sleep is enough? National Heart Lung and Blood Institute; 2012. https://www.nhlbi.nih.gov/health/health-topics/topics/sdd/howmuch.

84. Iglowstein I, Jenni OG, Molinari L, Largo RH. Sleep duration from infancy to adolescence: reference values and generational trends. Pediatrics. 2003;111(2):302–7 [see comment].

85. National Sleep Foundation. National Sleep Foundation: Sleep in America Poll. Sleep and children. Washington, DC: National Sleep Foundation; 2004.

86. National Sleep Foundation. National Sleep Foundation: Sleep in America Poll. Sleepy Teens. Washington, DC: National Sleep Foundation; 2006.

Chapter 9
Pregnancy-Related Sleep Disturbances and Sleep Disorders

Beth Ann Ward

Abstract Pregnancy is a time characterized by vast hormonal and physiologic changes. The dramatic increase in estrogen and progesterone impacts sleep architecture and produces systemic effects that may disrupt sleep. As pregnancy progresses, women experience a progressive increase in both the number and duration of nocturnal awakenings. The awakenings arise from a myriad of causes, including nocturia, nausea, heartburn, pain, and anxiety. Short sleep duration and poor quality sleep during pregnancy have been associated with a multitude of adverse outcomes, including maternal depression, gestational diabetes, prolonged labors, higher rate of cesarean deliveries, preterm birth, and low-birth-weight infants. Restless leg syndrome (RLS) and sleep-disordered breathing (SDB) are two of the most common sleep disorders during pregnancy. Both of these disorders may cause significant sleep disruption and daytime fatigue. RLS has been associated with an increased risk for maternal depression, preeclampsia, and need for cesarean delivery. Treatment of RLS during pregnancy is focused on repletion of iron stores, elimination of factors that may exacerbate RLS, and management of symptoms with behavioral techniques. SDB may increase the risk for intrauterine growth retardation, gestational diabetes, pregnancy-induced hypertension, and preeclampsia. CPAP has been demonstrated to be safe and effective for treatment of SDB during pregnancy. By optimizing sleep hygiene, utilizing cognitive behavioral therapy, and employing measures to reduce discomfort, heartburn, and nocturia, clinicians may improve a woman's sleep. Due to concerns of risk to the fetus, pharmacologic treatment of insomnia during pregnancy is reserved for women with severe symptoms refractory to conservative measures.

B.A. Ward, M.D. (✉)
Department of Sleep Medicine, St. Luke's Sleep Medicine and Research Center,
232 S. Woods Mill Road, Chesterfield, MO 63017, USA
e-mail: Beth.Ward@stlukes-stl.com

© Springer International Publishing Switzerland 2017
H.P. Attarian (ed.), *Clinical Handbook of Insomnia*, Current Clinical Neurology,
DOI 10.1007/978-3-319-41400-3_9

Keywords Pregnancy • Nocturnal awakenings • Restless leg syndrome • Sleep-disordered breathing • Obstructive sleep apnea • Insomnia

Introduction

Pregnancy is a time of extensive physiologic, physical, and hormonal changes. These changes can significantly disrupt a woman's sleep and may predispose to the development of a sleep disorder or may exacerbate pre-existing sleep disorders.

Sleep disruption during pregnancy is a nearly universal experience and may result in symptoms of daytime sleepiness and fatigue [1, 2]. Understanding how sleep is altered during pregnancy and recognizing sleep disorders that commonly develop during pregnancy may enable healthcare professionals to identify and treat sleep problems. Sleep is vital to the health and well-being of pregnant women. Emerging data suggests that both sleep deprivation and sleep disorders during pregnancy may increase the risk for adverse pregnancy outcomes, including increased risk for gestational diabetes, preterm birth, and postpartum depression [1, 3–6]. By counseling women on strategies to optimize sleep, healthcare professionals may improve the quality of nighttime sleep and reduce daytime sleepiness and fatigue.

Influence of Hormonal Changes on Sleep

The vast changes in hormonal levels that occur during pregnancy may impact sleep architecture and may cause physiologic changes that result in sleep disruption. Most notably, progesterone and estrogen levels steadily rise throughout the pregnancy [7]. Progesterone has been shown to have a sedating effect, and has been demonstrated to decrease sleep latency and increase non-REM sleep [8, 9]. Daytime sleepiness and fatigue are often one of the first symptoms of pregnancy, and these symptoms may be directly attributable to the soporific effects of progesterone [10]. Estrogen, conversely, appears to have alerting effects and has been shown to suppress REM sleep [11–14]. In addition to the direct effects of estrogen and progesterone on the central nervous system, these hormones have systemic effects that may impact sleep. For example, progesterone relaxes smooth muscle, which can lead to increased urination, even in the first trimester of pregnancy [10]. Estrogen can cause vasomotor rhinitis, characterized by nasal and pharyngeal mucosal edema, with resultant airway narrowing and increased airflow resistance [15]. These direct effects of estrogen can lead to snoring, and may predispose to obstructive sleep apnea.

In addition to the dramatic increases in estrogen and progesterone observed during pregnancy, many other hormonal levels are impacted by pregnancy, which may affect a woman's sleep. For example, progesterone and cortisol compete for binding sites on corticosteroid-binding globulin. Thus, as progesterone levels increase during pregnancy, free cortisol levels also increase, and elevated cortisol levels lead to increased arousals [16]. Secretion of oxytocin, a hormone that causes uterine contractions, has been demonstrated to display a circadian rhythm, with levels peaking at night. Thus, increasing oxytocin levels at the end of pregnancy may contribute to increased sleep fragmentation in the third trimester [17].

Changes in Sleep Patterns and Sleep Architecture During Pregnancy

Pregnancy profoundly impacts both the quantity and quality of a woman's sleep. During the first trimester, sleep duration increases. A longitudinal study of 33 American women, using in-home polysomnography to assess sleep patterns throughout pregnancy, demonstrated that total sleep time increases by an average of 0.6 h during the first trimester, as compared with prior to pregnancy [18]. Similarly, a survey study of 325 Finnish women revealed that women report an increase in sleep time by an average of 0.4 h during the first trimester, as compared with prior to pregnancy [19]. However, despite the increase in sleep time, women describe a decrease in the quality of their sleep and an increase in nocturnal awakenings [19–21]. A prospective study of 25 pregnant women demonstrated a 1.4-fold increase in nocturnal arousals during the first trimester as compared to prior to conception [22]. Moreover, during the first trimester many women complain of increased daytime sleepiness and fatigue, likely due to both the increased nocturnal awakenings and the soporific effect of high progesterone levels [17].

During the second trimester, sleep duration starts to decrease [1, 18, 19], but several studies suggest that sleep efficiency improves during the second trimester, and women have less wakefulness after sleep onset (WASO) [23–25]. Improvement in both energy levels and alertness during the second trimester has been widely reported in popular literature, leading to the second trimester being dubbed as the "honeymoon" phase of pregnancy [26]. However, there is little support in the scientific literature to support the assertion that energy levels improve during the second trimester. In a longitudinal study of 33 pregnant women, there was a slight decrease in the level of the fatigue reported in the second trimester, but this decrease did not meet statistical significance [27]. Conversely, in a cross-sectional survey of 2427 women, significant daytime sleepiness, increased fatigue, and decreased energy levels were reported in all months of pregnancy, without any clear improvement during the second trimester [1]. Similarly, in a cross-sectional survey of 127 pregnant women, women reported a moderate amount of sleepiness throughout the pregnancy, with no significant differences found between the trimesters [21].

The third trimester represents the period of most disturbed sleep for pregnant women. The average duration of nighttime sleep continues to decrease [1, 18, 19, 28], with total sleep duration returning to pre-pregnancy levels [18, 19]. The greatest change in the sleep patterns at this time is due to increased wakefulness after sleep onset [1, 18, 23, 29, 30]. During the third trimester both the number and duration of nocturnal awakenings increase [1, 20]. Several studies have demonstrated that over 90 % of women experience nocturnal awakenings during the third trimester [1, 19–21]. On average women have 2–5 awakenings per night [1, 21, 23], and during the third trimester women remain awake for an average of 20 min with each arousal [22]. In a cross-sectional study of 2427 women, women who were at least 8 months pregnant reported that the total duration of their awakenings resulted in an average of 80 min of wakefulness during the night [1]. As the pregnancy progresses women also experience longer sleep-onset latencies, with the average sleep latency in the third trimester being greater than 50 min [1, 21]. Women in the third trimester of pregnancy are twice as likely to have insomnia as compared with women in the first or second trimester [31]. With increased sleep disruption, the proportion of women who report overall short sleep duration increases as the pregnancy progresses [1, 28]. In a prospective study of 189 women, 40 % of the women slept less than 7 h per night during the third trimester [28]. A cross-sectional study of 2427 revealed even more dramatic sleep restriction, with 51.4 % of women who were at least 8 months pregnant obtaining 6 h or less of sleep per night [1]. Although many women nap during pregnancy, this may not sufficiently compensate for the nocturnal sleep disruption, as 33.1 % of women at the end of pregnancy obtain less than 6 h of sleep in a 24-h period [1].

The nearly universal sleep disruption that is present during pregnancy is often accompanied by complaints of daytime sleepiness and fatigue, with approximately 50 % of women reporting significant daytime sleepiness [1, 32]. Subjective quality of sleep declines as the pregnancy progresses, with studies finding that by the third trimester 54–83.5 % of women rate their quality of sleep as poor [1, 28]. Factors associated with increased risk for poor quality of sleep include advanced stage of pregnancy, maternal age, lower level of education, and lower income level [1]. Polysomnographic studies designed to assess changes in sleep architecture during pregnancy have been limited by small sample size, limited nights of polysomnography, and a paucity of longitudinal data. Most of these studies have found a decrease in slow-wave sleep as well as a slight decrease or no change in REM sleep as pregnancy progresses [18, 23, 29, 30], although these findings have not been fully consistent.

Causes of Nocturnal Arousals During Pregnancy

Many of the physical and hormonal changes that occur during pregnancy can account for the fragmented sleep that women experience. The causes of the frequent nocturnal arousals change as the pregnancy progresses. Nocturia is the most common cause of nocturnal arousals throughout the pregnancy [1, 22, 33]. In a cross-sectional study of 2427 women, 72.3 % of women less than 2 months pregnant reported that nocturia disrupted their sleep; the prevalence of nocturia increased throughout the pregnancy, with 91.9 % of women who were at least 8 months pregnant identifying nocturia as a cause for awakenings [1]. Nausea and vomiting frequently disrupt sleep in the first trimester, but these symptoms tend to improve and care less likely to cause awakenings as the pregnancy progresses [1, 22]. Back pain, hip pain, and general discomfort are cited as a cause for sleep disruption throughout the pregnancy, but these symptoms become more common toward the end of pregnancy, likely due to weight gain and increased abdominal size [1, 22, 29, 33–35]. Throughout pregnancy 79 % of women report that their sleep is disrupted because they are unable to find a comfortable position, but this is a nearly ubiquitous occurrence by the end of pregnancy, with 94 % of women who are at least 8 months pregnant noting that the inability to find a comfortable position interrupts their sleep [1, 21, 35]. Other discomforts, such as itchy skin [1] or the sensation of being too hot or perspiring [35], may impair a woman's ability to sleep.

Heartburn and reflux are also common sources of nocturnal awakenings [1, 22, 33]. The enlarging uterus displaces the intestines and lower esophageal sphincter, and the lower esophageal sphincter pressure progressively declines throughout the pregnancy [36]. Thus, heartburn and gastroesophageal reflux become more common and more bothersome in the third trimester, and may fragment sleep [1, 22]. Fetal movements and Braxton-Hicks contractions also become more likely to disrupt sleep as the pregnancy progresses [21, 22, 33].

Anxiety and insomnia have been tightly linked in the general population. Similarly, pregnant women often report anxiety as a source for their awakenings [1]. Worries about the baby, worries about labor and delivery, and worries about impending lifestyle changes after the birth of their child may all contribute to sleep disruption during pregnancy [1, 32, 33, 35]. Several studies have also identified vivid and frightening dreams as a frequently reported cause for nocturnal awakening during pregnancy [1, 22, 29, 34]. Environmental factors, such as older children and outside noises, may also interrupt a woman's sleep during pregnancy [1, 22].

Leg discomfort often disturbs sleep in pregnant women. The frequency of women who awaken due to leg cramps steadily increases during the pregnancy, affecting 12–21 % of women in the first trimester, and impacting up to 75 % of women during the third trimester [33, 37]. Furthermore, women are at an increased risk for developing restless leg syndrome (RLS) during pregnancy. Studies reveal that the prevalence of RLS during pregnancy varies between 10 and 33 %, with symptoms being most prevalent in the third trimester [1, 20, 28, 33, 38–43]. Restless leg syndrome is one of the most common causes of insomnia in pregnant women [30], as restless leg symptoms and associated periodic limb movements in sleep may cause prolonged sleep-onset latencies [20, 43] and frequent nocturnal awakenings [44]. Because restless leg syndrome is such a common cause of insomnia during pregnancy, this will be discussed in more detail below.

Pregnancy increases a woman's risk for snoring, which may disrupt a woman's sleep and cause awakenings. The prevalence of snoring increases as the pregnancy progresses; by the third trimester 16–35 % of women report snoring [1, 28, 45–47]. Snoring is also one of the most common symptoms of obstructive sleep apnea [48]. Obstructive sleep apnea may lead to multiple nocturnal awakenings and may predispose a woman to adverse pregnancy outcomes. This is discussed in detail below. Shortness of breath is also a commonly cited source of arousals, likely due to elevation of diaphragm by the expanding uterus, which reduces lung capacity [22, 35].

Restless Leg Syndrome in Pregnancy

Restless leg syndrome (RLS) is a neurologic disorder characterized by an overwhelming urge to move the legs, usually associated with an uncomfortable or painful sensation in the legs [49]. The urge to move the legs is worse at night, worse at rest, and relieved with movement [49]. The prevalence of RLS in the general population has been estimated to be 3.9–14.5% [50]. Restless leg syndrome occurs at a prevalence two to three times higher during pregnancy than it does in the general population, and most studies indicate that the prevalence increases as the pregnancy progresses, with symptoms peaking in the 7th to 8th month of pregnancy [51]. Large-scale studies assessing the prevalence of RLS during pregnancy have indicated that the prevalence may vary between 10 and 33% [1, 20, 28, 33, 38–42]. In a cross-sectional study of 2427 pregnant American women, 24.4% of women were found to have RLS based on the International Restless Legs Syndrome Study Group criteria (IRLSSG), with symptoms being most common during the 6th month of pregnancy (33.3% of women reported RLS symptoms during the 6th month of pregnancy) [1]. In a prospective study of 500 pregnant women in Sweden, 17% of women in the first trimester, 27.1% of women in the second trimester, and 29.6% of women in the third trimester were found to have RLS based on the IRLSSG criteria; 32% of the women surveyed reported RLS symptoms at some point during the pregnancy [40]. A larger study surveyed 1428 pregnant Swedish women at 32 weeks' gestation and found that 18.5% of the women met the criteria for RLS based on the IRLSSG criteria; the prevalence decreased to 9.4% based on the Cambridge-Hopkins Restless Legs Syndrome Short Form 2 diagnostic criteria, which attempts to eliminate RLS-mimics, such as nocturnal leg cramps or positional discomfort [41]. In a sample of 189 American women, 17.5% were found to have RLS based on the IRLSSG criteria during an initial survey between 6 and 20 weeks' gestation; by the third trimester 31.2% of the women had symptoms of RLS [28]. Other studies have reported lower prevalence of RLS in pregnancy; in a study of 461 pregnant women in Taiwan the prevalence of RLS was found to be 10.4% and in a study of 501 pregnant women in Switzerland the prevalence of RLS was 12% [38, 39]. The differences in reported prevalence may be due to differences in maternal age, ethnicity, number of previous pregnancies, level of iron stores prior to pregnancy, and family history of RLS in the populations studied. The method of data collection and rigor of the scales used to diagnose RLS may also have impacted the findings. Taken together, however, these studies demonstrate that RLS commonly occurs in pregnancy, and generally becomes more common as pregnancy progresses.

Restless leg syndrome is more likely to develop during pregnancy in women with a prior history of RLS, a history of RLS during a previous pregnancy, or a family history of RLS [33, 39]. The risk of developing RLS during pregnancy increases with mulitparity [39, 41]. Both tobacco use and coffee consumption, both prior to the pregnancy and during the pregnancy, have been associated with an increased risk for RLS [20, 38–41]. Short sleep duration has also been associated with RLS, with sleep duration of less than 7 h reported as a risk factor for the development of RLS in a cross-sectional study of approximately 16,500 pregnant women in Japan [20] and sleep duration of less than 6 h reported as a risk factor for the development of RLS in a study of 1428 pregnant women in Sweden [41].

The pathophysiology of restless leg syndrome is not fully understood, but it is thought to be related to deficiency of iron stores in the brain and dysfunction of central nervous system dopaminergic regulation [49, 52]. It is not clear why the risk of RLS significantly increases during pregnancy. Iron deficiency is a risk factor for the development of RLS in the general population, with ferritin levels less than 50 ng/mL correlating with more severe symptoms [53, 54]. Given the high metabolic demand for iron during pregnancy, iron deficiency has been suspected to play a role in the increased prevalence of RLS during pregnancy. Some studies have indeed found that women who develop RLS during pregnancy have lower ferritin levels than women who do not develop RLS [33], but other studies have failed to demonstrate this relationship [39, 43]. Several studies have revealed that women who develop RLS during pregnancy are more likely to have anemia or are likely to have lower hemoglobin than women who do not develop RLS during pregnancy [33, 38, 55], and tend to have lower use of iron supplementation [38, 41], although, again, these are not consistent findings [39–41]. The fact that RLS tends to resolve within days to weeks after the delivery of the baby [33, 38–40], whereas it can take months to replenish iron stores following a pregnancy [4], raises doubt that iron deficiency could be the primary factor driving the increased prevalence of RLS during pregnancy. The conflicting findings regarding the role of iron deficiency in the development of RLS during pregnancy suggest that, while iron deficiency may play a role, other factors must also be involved.

The elevated estrogen levels that occur during pregnancy have been proposed as an etiologic factor for the increased prevalence of RLS during pregnancy. Estrogen modulates dopaminergic transmission in the ventral striatum [56]. Estrogen levels steadily increase throughout pregnancy and then rapidly decrease after delivery, a pattern that corresponds well to the increased prevalence of RLS observed as the pregnancy progresses followed by the swift improvement in symptoms after the birth of the child [33, 40]. A small study found that estradiol levels were significantly higher in pregnant women with RLS than in pregnant women without RLS [56], but a subsequent study failed to find any significant difference in estrogen levels among women with RLS and women without RLS [39]. Thus, further studies are needed to explore the role that estrogen may be playing in the development of RLS symptoms during pregnancy.

Folate deficiency has been implicated in the development of RLS during pregnancy. One study revealed that women who developed restless leg syndrome had consistently lower folate levels than women who did not develop restless leg syndrome [43], although a subsequent study failed to confirm this finding [57].

Nevertheless, studies of RLS in pregnancy have demonstrated that women who develop RLS tend to have lower rates of folate supplementation [38, 57, 58]. Prolactin has also been proposed as an etiologic factor in the development of RLS through its modulation of dopaminergic activity, given that the circadian rhythm of prolactin secretion results in peak prolactin levels in the evening, corresponding to when RLS symptoms are most prominent [59]. However, the fact that RLS symptoms rapidly abate following the birth of a child, even among lactating mothers, argues against prolactin playing a significant role in the development of RLS. Further research is needed to elucidate the mechanism by which RLS develops during pregnancy. Although findings have been inconsistent regarding the various proposed etiological factors studied to date, it is possible that the development of RLS depends on the interaction of multiple factors, and thus, iron, folate, estrogen, and prolactin may all play a role.

The impact of restless leg syndrome during pregnancy can be profound. Restless leg syndrome is one of the most common causes of insomnia in pregnant women [31]. Women with RLS during pregnancy have more difficulty falling asleep, more frequent nocturnal arousals, poorer quality of sleep, and shorter sleep duration [20, 33, 38, 39, 60]. Women with RLS during pregnancy report greater fatigue and more significant daytime sleepiness [40, 57]. Women with restless leg syndrome have also been demonstrated to have higher rates of depression, both during the pregnancy and in postpartum period [41, 61]. Recent studies have suggested that RLS may be associated with adverse pregnancy outcomes, including increased risk for preeclampsia and increased risk for cesarean delivery [60, 62]. The development of RLS during pregnancy places women at higher risk of developing RLS during subsequent pregnancies [63] as well as at higher risk of developing idiopathic RLS independent of pregnancy in the future [40, 64, 65].

Prior to conception, women who are at high risk for RLS during pregnancy should be identified and provided counseling. This would include women who have idiopathic RLS prior to a pregnancy, women who have experienced RLS during a previous pregnancy, and women with a family history of RLS [33, 39, 63, 64]. Given that it is very difficult to replenish iron stores during pregnancy and given the potential role that iron deficiency plays in the development of RLS during pregnancy, it has been recommended that all women with RLS present prior to a planned pregnancy undergo evaluation for iron deficiency and receive iron supplementation if the ferritin level is less than 75 ng/mL [51]. Likewise, it would be reasonable to assess iron stores prior to conception in any women at risk for developing RLS during pregnancy, as well as in any pregnant women who develops RLS. Oral iron supplementation is recommended with ferrous sulfate 325 mg (65 mg of elemental iron) one to two times per day if the ferritin level is less than 50–75 ng/mL. A ferritin level should be repeated 6–8 weeks after starting iron supplementation. If the ferritin level remains less than 30 ng/mL, treatment with IV iron infusion may be considered after the first trimester in pregnant women with severe RLS symptoms that cannot be sufficiently controlled with non-pharmacologic treatment modalities [51, 66], although IV iron infusion does carry a risk of anaphylaxis [67]. A decrease in maternal blood pressure may occur during the infusion, although whether this poses any risk to the fetus is not known [66].

When RLS develops during pregnancy, management of symptoms should begin with non-pharmacologic therapy. An effort should be made to eliminate any factors that could cause or exacerbate RLS symptoms, such as avoiding situations that require prolonged immobility, limiting the use of caffeine, and when possible eliminating the use of medications that can aggravate RLS, such as SSRI antidepressants, antiemetics, antipsychotics, and antihistamines. Studies have demonstrated that moderate-intensity exercise can reduce RLS symptoms, and thus, if there are no contraindications to physical activity, moderate physical exercise (such as brisk walking, water aerobics, gardening) has been recommended for management of RLS during pregnancy. Other non-pharmacologic treatment modalities that have been shown to be of some benefit in treatment of RLS include yoga, massage, and pneumatic compression devices [51]. Anecdotally, stretching, applying heat to the limbs, performing relaxation techniques, or engaging in mental activities that may serve as a distraction from the symptoms have all been reported to reduce symptoms, although there is less data to support these treatments [51]. Women should be reminded to dedicate an adequate amount of time for sleep, as total sleep duration less than 7 h is associated with restless leg syndrome [20]. Alcohol and tobacco use are both associated with an increased risk of RLS during pregnancy, and pose other risks to the developing fetus, and thus women should be counseled to abstain from both during pregnancy [20]. Untreated obstructive sleep apnea may exacerbate RLS symptoms, as well as increase the risk for other adverse pregnancy outcomes, and so treatment should be provided for sleep-disordered breathing, when present.

The effectiveness of folate supplementation in reducing or preventing RLS is unclear. A recent consensus paper regarding the management of RLS during pregnancy noted that there is insufficient evidence to recommend folate for treatment of RLS during pregnancy [51]. However, supplementation of 400–800 mcg daily is recommended for all women for prevention of neural tube defects, and various studies have observed that women who regularly take prenatal vitamins containing folate are less likely to have restless leg syndrome. Thus, in managing the care of a pregnant woman with RLS, it is reasonable to ensure that she is receiving adequate folate supplementation.

If RLS symptoms are moderate–severe, consideration may be given to the use of pharmacologic agents. A 2015 consensus guideline for the treatment of RLS during pregnancy asserts that medications should only be considered after an adequate attempt at iron supplementation and the use of at least one non-pharmacologic therapy have failed [51]. Moreover, when medications are considered, the lowest effective dose should be used, and treatment should be limited to the shortest duration necessary, with regular reassessments made to consider whether continued use of the medication is needed [51].

For individuals who are not pregnant, dopamine agonists, such as ropinirole, pramipexole, and rotigotine, are considered the treatment of choice for RLS [68]. However, little is known about the teratogenic effects of these medications in humans. These medications are all classified by the Food and Drug Administration (FDA) as Class C in pregnancy, indicating that they are of uncertain safety in humans. Limited case reports and case series regarding the use of ropinirole, prami-pexole, and rotigotine during pregnancy have not revealed any increased risk of major malformations, but the data is very meager [69]. As a result, the 2015 consensus statement by the International Restless Legs Syndrome Study Group (IRLSSG) noted that there was "insufficient evidence to reach consensus" on the use of these medications in pregnancy. Given that there is more safety data available for the use of carbidopa/levodopa, the use of carbidopa/levodopa is recommended rather than the dopamine agonists [51]. Other pharmacologic treatment options could include clonazepam, opioids, gabapentin, gabapentin enacarbil, or clonidine; more data exists for these medications regarding their use during pregnancy, but none of these are recommended as standard therapy in the non-pregnant population for treatment of restless leg syndrome [68]. The IRLSSG 2015 consensus committee deemed the use of clonazepam reasonable during the second or third trimester based on the safety data available, but counseled against the use of clonazepam during the first trimester to reduce the risk of congenital malformations [15]. Opioids have been demonstrated to be effective in the treatment of RLS symptoms refractory to other medications [68]. Based on the safety and efficacy data available, the IRLSSG 2015 consensus committee recommends low-dose oxycodone be used during pregnancy only in women with very severe RLS symptoms after attempts to manage the symptoms with iron supplementation, non-pharmacologic therapy, and at least one non-opioid medication have all failed. Furthermore, oxycodone should not be used in the first trimester, due to the risk of birth defects. The use of opioids during pregnancy may increase the risk for respiratory depression as well as opioid withdrawal in neonates exposed in utero, and thus consideration should be given to discontinuing the use of opioids as the pregnancy approaches term [51, 59]. Gabapentin, gabapentin enacarbil, and clonidine are all listed as Class C in pregnancy (uncertain safety), and there is insufficient data regarding the safety and efficacy of these medications during pregnancy to recommend the use of these medications during pregnancy.

Sleep-Disordered Breathing in Pregnancy

Sleep-disordered breathing (SDB) is a general term used to describe respiratory disturbances in sleep; this can include primary snoring, upper-airway resistance syndrome, obstructive sleep apnea (OSA), central sleep apnea, and obesity hypoventilation syndrome. Many of the physiologic changes that occur during pregnancy may precipitate the development of SDB. Excess body weight is the strongest risk factor for obstructive sleep apnea in the general population, with the risk of sleep apnea increasing relative to the degree of excess weight [49, 70]. The average weight gain during pregnancy is 25–35 pounds, often resulting in an increase of 20% or more of the total body weight. This degree of weight change, over a relatively short period of time, may predispose to the development of SDB. The anatomic and physiologic changes of pregnancy result in elevation of the diaphragm, increased intrathoracic pressure, and reduced functional residual capacity [71]. Elevated estrogen levels during pregnancy can cause vasomotor rhinitis, nasopharyngeal hyperemia, and mucosal edema [59]. These changes can result in airway narrowing, increased resistance to airflow, increased collapsibility, and ultimately, airway obstruction. The increase in nocturnal awakenings and sleep fragmentation that occurs during pregnancy may also augment the risk for SDB. Sleep onset is associated with an irregular ventilatory pattern, typically characterized by oscillating, periodic breathing [72, 73]. When sleep is fragmented, the increased frequency of wake-sleep transitions can amplify this unstable breathing pattern, heightening the risk for SDB.

Many studies have demonstrated that snoring increases in frequency and severity during pregnancy; by the third trimester, snoring is reported in 16–35 % of women [1, 28, 45–47, 74]. Obese women are more likely to snore during pregnancy than women who are not obese [48], and it has been suggested that both the initial BMI and the amount of weight gain during the pregnancy impact whether sleep-disordered breathing develops [75]. Snoring may contribute to sleep complaints, as it can lead to arousals and fragmented sleep. Moreover, snoring is one of the most common symptoms of obstructive sleep apnea [48], and thus the onset of snoring may herald the development of sleep apnea.

The true prevalence of obstructive sleep apnea in pregnancy is not known, as large population-based studies utilizing polysomnography to evaluate for sleep apnea have not been performed. Many early studies attempted to estimate the prevalence of OSA during pregnancy based on surveys assessing symptoms of OSA (snoring, gasping, excessive daytime sleepiness, etc.). These studies consistently reported an increase in symptoms of OSA as pregnancy progresses [28, 75, 76], and revealed that 10–29 % of pregnant women have symptoms of OSA [1, 77, 78]. However, recent studies using objective assessments of OSA (based on out-of-center sleep testing or full polysomnography) have demonstrated that symptom-based surveys, such as the Berlin Questionnaire for Sleep Disordered Breathing, have low specificity when used to identify OSA in pregnant women [79–81]. Thus, attempting to estimate the prevalence of OSA in pregnant women based on symptoms alone is problematic, and objective assessment is needed. Currently, most studies using objective assessments of OSA in pregnant women have been done in populations at an increased risk for developing sleep apnea. For example, Louis et al. performed out-of-center sleep testing (OCST) in a cohort of 175 obese pregnant women and found that 15.4 % of the women had OSA [82]. Facco et al. performed OCSTs in 182 high-risk pregnant women (risk factors included obesity, chronic hypertension, pregestational diabetes, prior preeclampsia, and twin gestation). In this cohort, 30 % of the women were found to have OSA in early pregnancy (prior to 20 weeks), and 47 % of the women were found to have OSA by the third trimester [83]. These studies of high-risk women demonstrate that the OSA does indeed occur during pregnancy, and highlight the need for objective population-based studies to assess the true prevalence of OSA during pregnancy.

   Much research has been done in recent years exploring the impact of SDB during
pregnancy on both maternal and fetal health outcomes, with particular emphasis on
the link between SDB during pregnancy and intrauterine growth retardation (IUGR),
gestational diabetes, pregnancy-induced hypertension, and preeclampsia, and it is
thus worth reviewing this literature here. A prospective longitudinal study of 41
pregnant women, evaluated for OSA using a portable monitoring device, found evidence of fetal growth impairment in 43 % of the women with OSA, whereas only
11 % of the women without OSA had evidence of impaired fetal growth [79]. Of
note, the majority of the women with OSA in this study had mild sleep apnea (with
a median RDI of 7.9), thus emphasizing that even mild OSA may result in adverse
fetal outcomes. Further support for the idea that OSA during pregnancy may impair
fetal growth was provided by a large retrospective study of 791 pregnant women
with OSA, which demonstrated that these women were at higher risk for having a
baby with a low birth weight or one that was small for gestational age [84]. Although
other studies have failed to confirm the relationship between OSA in pregnancy and
impaired fetal growth, many of the negative studies were smaller, retrospective
studies, thus highlighting the need for additional large, prospective studies.
   Obstructive sleep apnea in pregnancy also appears to increase the risk of gestational diabetes. A prospective study of 182 pregnant women who underwent out-of-
center sleep testing for evaluation of OSA found that obstructive sleep apnea in
early pregnancy is an independent risk factor for the development of gestational
diabetes [83]. Moreover, this study demonstrated that the risk of developing gestational diabeteses was directly proportional to the severity of the obstructive sleep
apnea. The link between obstructive sleep apnea in pregnancy and gestational diabetes has been further supported by several large-scale studies demonstrating that
women with symptoms of SDB are at a 2–3-fold increased risk of developing gestational diabetes [85–89].
   Obstructive sleep apnea in pregnancy increases the risk for pregnancy-induced
hypertension and preeclampsia. There have been two studies to date that have utilized objective assessments of OSA to investigate the link between OSA during
pregnancy and preeclampsia. The first study, a retrospective case-control study of
57 pregnant women with OSA (diagnosed by full polysomnography) and 114 controls, found that the women with OSA were more likely to develop preeclampsia, as
compared with normal-weight pregnant controls [90]. The second study, a prospective, observational study of 175 obese pregnant women, similarly demonstrated that
women with OSA were more likely to develop preeclampsia [82]. Many other studies have explored the relationship between symptoms of SDB and hypertensive disease in pregnancy. Although these studies likely included both women with OSA
and women with just snoring (given the low specificity of symptom-based surveys
in identifying women with OSA during pregnancy), the findings of several large-
scale studies and two meta-analyses have demonstrated that women with symptoms
of SDB are at higher risk for developing pregnancy-induced hypertension and preeclampsia [45, 47, 85, 86, 88, 91, 92]. An interesting finding in O'Brien's study of
1719 pregnant women was that new onset of habitual snoring during pregnancy
increased the risk of gestational hypertension and preeclampsia, whereas the pres-

ence of chronic habitual snoring prior to pregnancy was not found to be associated with increased risk. Given that the large-scale studies done to date have identified women with SDB based on reports of symptoms alone, further large studies that utilize objective measures to assess for OSA are needed, to determine whether it is snoring alone or obstructive sleep apnea that places women at increased risk for pregnancy-induced hypertension and preeclampsia.

Other adverse outcomes reported to be associated with SDB during pregnancy include preterm birth [46, 84, 85, 88, 90], cesarean delivery [82], and NICU admission [82], although the studies investigating the link between SDB and these outcomes are not as robust. Women with sleep-disordered breathing during pregnancy may have a higher maternal mortality rate. Review of pregnancy-related hospital discharges in the USA from 1998 through 2009 found that women with a diagnosis of OSA experienced approximately a fivefold higher rate of death prior to discharge [85]. Sleep-disordered breathing during pregnancy may also have implications for maternal health risks extending beyond the pregnancy. It has been suggested that SDB during pregnancy increases a woman's risk for future development of cardiovascular disease [93], but more studies are needed to explore this possible relationship.

Given the compelling evidence that sleep-disordered breathing during pregnancy increases the risk for intrauterine growth retardation, gestational diabetes, pregnancy-induced hypertension, and preeclampsia, it is important that clinicians identify women who are at risk for developing sleep-disordered breathing. Risk factors for developing obstructive sleep apnea during pregnancy include obesity, Mallampati Class III and Class IV airways, large neck circumferences (neck circumferences greater than 42 cm or 16.5 in.), and a small or crowded posterior oropharynx [17, 94]. Consideration should be given to evaluating for obstructive sleep apnea in women with these risk factors, particularly if these women report habitual snoring or have a history of hypertension prior to pregnancy [4, 17]. Because standardized screening questionnaires such as the Berlin Questionnaire for Sleep Disordered Breathing have been demonstrated to have a low specificity in identifying obstructive sleep apnea in pregnant women, Facco et al. [95] have developed a four-variable model to predict sleep apnea in pregnant women, which utilizes the presence of habitual snoring, chronic hypertension, age, and body mass index to identify women at risk for developing obstructive sleep apnea during pregnancy.

CPAP, the most effective treatment of OSA in the general population, has been demonstrated to be safe and effective in pregnant women [96, 97]. The rapid weight gain and changes in respiratory physiology that occur during the pregnancy may cause pressure needs to increase as the pregnancy progresses, and thus patients may benefit from the use of an auto-titrating CPAP device. Women on a fixed CPAP setting may require a repeat titration in the second or third trimester [97]. These women should be followed closely for symptoms of recurrent snoring, waking up gasping for air, witnessed apneas, or increased daytime sleepiness, as these symptoms may indicate that the current CPAP settings are suboptimal. The benefit of CPAP has been well documented in the general population, with the use of CPAP leading to decreased daytime sleepiness and improved quality of life [98–100]. The impact of CPAP during pregnancy has not been as well studied, but several small studies have suggested that the use of CPAP during pregnancy in women with hypertension or preeclampsia may improve pregnancy outcomes. In a small randomized-controlled study of pregnant women with hypertension and chronic snoring (but not found to have OSA on polysomnography), treatment with CPAP led to improved blood pressure control [101]. A case report of a woman with severe OSA and preeclampsia treated with CPAP documented improvement in both clinical and biochemical markers of preeclampsia; the significant improvement in preeclampsia enabled the pregnancy to be safely prolonged by 30 days [102]. CPAP has also been investigated as a treatment option for women with preeclampsia independent of whether SDB is present. A study of 11 women with preeclampsia demonstrated that the use of CPAP during a single night of polysomnography led to significantly lower blood pressure levels, as compared to the previous night when CPAP was not used [103]. Similarly, a small randomized study of women with preeclampsia found that the use of CPAP during a single night of polysomnography led to significantly less reduction in cardiac output and smaller increases in total peripheral resistance as compared with women who did not receive treatment [104]. The women in this study were selected based on the presence of preeclampsia alone and were randomized to treatment with CPAP, regardless of whether they met the criteria for OSA. Of note, however, all of the women with preeclampsia were found to have flow limitation, and many of them met the criteria for OSA (the mean RDI in the group treated with CPAP was 19; the mean RDI in the group not treated with CPAP was 22). In a small group of women with preeclampsia (all of whom had evidence of flow limitation and many of whom met the criteria for OSA, with the group having a mean AHI of 8.9), the use of auto-titrating CPAP resulted in improvement in fetal movement [105]. Collectively, these studies demonstrate that the use of CPAP during pregnancy may provide benefits to both the mother and fetus, at least for women with preeclampsia or hypertension. Larger prospective studies are needed to assess whether the use of CPAP during pregnancy for the treatment of obstructive sleep apnea may reduce the risk of developing the adverse pregnancy outcomes discussed above.

Alternate treatment options for obstructive sleep apnea have not been studied in pregnant women, and thus, the effectiveness of alternate treatment options during pregnancy is not known. The lower reported efficacy of the oral appliance as compared with CPAP in the general population, and the delay in treatment that may occur due to the time needed to make and sufficiently advance the device, causes the oral appliance to be a less optimal treatment option [4]. Likewise, the potential risks of upper airway surgery in pregnant women, the lower efficacy of surgery as compared with CPAP, and the fact that OSA may resolve following the pregnancy do not support the use of surgery as a treatment option in pregnant women [2, 4]. Conservative treatment measures such as avoiding excessive weight gain, abstaining from alcohol, and restricting sleep in the supine position may be prudent, particularly in women who are obese prior to conception or have other risk factors for SDB, but again, data on the efficacy of these measures when used during pregnancy is lacking.

Implications of Insomnia During Pregnancy

Insomnia during pregnancy can cause sleep disruption and may lead to sleep deprivation, both of which may increase the risk for adverse pregnancy outcomes. In a prospective study of 131 women during the last month of pregnancy, women who averaged less than 6 h of sleep per night were found to have significantly longer labors and were 4.5 times more likely to require a cesarean delivery as compared with women who averaged at least 7 h of sleep per night [106]. Similarly, short sleep on the night prior to labor has been associated with the perception of greater pain and discomfort during labor [107]. Emerging data also suggests that sleep deprivation and poor quality of sleep may be a risk for preterm birth. In a prospective study of 1091 women, those women who reported obtaining 5 h or less of sleep per day were observed to have a higher risk of preterm birth [108]. Several cross-sectional and observational studies have likewise demonstrated that disturbed sleep during pregnancy (as measured by the Pittsburgh Sleep Quality Index or assessed through sleep questionnaires) is a risk factor for preterm birth [109–111]. Poor-quality sleep during pregnancy has also been associated with increased risk for the development of depression later in the pregnancy [112]. Furthermore, insomnia during pregnancy is a risk factor for the development of postpartum depression, at least in women with a prior history of depression [5, 6]. Recent evidence suggests that short sleep duration may be a risk factor for gestational diabetes. In a prospective study of 63 women, short sleep time in mid-pregnancy, as measured by wrist actigraphy, was associated with higher risk for maternal hyperglycemia (measured by a 1-h oral glucose tolerance test at the beginning of the third trimester) [113]. Larger cross-sectional studies have also found that self-reported short sleep duration during the second trimester is associated with a higher risk for developing gestational diabetes [89, 114]. Finally, short sleep duration has been shown to increase the risk for low birth weight [115, 116]. Although the exact mechanism whereby insomnia and sleep disruption lead to these various adverse outcomes is not known, current research is exploring the role that pro-inflammatory cytokines may play, given that higher levels of pro-inflammatory cytokines are found in individuals with insomnia and are also found in women with preterm birth and postpartum depression [2, 3, 46, 117].

Treatment of Insomnia During Pregnancy

Given the impact that sleep problems can have on the health and well-being of individuals, healthcare professionals should inquire about symptoms of disturbed sleep during pregnancy. Pregnant women should be instructed on principles of good sleep hygiene. Women should be advised to dedicate sufficient time for sleep and to ensure that their sleep environment is quiet and conducive to sleep. During the first and third trimesters, when nocturia is one of the most common causes of nighttime awakenings, women should be counseled to limit fluid intake for several hours prior to bedtime. Women should avoid food that is likely to provoke heartburn, and limit food intake several hours prior to bedtime to reduce gastroesophageal reflux. Supportive pillows may be used to help women sleep comfortably. Massage and local heat application may also help reduce low back pain. Cognitive behavioral therapy, which has been demonstrated to be effective in the treatment of insomnia in the general population, may also be helpful, although this has not been specifically studied in pregnant women. Healthcare professionals should screen for symptoms of restless leg syndrome or sleep-disordered breathing; when symptoms are present the appropriate diagnostic workup and treatment should be provided, as detailed above.

If symptoms of insomnia are severe and are refractory to conservative measures, consideration can be given to short-term pharmacologic treatment, although research regarding the safety of sleep-promoting medications is limited. A recent review of the current research available regarding the safety of sleep-promoting medications during pregnancy found no clear evidence of increased risk of congenital malformations among women who had used benzodiazepines, benzodiazepine receptor agonists, antidepressants, or antihistamines during pregnancy [118]. However, some studies have reported that the use of benzodiazepines and benzodiazepine receptor agonists is associated with an increased risk of low-birth-weight infants and preterm birth [118–120]. It should be noted that not all studies have confirmed the increased risk of low birth weight and preterm birth with benzodiazepine receptor agonists [118, 120, 121]. Furthermore, insomnia and short sleep have been associated with increased risk of low-birth-weight infants and preterm birth [108, 115, 116]; thus, it is not clear if the increased risk is attributable to the medication usage or to the disease process itself. Nevertheless, if pharmacologic treatment of insomnia is considered, the risks and benefits of treatment should be discussed in detail with the patient.

References

1. Mindell JA, Cook RA, Nikolovski J. Sleep patterns and sleep disturbances across pregnancy. Sleep Med. 2015;16:483–8.
2. Nodine PM, Matthews EE. Common sleep disorders: management strategies and pregnancy outcomes. J Midwifery Womens Health. 2013;58:368–77.
3. Palagini L, Gemignani A, Banti S, Manconi M, Mauri M. Chronic sleep loss during pregnancy as a determinant of stress: impact on pregnancy outcome. Sleep Med. 2014;15:853–9.
4. Abbott SM, Attarian H, Zee PC. Sleep disorders in perinatal women. Best Pract Res Clin Obstet Gynaecol. 2014;28:159–68.
5. Dorheim SK, Bjorvatn B, Eberhard-Gran M. Can insomnia in pregnancy predict postpartum depression? A longitudinal, population-based study. PLoS One. 2014;9:e94674.
6. Marques M, Bos S, Soares MJ, Maia B, Pereira AT, Valente J, Gomes AA, Macedo A, Azevedo MH. Is insomnia in late pregnancy a risk factor for postpartum depression/depressive symptomatology? Psychiatry Res. 2011;186:272–80.

7. Torrealday S, Taylor HS, Burney RO, Mooney SB, Giudice LC. Endocrinology of pregnancy. In: De Groot LJ, Beck-Peccoz P, Chrousos G, Dungan K, Grossman A, Hershman JM, Koch C, McLachlan R, New M, Rebar R, Singer F, Vinik A, Weickert MO, editors. Endotext. South Dartmouth, MA: MD Text.com, Inc.; 2012.
8. Manber R, Armitage R. Sex, steroids, and sleep: a review. Sleep. 1999;22:540–55.
9. Lancel M, Faulhaber J, Holsboer F, Rupprecht R. Progesterone induces changes in sleep comparable to those of agonistic GABAA receptor modulators. Am J Physiol. 1996;271:E763–72.
10. Lee KA. Alterations in sleep during pregnancy and postpartum: a review of 30 years of research. Sleep Med Rev. 1998;2:231–42.
11. Colvin GB, Whitmoyer DI, Lisk RD, Walter DO, Sawyer CH. Changes in sleep-wakefulness in female rats during circadian and estrous cycles. Brain Res. 1968;7:173–81.
12. Kleinlogel H. The female rat's sleep during oestrous cycle. Neuropsychobiology. 1983;10:228–37.
13. Branchey M, Branchey L, Nadler RD. Effects of estrogen and progesterone on sleep patterns of female rats. Physiol Behav. 1971;6:743–6.
14. Hadjimarkou MM, Benham R, Schwarz JM, Holder MK, Mong JA. Estradiol suppresses rapid eye movement sleep and activation of sleep-active neurons in the ventrolateral preoptic area. Eur J Neurosci. 2008;27:1780–92.
15. Marbry RL. Rhinitis of pregnancy. South Med J. 1986;79:965–71.
16. Teran-Perez G, Arana-Lechuga Y, Esqueda-Leon E, Santana-Miranda R, Rojas-Zamorano JA, Moctezuma JV. Steroid hormones and sleep regulation. Mini Rev Med Chem. 2012;12:1040–8.
17. Izci-Balaserak B, Lee K. Sleep disturbances and sleep-related disorders in pregnancy. In: Kryger MH, Roth T, Dement WC, editors. Principles and practices of sleep medicine. 5th ed. St. Louis, MO: Elsevier Saunders; 2010. p. 1572–86.
18. Lee KA, Zaffke ME, McEnany G. Parity and sleep patterns during and after pregnancy. Obstet Gynecol. 2000;95:14–8.
19. Hedman C, Pohjasvaara T, Tolonen U, Suhonen-Malm AS, Myllyla VV. Effects of pregnancy on mother's sleep. Sleep Med. 2002;3:37–42.
20. Suzuki S, Dennerstein L, Greenwood KM, Armstrong SM, Satohisa E. Sleeping patterns during pregnancy in Japanese women. J Psychosom Obstet Gynecol. 1994;15:19–26.
21. Mindell JA, Jacobson BJ. Sleep disturbances during pregnancy. J Obstet Gynecol Neonatal Nurs. 2000;29:590–7.
22. Baratte-Beebe KR, Lee K. Sources of midsleep awakenings in childbearing women. Clin Nurs Res. 1999;8:386–97.
23. Brunner DP, Munch M, Biedermann K, Huch R, Huch A, Borbeley AA. Changes in sleep and sleep electroencephalogram during pregnancy. Sleep. 1994;17:576–82.
24. Signal TL, Gander PH, Sangalli MR, Travier N, Firestone RT, Tuohy JF. Sleep duration and quality in healthy nulliparous and multiparous women across pregnancy and post-partum. Aust N Z J Obstet Gynaecol. 2007;47:16–22.
25. Coble PA, Reynolds 3rd CF, Kupfer DJ, Houck PR, Day NL, Giles DE. Childbearing in women with and without a history of affective disorder. II. Electroencephalographic sleep. Compr Psychiatry. 1994;35:215–24.
26. Murkoff HE, Mazel S. What to expect when you're expecting. 4th ed. New York: Workman Pub; 2008.
27. Lee KA, Zaffke ME. Longitudinal changes in fatigue and energy during pregnancy and the postpartum period. J Obstet Gynecol Neonatal Nurs. 1999;28:183–91.
28. Facco FL, Kramer J, Ho KH, Zee PC, Grobman WA. Sleep disturbances in pregnancy. Obstet Gynecol. 2010;115:77–83.
29. Hertz G, Fast A, Feinsilver SH, Albertario CL, Shulman H, Fein AM. Sleep in normal late pregnancy. Sleep. 1992;15:246–51.
30. Driver HS, Shapiro CM. A longitudinal study of sleep stages in young women during pregnancy and postpartum. Sleep. 1992;15:449–53.

31. Kızılırmak A, Timur S, Kartal B. Insomnia in pregnancy and factors related to insomnia. ScientificWorldJournal. 2012;2012:197093.
32. National Sleep Foundation. Women and sleep poll. Washington, DC: National Sleep Foundation; 2007.
33. Manconi M, Govoni V, De Vito A, Economou NT, Cesnik E, Casetta I, Mollica G, Ferini-Strambi L, Granieri E. Restless legs syndrome and pregnancy. Neurology. 2004;63:1065–9.
34. Schweiger MS. Sleep disturbance in pregnancy. A subjective survey. Am J Obstet Gynecol. 1972;114:879–82.
35. Wolfson AR, Crowley SJ, Anwer U, Bassett JL. Changes in sleep patterns and depressive symptoms in first-time mothers: last trimester to 1-year postpartum. Behav Sleep Med. 2003;1:54–67.
36. Van Thiel DH, Gavaler JS, Joshi SN, Sara RK, Stremple J. Heartburn of pregnancy. Gastroenterology. 1977;72:666–8.
37. Gupta MA, Schork MJ, Gay C. Nocturnal leg cramps of pregnancy: a prospective study of clinical features. Sleep Res. 1992;21:294.
38. Chen P-H, Liou K-C, Chen C-P, Cheng S-J. Risk factors and prevalence rate of restless legs syndrome among pregnant women in Taiwan. Sleep Med. 2012;13:1153–7.
39. Hubner A, Krafft A, Gadient S, Werth E, Zimmerman R, Bassetti C. Characteristics and determinants of restless legs syndrome in pregnancy: a prospective study. Neurology. 2013;80:738–42.
40. Sarberg M, Josefsson A, Wirehn A-B, Svanborg E. Restless legs syndrome during and after pregnancy and its relation to snoring. Acta Obstet Gynecol Scand. 2012;91:850–5.
41. Wesstrom J, Skalkidou A, Manconi M, Fulda S, Sundstrom-Poromaa I. Pre-pregnancy restless legs syndrome (Willis-Ekbom disease) is associated with perinatal depression. J Clin Sleep Med. 2014;10:527–33.
42. Alves DA, Carvalho LB, Morais JF, Prado GF. Restless legs syndrome during pregnancy in Brazilian women. Sleep Med. 2010;10:1049–54.
43. Lee KA, Zaffke ME, Baratte-Beebe K. Restless legs syndrome and sleep disturbance during pregnancy: the role of folate and iron. J Womens Health Gend Based Med. 2001;10:335–41.
44. Nikkola E, Ekblad U, Ekholm E, Mikola H, Polo O. Sleep in multiple pregnancy: breathing patterns, oxygenation, and periodic leg movements. Am J Obstet Gynecol. 1996;174:1622–5.
45. O'Brien LM, Bullough AS, Owusu JT, Tremblay KA, Brincat CA, Chames MC, Kalbfleish JD, Chervin RD. Pregnancy-onset habitual snoring, gestational hypertension, and pre-eclampsia: prospective cohort study. Am J Obstet Gynecol. 2012;207:487.e1–9.
46. Facco FL, Grobman WA, Dramer J, Ho KH, Zee PC. Self-reported short sleep duration and frequent snoring in pregnancy: impact on glucose metabolism. Am J Obstet Gynecol. 2010;203:142.e1–5.
47. Perez-Chada D, Videla AJ, O'Flaherty ME, Majul C, Catalini AM, Caballer CA, Franklin KA. Snoring, witnessed sleep apnoeas and pregnancy-induced hypertension. Acta Obstet Gynecol Scand. 2007;86:788–92.
48. Guilleminault C, Tilkian A, Dement WC. The sleep apnea syndromes. Annu Rev Med. 1976;27:465–84.
49. Sateia M, editor. The international classification of sleep disorders. Diagnostic & coding manual. 3rd ed. Darien, IL: American Academy of Sleep Medicine; 2014.
50. Ohayon MM, O'Hara R, Vitiello MV. Epidemiology of restless legs syndrome: a synthesis of the literature. Sleep Med Rev. 2012;16:283–95.
51. Picchietti DL, Hensley JG, Bainbridge JL, Lee KA, Manconi M, McGregor JA, Silver RM, Trenkwalder C, Walters AS. Consensus clinical practice guidelines for the diagnosis and treatment of restless legs syndrome/Willis-Ekbom disease during pregnancy and lactation. Sleep Med Rev. 2015;22:64–77.
52. Earley CJ, Connor J, Garcia-Borreguero D, Jenner P, Winkelman J, Zee PC, Allen R. Altered brain iron homeostasis and dopaminergic function in restless legs syndrome (Willis-Ekbom disease). Sleep Med. 2014;15:1288–301.

53. Aul EA, Davis BJ, Rodnitzky RL. The importance of formal serum iron studies in the assessment of restless legs syndrome. Neurology. 1998;51:912.
54. Sun ER, Chen CA, Ho G, Earley CJ, Allen RP. Iron and the restless legs syndrome. Sleep. 1998;21:371–7.
55. Sikandar R, Khealani BA, Wasay M. Predictors of restless legs syndrome in pregnancy: a hospital based cross sectional survey from Pakistan. Sleep Med. 2009;10:676–8.
56. Dzaja A, Wehrle R, Lancel M, Pollmächer T. Elevated estradiol plasma levels in women with restless legs during pregnancy. Sleep. 2009;32:169–74.
57. Tunç T, Karadağ YS, Doğulu F, Inan LE. Predisposing factors of restless legs syndrome in pregnancy. Mov Disord. 2007;22:627–31.
58. Botez MI, Lambert B. Folate deficiency and restless legs syndrome in pregnancy. N Engl J Med. 1977;297:670.
59. Oyiengo D, Louis M, Hott B, Bourjeily G. Sleep disorders in pregnancy. Clin Chest Med. 2014;35:571–87.
60. Vahdat M, Sariri E, Miri S, Rohani M, Kashanian M, Sabet A, Zamani B. Prevalence and associated features of restless legs syndrome in a population of Iranian women during pregnancy. Int J Gynaecol Obstet. 2013;123:46–9.
61. Li Y, Mirzaei F, O'Reilly EJ, Winkelman J, Malhotra A, Okereke OI, Ascherio A, Gao X. Prospective study of restless legs syndrome and risk of depression in women. Am J Epidemiol. 2012;176:279–88.
62. Ramirez JO, Cabrera SA, Hidalgo H, Cabrera SG, Linnebank M, Bassetti CL, Kallweit U. Is preeclampsia associated with restless legs syndrome? Sleep Med. 2013;14:894–6.
63. Manconi M, Ulfberg J, Berger K, Ghorayeb I, Wesström J, Fulda S, Allen RP, Pollmächer T. When gender matters: restless legs syndrome. Report of the "RLS and woman" workshop endorsed by the European RLS Study Group. Sleep Med Rev. 2012;16:297–307.
64. Cesnik E, Casetta I, Turri M, Govoni V, Granieri E, Ferini Strambi L, Manconi M. Transient RLS during pregnancy is a risk factor for the chronic idiopathic form. Neurology. 2010;75:2117–20.
65. Berger K, Luedemann J, Trenkwalder C, John U, Kessler C. Sex and the risk of restless legs syndrome in the general population. Arch Intern Med. 2004;164:196–202.
66. Schnieder J, Krafft A, Bloch A, Hubner A, Raimondi M, Baumann C, Werth E, Bassetti C. Iron infusion in restless legs syndrome in the third trimester of pregnancy. Sleep Med. 2011;12:S17–8.
67. Wang C, Graham DJ, Kane RC, Xie D, Wernecke M, Levenson M, MaCurdy TE, Houstoun M, Ryan Q, Wong S, Mott K, Sheu TC, Limb S, Worrall C, Kelman JA, Reichman ME. Comparative risk of anaphylactic reactions associated with intravenous iron products. JAMA. 2015;314:2062–8.
68. Aurora RN, Kristo DA, Bista SR, Rowley JA, Zak RS, Casey KR, Lamm CI, Tracy SL, Rosenberg RS. The treatment of restless legs syndrome and periodic limb movement disorder in adults—an update for 2012: practice parameters with an evidence-based systematic review and meta-analysis: an American Academy of Sleep Medicine Clinical Practice Guideline. Sleep. 2012;35:1039–62.
69. Dostal M, Weber-Schoendorfer C, Sobesky J, Schaefer C. Pregnancy outcome following use of levodopa, pramipexole, ropinirole, and rotigotine for restless legs syndrome during pregnancy: a case series. Eur J Neurol. 2013;20:1241–6.
70. Peppard PE, Young T, Palta M, Dempsey J, Skatrud J. Longitudinal study of moderate weight change and sleep-disordered breathing. JAMA. 2000;284:3015–21.
71. Wise RA, Polito AJ, Krishnan V. Respiratory physiology in pregnancy. Immunol Allergy Clin North Am. 2006;26:1–12.
72. Douglas NJ. Respiratory physiology: understanding the control of ventilation. In: Kryger MH, Roth T, Dement WC, editors. Principles and practices of sleep medicine. 5th ed. St. Louis, MO: Elsevier Saunders; 2010. p. 250–8.
73. Thomson S, Morrell MJ, Cordingley JJ, Semple SJ. Ventilation is unstable during drowsiness before sleep onset. J Appl Physiol. 2005;99:2036–44.

74. O'Brien LM, Bullough AS, Owusu JT, Tremblay KA, Brincat CA, Chames MC, Kalbfleisch JD, Chervin RD. Snoring during pregnancy and delivery outcomes: a cohort study. Sleep. 2013;36:1625–32.
75. Pien GW, Schwab RJ. Sleep disorders during pregnancy. Sleep. 2004;27:1405–17.
76. Sahota PD, Jain SS, Dhand R. Sleep disorders in pregnancy. Curr Opin Pulm Med. 2003;9:477–83.
77. Pien GW, Fife D, Pack AI, Nkwuo E, Schwab RJ. Changes in symptoms of sleep-disordered breathing during pregnancy. Sleep. 2005;28:1299–305.
78. Olivarez SA, Ferres M, Antony K, Mattewal A, Maheshwari B, Sangi-Haghpeykar H, Aagaard-Tillery K. Obstructive sleep apnea screening in pregnancy, perinatal outcomes, and impact of maternal obesity. Am J Perinatol. 2011;28:651–8.
79. Fung AM, Wilson DL, Lappas M, Howard M, Barnes M, O'Donoghue F, Tong S, Esdale H, Fleming G, Walker SP. Effects of maternal obstructive sleep apnoea on fetal growth: a prospective cohort study. PLoS One. 2013;8:e68057.
80. Wilson DL, Walker SP, Fung AM, O'Donoghue F, Barnes M, Howard M. Can we predict sleep-disordered breathing in pregnancy? The clinical utility of symptoms. J Sleep Res. 2013;22:670–8.
81. Olivarez SA, Maheshwari B, McCarthy M, Zacharias N, van den Veyver I, Casturi L, Sangi-Haghpeykar H, Aagaard-Tillery K. Prospective trial on obstructive sleep apnea in pregnancy and fetal heart rate monitoring. AM J Obstet Gynecol. 2010;202:552.e1–7.
82. Louis J, Auckly D, Miladinovic B, Shepherd A, Mencin P, Kumar D, Mercer B, Redline S. Perinatal outcomes associated with obstructive sleep apnea in obese pregnant women. Obstet Gynecol. 2012;120:1085–92.
83. Facco FL, Ouyang DW, Zee PC, Strohl AE, Gonzalez AB, Lim C, Grobman GA. Implications of sleep-disordered breathing in pregnancy. Am J Obstet Gynecol. 2014;210:559.e1–6.
84. Chen YH, Kang JH, Lin CC, Wang IT, Keller JJ, Lin HC. Obstructive sleep apnea and the risk of adverse pregnancy outcomes. Am J Obstet Gynecol. 2012;206:136.e1–5.
85. Louis JM, Mogos MF, Salemi JL, Redline S, Salihu HM. Obstructive sleep apnea and severe maternal-infant morbidity/mortality in the United States, 1998–2009. Sleep. 2014;37:843–9.
86. Pamidi S, Pinto LM, Marc I, Benedetti A, Schwartzman K, Kimoff RJ. Maternal sleep-disordered breathing and adverse pregnancy outcome: a systemic review and metaanalysis. Am J Obstet Gynecol. 2014;201:52.e1–14.
87. Izci-Balserak B, Jackson N, Ratcliffe SA, Pack AI, Pien GW. Sleep-disordered breathing and daytime napping are associated with maternal hyperglycemia. Sleep Breath. 2013;17:1093–102.
88. Bourjeily G, Raker CA, Chalhoub M, Miller MA. Pregnancy and fetal outcomes of symptoms of sleep-disordered breathing. Eur Respir J. 2010;36:849–55.
89. Reutrakul S, Zaidi N, Wroblewski K, Kay HH, Ismail M, Ehrmann DA, Van Cauter E. Sleep disturbances and their relationship to glucose tolerance in pregnancy. Diabetes Care. 2011;34:2454–7.
90. Louis JM, Auckley D, Sokol RJ, Mercer BM. Maternal and neonatal morbidities associated with obstructive sleep apnea complicating pregnancy. Am J Obstet Gynecol. 2010;202:261.e1–5.
91. Antony KM, Agrawal A, Arndt ME, Murphy AM, Alapat PM, Guntupalli KK, Aagaard KM. Association of adverse perinatal outcomes with screening measures of obstructive sleep apnea. J Perinatol. 2014;34:441–8.
92. Ding XX, Wu YL, Xu SJ, Zhang SF, Jia XM, Zhu RP, Hao JH, Tao FB. A systematic review and quantitative assessment of sleep-disordered breathing during pregnancy and perinatal outcomes. Sleep Breath. 2014;18:703–13.
93. Dunietz GL, Chervin RD, O'Brien LM. Sleep-disordered breathing during pregnancy: future implications for cardiovascular health. Obstet Gynecol Surv. 2014;69:164–76.
94. Jones CR. Diagnostic and management approach to common sleep disorders during pregnancy. Clin Obstet Gynecol. 2013;56:360–71.

95. Facco FL, Ouyang DW, Zee PC, Grobman WA. Development of a pregnancy-specific screening tool for sleep apnea. J Clin Sleep Med. 2012;8:389–94.
96. Guilleminault C, Kreutzer M, Chang JL. Pregnancy, sleep disordered breathing and treatment with nasal continuous positive airway pressure. Sleep Med. 2004;5:43–51.
97. Guilleminault C, Palombini L, Poyares D, Takaoka S, Huynh NT, El-Sayed Y. Pre-eclampsia and nasal CPAP: part 1. Early intervention with nasal CPAP in pregnant women with risk-factors for pre-eclampsia: preliminary findings. Sleep Med. 2007;9:9–14.
98. Montserrat JM, Ferrer M, Hernandez L, Farré R, Vilagut G, Navajas D, Badia JR, Carrasco E, De Pablo J, Ballester E. Effectiveness of CPAP treatment in daytime function in sleep apnea syndrome: a randomized controlled study with an optimized placebo. Am J Respir Crit Care Med. 2001;164:608–13.
99. Engleman HM, Martin SE, Deary IJ, Douglas NJ. Effect of continuous positive airway pressure treatment on daytime function in sleep apnoea/hypopnoea syndrome. Lancet. 1994;343:572–5.
100. Jenkinson C, Davies RJ, Mullins R, Stradling JR. Comparison of therapeutic and subtherapeutic nasal continuous positive airway pressure for obstructive sleep apnoea: a randomised prospective parallel trial. Lancet. 1999;353:2100–5.
101. Poyares D, Guilleminault C, Hachul H, Fujita L, Takaoka S, Tufik S, Sass N. Pre-eclampsia and nasal CPAP: part 2. Hypertension during pregnancy, chronic snoring, and early nasal CPAP intervention. Sleep Med. 2007;9:15–21.
102. Whitehead C, Tong S, Wilson D, Howard M, Walker SP. Treatment of early-onset preeclampsia with continuous positive airway pressure. Obstet Gynecol. 2015;125:1106–9.
103. Edwards N, Blyton DM, Kirjavainen T, Kesby GJ, Sullivan CE. Nasal continuous positive airway pressure reduces sleep-induced blood pressure increments in preeclampsia. Am J Respir Crit Care Med. 2000;162:252–7.
104. Blyton DM, Sullivan CE, Edwards N. Reduced nocturnal cardiac output associated with pre-eclampsia is minimized with the use of nocturnal nasal CPAP. Sleep. 2004;27:79–84.
105. Blyton DM, Skilton MR, Edwards N, Hennessy A, Celermajer DS, Sullivan CE. Treatment of sleep disordered breathing reverses low fetal activity levels in preeclampsia. Sleep. 2013;36:15–21.
106. Lee KA, Gay CL. Sleep in late pregnancy predicts length of labor and type of delivery. Am J Obstet Gynecol. 2004;6:2041–6.
107. Beebe KR, Lee KA. Sleep disturbance in late pregnancy and early labor. J Perinat Neonatal Nurs. 2007;21:103–8.
108. Micheli K, Komninos I, Bagkeris E, Roumeliotaki T, Koutis A, Kogevinas M, Chatzi L. Sleep patterns in late pregnancy and risk of preterm birth and fetal growth restriction. Epidemiology. 2011;22:738–44.
109. Strange LB, Parker KP, Moore ML, Strickland OL, Bliwise DL. Disturbed sleep and preterm birth: a potential relationship? Clin Exp Obstet Gynecol. 2009;36:166–8.
110. Okun ML, Schetter CD, Glynn LM. Poor sleep quality is associated with preterm birth. Sleep. 2011;34:1493–8.
111. Okun ML, Luther JF, Wisniewski SR, Sit D, Prairie BA, Wisner KL. Disturbed sleep, a novel risk factor for preterm birth? J Womens Health. 2012;21:54–60.
112. Skouteris H, Germano C, Wertheim EH, Paxton SJ, Milgrom J. Sleep quality and depression during pregnancy: a prospective study. J Sleep Res. 2008;17:217–20.
113. Herring SJ, Nelson DB, Pien GW, Homko C, Goetzl LM, Davey A, Foster GD. Objectively measured sleep duration and hyperglycemia in pregnancy. Sleep Med. 2014;15:51–5.
114. Qiu C, Enquobahrie D, Frederick IO, Abetew D, Williams MA. Glucose intolerance and gestational diabetes risk in relation to sleep duration and snoring during pregnancy: a pilot study. BMC Womens Health. 2010;10:17.
115. Abeysena C, Jayawardana P, Seneviratne RA. Effect of psychosocial stress and physical activity on low birthweight: a cohort study. J Obstet Gynaecol Res. 2010;36:296–303.

116. Zafarghandi N, Hadavand S, Davati A, Mohseni SM, Kimiaiimoghadam F, Torkestani F. The effects of sleep quality and duration in late pregnancy on labor and fetal outcome. J Matern Fetal Neonatal Med. 2012;25:535–7.

117. Chang JJ, Pien GW, Duntley SP, Macones GA. Sleep deprivation during pregnancy and maternal and fetal outcomes: is there a relationship? Sleep Med Rev. 2010;14:107–14.

118. Okun ML, Ebert R, Saini B. A review of sleep-promoting medications used in pregnancy. Am J Obstet Gynecol. 2015;212:428–41.

119. Wang LH, Lin HC, Lin CC, Chen YH, Lin HC. Increased risk of adverse pregnancy outcomes in women receiving zolpidem during pregnancy. Clin Pharmacol Ther. 2010;88:369–74.

120. Wikner BN, Stiller CO, Bergman U, Asker C, Källén B. Use of benzodiazepines and benzodiazepine receptor agonists during pregnancy: neonatal outcome and congenital malformations. Pharmacoepidemiol Drug Saf. 2007;16:1203–10.

121. Juric S, Newport DJ, Ritchie JC, Galanti M, Stowe ZN. Zolpidem (Ambien) in pregnancy: placental passage and outcome. Arch Womens Ment Health. 2009;12:441–6.

Chapter 10
Insomnia and Menopause

Helena Hachul, Andréia Gomes Bezerra, and Monica Levy Andersen

Abstract Global life expectancy has increased substantially over the last century. For women, this means that they now live nearly one-third of their lives in the climacteric period with the undesirable effects of hypoestrogenism. The consequences of this decrease in estrogen may occur in the short or long term. Among the early manifestations, the most important are vasomotor symptoms, insomnia, increased irritability, anxiety, depression, and loss of memory. Hormonal changes can be responsible for insomnia in the menopause transition and postmenopause, but it can also be caused by biopsychological changes that often happen in women's lives. Many women retire during this time, and may pass through social and health changes. Women can develop "empty nest syndrome," when their children leave home. These changes can lead to depression, a factor which is closely linked to insomnia. In addition, other consequences of hypoestrogenism, such as genital atrophy, nocturia, body pain, and other changes, can lead to sleep fragmentation. The aim of this chapter is not only to review the current literature on the subject but also to describe the pathophysiology of insomnia in postmenopause and the care that can be given by a multidisciplinary team. We highlight the importance of evaluating the patient as a whole, in an individualized and personalized manner. In our view, looking at both the body and the mind, from a hormonal to a biopsychosocial context, is the best approach to effective treatment.

Keywords Sleep disorders • Postmenopause • Menopausal transition • Hormonal therapy • Antidepressants • Sedatives • Hypnotics • Complementary and alternative medicine

H. Hachul, M.D., Ph.D. (✉)
Departments of Gynecology and Psychobiology, Head of the Women's Sleep Division,
Universidade Federal de São Paulo, Rua Napoleão de Barros, 925, São Paulo,
SP 04021-002, Brazil
e-mail: helena.hachul@hotmail.com

A.G. Bezerra, M.Sc. • M.L. Andersen, Ph.D.
Department of Psychobiology, Universidade Federal de São Paulo, Rua Napoleão de Barros,
925, São Paulo, SP 04021-002, Brazil
e-mail: andreia.gomes@unifesp.br; ml.andersen12@gmail.com

© Springer International Publishing Switzerland 2017
H.P. Attarian (ed.), *Clinical Handbook of Insomnia*, Current Clinical Neurology,
DOI 10.1007/978-3-319-41400-3_10

Basic Concepts

Menopause

Menopause is commonly defined as the moment when women's menstrual cycles and periods cease permanently, as a result of regressive modifications, including lack of ovulation and sexual hormonal synthesis impairment. According to the World Health Organization [1], the menopause transition begins with a decrease in reproductive capacity at around 40 years of age, and represents the change from the reproductive (menacme) to the non-reproductive life stages. Thus, we can assume that menopause is a sectional period, or a transversal event in women's lives, most specifically represented by the date of the last menstruation. It is confirmed after 12 consecutive months of amenorrhea (i.e., lack of menstruation).

The most important concepts, based on the definitions of the International Menopause Society and the World Health Organization [1, 2], are the following:

- Perimenopause: the period around menopause, both immediately before and the first year after menopause.
- Menopausal transition: the period before menopause characterized by marked variability in the menstrual cycle.
- Climacteric: the period marking the transition from the reproductive to non-reproductive phase. It encompasses longer periods than perimenopause (both before and after) and when associated with symptoms is known as climacteric syndrome.
- Premenopause: the period before menopause. It encompasses the entire reproductive period up to the definitive cessation of menstruation.
- Postmenopause: the period after menopause.
- Early postmenopause: the first 5 years after menopause.
- Late postmenopause: more than 5 years after menopause.

There are symptoms in each phase of postmenopause related to hypoestrogenism, due to the short-term or long-term absence of estrogen [3].

Pathophysiology of Menopausal Transition and Postmenopausal Period

At birth, the ovaries have about 2 million follicles. The number of follicles decays over women's lives. With this reduction, there is greater activation of the pituitary-gonadal axis and increased production of the follicle-stimulating hormone (FSH). Currently, measures of FSH and luteinizing hormone (LH) are considered reliable in terms of confirming the reproductive stage of women (reproductive period, menopausal transition, and postmenopause) [3]. Nevertheless, the report of last menstrual cycle is still the most important point in regard to diagnosing menopausal transition and postmenopause (Fig. 10.1).

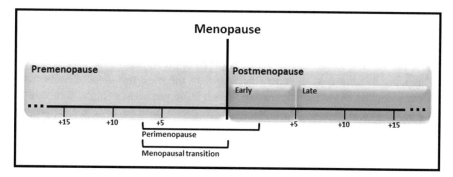

Fig. 10.1 Women's life-span and perimenopausal events [3]. The *horizontal bar* represents life-span

The rise in FSH levels leads to an increase in the recruitment of follicles, resulting in acceleration of follicular maturation, with a consequent shortening of the follicular phase of the menstrual cycle. Follicular atresia, the breakdown of the ovarian follicles, is also related to the reduction in estrogen, since the follicles are responsible for its production.

Clinical Manifestations

The physiological changes described above are responsible for the clinical manifestations arising from the transition to the postmenopausal period. The regularity of the menstrual cycle depends on the number of follicles. Usually, women present shorter cycles and then longer ones as a consequence of fluctuating hormone levels. Women can present different patterns of irregularity, such as interruption of the menstrual cycle, and so be in periods of amenorrhea until postmenopause is established. The period when women become affected by hypoestrogenism leads to physiological changes in the short and long terms.

Among the early manifestations, the most important are the presence of vasomotor symptoms (with hot flashes and increased sweating), which occur in nearly 70 % of women [4], insomnia, increased irritability, anxiety and depression, loss of memory, and decreased libido. As time passes, women suffer from the consequences of longer term absence of estrogen. Late-menopause manifestations can be found in the cardiovascular system (such as increases in low-density lipoprotein), in bone (osteoporosis), skin (loss of collagen), and the urogenital system (atrophy and vaginal dryness) [4].

Insomnia in the Climacteric

According to the most recent version of the Diagnostic and Statistical Manual of Mental Disorders/DSM-V [5], insomnia is defined as difficulties initiating and/or maintaining sleep or early-morning awakening accompanied by daytime impairment. Population-based studies indicate that about one-third of adults report insomnia symptoms, with objective prevalence estimates being higher than the prevalence according to subjective measures [6]. Insomnia has a multifactorial profile, with several social, environmental, psychological, and physiological factors influencing its course, with gender being one of the most prominent factors influencing insomnia among adults. Insomnia is a more prevalent complaint in women than men, and it is usually associated with menopause in middle-age women. According to epidemiological studies, the prevalence of insomnia in women is usually higher than in men, regardless of age and life period. As observed in a Brazilian sample, 40 % of women complain of insomnia, while the condition is observed in only 25 % of men [7]. Additionally, aging is a significant risk factor for the development of insomnia: a large US population study has demonstrated that about 30 % of individuals over the age of 65 have some degree of difficulty in maintaining sleep [8]. Our previous studies showed that menopause itself exerts a modest, but important influence on objective sleep patterns, independent of age [9]. Considering that both female gender and aging are significantly associated with insomnia, the high prevalence of this sleep disorder becomes important in postmenopausal women. Indeed the prevalence of insomnia rises during the postmenopausal period, ranging between 28 and 63 %, according to different studies [10–12]. Women frequently report disrupted sleep and awakenings when hot flashes occur during the night [13]. Sleep impairment in menopausal women, however, can persist even after associated symptoms, such as hot flashes, have resolved [14] and remains highly prevalent in postmenopause. Although early menopause is associated with several symptoms, complaints related to sleep are higher in the late postmenopausal group [15].

Another consequence of hypoestrogenism is the atrophy of the lower genital urinary tract that frequently results in nocturia (i.e., the need to wake in the middle of the night to urinate) [16]. Because the individual constantly wakes up, nocturia ultimately leads to sleep fragmentation, resulting in an insomnia complaint. A recent literature review showed that nocturia was related to poorer quality of sleep due to the decrease in the number of hours of restful sleep, thereby affecting sleep quality [17]. These data become even more relevant in the current sociodemographic scenario. Global life expectancy has increased substantially in the last century, rising from about 50 years in 1900 to 64 years in 1990, and to 71 years in 2010 [18]. Together with the natural growth in world population, women now live longer after menopause and have to face sleep-related complications during the postmenopausal period. Climacteric-related sleep impairment is a significant public health issue due to the potential negative impact on mental health, quality of life, and productivity.

Clinical Evaluation of Insomnia in the Climacteric

Considering the multifactorial aspect of the peri- and postmenopausal periods, it is extremely important for this population to be evaluated by a multidisciplinary team. A proposed flowchart for the clinical evaluation can be found in Fig. 10.2. Insomnia

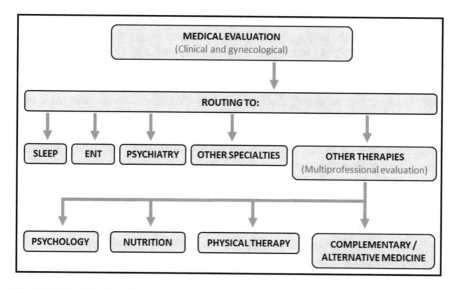

Fig. 10.2 Flowchart for the approach to a postmenopausal woman with insomnia. This flowchart assumes a primary evaluation at a gynecology clinic/service, since this is the most frequent service sought by postmenopausal women. Once the insomnia complaint is identified, the preferred option is to route the patient to a sleep clinic/service. Acknowledging the fact that this kind of service is not always available, the most specific possible specialty related to the patient's complaint should be identified, based on a potential differential diagnosis (ENT and psychiatry are often requested, due to sleep apnea and comorbid anxiety, respectively). Multidisciplinary treatment is desirable. Physical therapy plays an important role, especially when insomnia figures concomitantly with pain complaints. Lastly, complementary and alternative treatments may be useful as adjuvant treatments, especially acupuncture, yoga, and massage

can be associated with several comorbidities and life circumstances such as aging, vasomotor symptoms, climacteric syndrome, obesity, and psychiatric disorders [19–22], and this should be acknowledged in the clinical examination.

It is worth mentioning that the evaluation of the social context deserves further awareness. In addition to physical changes, this stage of life has marked social changes. Women can develop "empty nest syndrome," when their children leave home; this and other changes in life circumstances can lead to depression, which is closely linked to insomnia [23].

Because physiological and hormonal changes during the climacteric affect women's quality of life and sleep, the clinical evaluation of these women should also include a careful gynecological assessment. A decrease in estrogen levels during postmenopause leads to symptoms, such as hot flashes and excessive sweating that can also disrupt sleep. These vasomotor symptoms are often associated with psychological distress, increased anxiety, irritability, and depressive symptoms. Although these psychological outcomes may or may not be related to decreased estrogen levels, they can be a secondary cause of insomnia.

A clinical evaluation by a sleep medicine specialist is essential for the proper assessment of the patient. This is due to the common comorbidity between insomnia and other sleep disorders such as obstructive sleep apnea (OSA) and restless leg syndrome (RLS), which are highly prevalent in postmenopausal women [24–26]. The increased prevalence of OSA seems to be the result of a reduction in female hormones, particularly progesterone, considered a respiratory stimulant [27, 28]. Regarding RLS, it is known that this disease is more prevalent in women who present vasomotor symptoms during menopausal transition [24]. These conditions may therefore need to be considered as part of a differential diagnosis, since they can be a primary source of excessive daytime sleepiness, which can be confused with an insomnia complaint. In fact, a previous study indicated that 50 % of women who have a complaint of insomnia also have a diagnosis of sleep apnea [29]. In a cohort of 326 postmenopausal women with OSA, the prevalence of insomnia was 83 % [25, 26].

Considering the important comorbidity between insomnia and other sleep disorders, a careful sleep diagnosis is required. Polysomnography, the gold standard for the objective diagnosis of most sleep disorders, must be used whenever possible. In addition, standardized questionnaires such as the Pittsburgh Sleep Quality Index (PSQI), the Insomnia Severity Index (ISI), and Epworth Sleepiness Scale (ESS) are of great value in the screening of sleep conditions. Unfortunately, access to a sleep medicine clinic or service is not always available. In this case, the patient should be referred to the most appropriate medical specialist according to her insomnia complaints and related symptoms. Ear, nose, and throat (ENT) and psychiatric services stand out as the most important due to the high comorbidities between insomnia and OSA and psychiatric conditions. Other specialties may also be suggested, such as pulmonologists for a broader assessment of sleep-disordered breathing, and neurologists for a better assessment of RLS, among others.

Contributing to the final clinical screening, the evaluation of the patient by other health professionals such as physical therapists, nutritionists, and psychologists could also be useful. Physical therapy can be an important therapy for chronic pain, fibromyalgia, and arthritis, conditions that might be associated with insomnia and are often experienced by women in the climacteric [30, 31]. Nutritional care is important because of the high prevalence of obesity among postmenopausal women [32], as being overweight is closely associated with increased risk for sleep apnea. Weight loss can be beneficial, not only in reducing OSA, but also in consequently reducing sleep fragmentation, as well as reducing cardiovascular outcomes [33].

Beyond the physical and hormonal changes related to menopause, middle-age women are at a high risk of developing insomnia due to the stresses related to a multitask lifestyle that can include demands from work, family, and social life. Thus, the evaluation of women by a psychologist, and continuous psychological follow-up, can play an important role in preventing or reversing insomnia complaints. The increasing role of women in the labor force and involvement in socioeconomic activities has not necessarily been accompanied by a decrease in household and family responsibilities, leading to increasing levels of stress. In addition, for many women it is a time when their role in the family is changing as their children become less dependent on them and eventually leave home. As a result, sleep can be greatly affected by changes in the daily lives of contemporary women. Together with the fact that insomnia has been related to a higher prevalence of anxiety [34] and depression [22], psychological support by a health professional can be extremely important.

Treatment of Insomnia in Postmenopausal Woman

The whole context of postmenopause should be considered for optimal treatment, including not only the insomnia complaint, but other factors such as its source (primary or secondary), women's general and gynecological medical condition, hormonal profile, presence of musculoskeletal pain, presence of concomitant sleep disorders, presence of other comorbidities, and psychosocial context.

The literature is broad in regard to the various types of treatments and approaches for the treatment or management of insomnia in climacteric women. Several therapeutic options are currently available, ranging from hormonal therapies and pharmacological agents to non-pharmacological and behavioral treatments. Table 10.1 depicts the levels of evidence of the most used therapeutic methods for insomnia in climacteric women.

Table 10.1 Levels of evidence of the most used therapeutic methods for insomnia in climacteric women [36]

Treatment method	Recommendations	Evidence
Biomedical and pharmacological agents		
Hormone therapy		
Sedatives/hypnotics		
Zolpidem	Probably should not be considered	C
Eszopiclone	Suggested	B
Ramelteon	Probably should not be considered	C
Antidepressants		
Paroxetine and venlafaxine	Not available	
Escitalopram	Suggested	B
Citalopram	Probably should not be considered	C
Quetiapine	Probably should not be considered	C
Mirtazapine	Probably should not be considered	C
Gabapentin	Suggested	B
Herbal and nutritional supplements		
Isoflavones	Suggested	B
Valerian root	Suggested	B
Pycnogenol	Probably should not be considered	C
Phyto-female complex	Probably should not be considered	C
Kampo	Not recommended	A
Behavioral interventions		
Cognitive behavioral therapy		
For insomnia	Recommended	A
In general	Probably should not be considered	C
High-intensity exercise	Suggested	B
Hypnosis	Suggested	B
Yoga	Probably should not be considered	C
Massage	Probably should not be considered	C
Acupuncture	Probably should not be considered	C

Hormone Therapy

Due to the hormonal characteristics of the menopause transition and climacteric, hormone therapy stands out as one of the most important clinical treatments for menopausal syndrome [35]. It seems to be a useful therapeutic choice to manage and treat vasomotor symptoms. Consequently, it has been theoretically argued that hormone therapy can improve chronic insomnia indirectly, as vasomotor symptoms and insomnia complaints are closely associated [21]. The same efficacy observed in reducing vasomotor symptoms is not, however, observed in regard to climacteric-related insomnia. Several clinical trials have been performed to evaluate the use of hormone therapy in postmenopausal insomnia complaints, but the results acquired so far are inconsistent: while some trials report positive results, others show partial or negative effects [36]. Several factors account for these discrepancies, including the high heterogeneity within these studies and the variety of treatment protocols, dosages, and formulations.

Despite the aforementioned variability, hormone therapy is suggested, either in the forms of low-dose conjugated estrogen or low-dose progesterone. However, one must bear in mind the potential side effects of hormone therapy (especially thromboembolic events) whenever prescribing it to postmenopausal women [37]. This therapy should be considered when insomnia is refractory to other treatments and when it is comorbid with other distressing menopausal symptoms. Additionally, to justify its use the potential benefits of hormone therapy should outweigh the risks of continued hormonal exposure.

Sedatives/Hypnotics

In general, sedatives and hypnotics present good clinical efficacy in treating insomnia complaints. However, some important caveats should be borne in mind whenever these drugs are considered for climacteric women. First, caution in their use is advised considering the possible negative consequences of long-term use [38, 39]. It should also be taken into account that these drugs act only on insomnia symptoms and complaints, but may have no effect on the primary cause. Finally, it is unclear whether hypnotics show some degree of specificity to postmenopausal insomnia, or if they act generically.

Zolpidem

The use of Zolpidem for insomnia in regular patients has been the focus of many clinical studies, presenting successful clinical results and, consequently, has become a common therapeutic option. Only a single report on Zolpidem as a treatment for postmenopausal insomnia has been published [40]. Despite the positive effects found in this study, it should be noted that the dosage was twice that currently recommended for women, and that a non-standardized sleep measure was used.

Eszopiclone

Eszopiclone has proven to be effective in treating insomnia at a dose of 3 mg, based on the results of a number of randomized controlled trials [41, 42]. Moreover, this drug leads to a concomitant improvement in anxiety and depression symptoms [41], which may secondarily affect sleep quality. As a drawback, one may note that the Food and Drugs Administration (FDA) recommends a dose of 1 mg, based on potential residual impairment observed the morning after use.

Ramelteon

This drug, which is an MT1 and MT2 melatonin receptor agonist, has been indicated by the FDA as a useful alternative for the treatment of insomnia. However, it seems that the effects are clinically relevant only after 4 weeks of use [43].

Antidepressants

Paroxetine, Venlafaxine, and Desvenlafaxine

Several trials have been performed to evaluate the effects of these drugs on vasomotor symptoms, but none has been performed to evaluate their effects on sleep and insomnia complaints [36].

Escitalopram

Three trials employing escitalopram as a potential treatment for insomnia in perimenopausal women have shown positive results. These positive results were not restricted to sleep-related complaints, but also to vasomotor symptoms, mood, and quality of life [44–46].

Citalopram and Fluoxetine

Only one study has evaluated both these drugs as treatments for climacteric women. Insomnia improved only with the use of citalopram, while fluoxetine had no effect. The effects of citalopram were observed only on sleep-related complaints, but not on vasomotor symptoms [47].

Quetiapine

Positive effects were observed in a single study of 40 perimenopausal women with concomitant major depression and chronic insomnia [48].

Mirtazapine

Only a single case series has evaluated the effects of mirtazapine for insomnia, with good results. However, considering the low level of evidence, new and broader studies are needed in order to estimate the real potential of mirtazapine on the current topic [49].

Gabapentin

Gabapentin is a neurotherapeutic drug, originally thought to act as an anticonvulsant. Due to its clinical efficacy in previous case reports and clinical trials [50, 51], it is now considered as a first-line pharmacological treatment, mainly when strong vasomotor symptoms are associated with insomnia. Doses between 300 and 900 mg are indicated, based on previous studies.

Herbal and Nutritional Supplements

There are a wide variety of herbal and nutritional supplements with supposed beneficial effects in insomnia, but in general, the level of evidence on their use is low. Despite usually being safer than pharmacotherapy, natural supplements should be used with caution, and risk-benefit evaluations should be performed before any of these supplements can be prescribed. A useful alternative is to combine pharmacologicals with these supplements for the treatment of insomnia.

Isoflavones

Isoflavones are known phytoestrogens, with potential use as an alternative to hormone therapy. A number of studies have demonstrated positive results both on sleep complaints and on polysomnographic results. The dosage, presentation, and clinical protocols vary greatly among protocols [52, 53].

Valerian Root

The use of *Valeriana officinalis* has been reported for diverse purposes since ancient times. Traditionally, it is believed that valerian has hypnogenic and sedative properties, in a benzodiazepine-like effect. The mechanism for the action of these effects is inconclusive, but it is believed that some compounds found in valerian root, especially valerenic acids and sesquiterpenoids, have some effect on GABA-A receptors [54].

Several studies have been conducted into the use of valerian for sleep, with most finding positive effects [55]. Among postmenopausal women, it has been described as resulting in significant improvements on subjective sleep quality, despite being ineffective as a treatment for primary insomnia [56, 57].

Pycnogenol

This is a French maritime pine bark extract, which was the focus of a single randomized controlled trial [58]. Positive effects were observed on subjective sleep, but
more studies are needed for a higher evidence level.

Phyto-Female Complex

This is a commercial blend composed of extracts of several herbal products (extracts
of black cohosh, dong quai, milk thistle, red clover, American ginseng, chaste-tree
berry), intended for the relief of menopausal symptoms. A single trial was performed on the use of this product for insomnia in climacteric women, with a modest
improvement in self-rated sleep quality [59]. However, this was a cohort of limited
sample size with the participants not meeting criteria for chronic insomnia at baseline. Further studies are warranted for a higher evidence level.

Kampo

This form of herbal medicine, with its roots in traditional Chinese and Japanese
medicine, mainly relies on the prescription of specific herb blends for a variety of
disorders and complaints. Three trials were conducted with the use of Kampo for
insomnia in postmenopausal women, all of them providing negative results. Despite
its potential beneficial uses for other clinical conditions, Kampo should not be recommended for insomnia [36].

Cognitive Behavioral Therapy

Cognitive behavioral therapy stands as one of the most important non-
pharmacological treatments for several insomnia comorbidities, such as anxiety,
depression, and menopausal symptoms [60]. However, its effects on insomnia itself
and on sleep complaints in general are not so clear [60–62], mainly when evaluated
by means of subjective sleep assessment methods such as the Pittsburgh Sleep
Quality Index. Thus, generic cognitive behavioral therapy does not seem to be effective and should not be considered in cases of menopause-related insomnia.

On the other hand, cognitive behavioral therapy for insomnia (CBT-I) presents
remarkable results for these conditions. This is a multicomponent treatment targeting cognitive and behavioral factors specifically related to chronic insomnia, which
is currently considered as the first-line treatment for this condition according to the
clinical guidelines of the American Academy of Sleep Medicine [63]. Previous
studies demonstrated that up to 80 % of total patients who were subjected to CBT-I
present some benefit, while 40 % of the cases of insomnia resolve completely [64,
65]. Despite the lack of trials specifically devoted to postmenopausal women, the
positive results acquired through several other studies recommend CBT-I as a reliable tool for treatment of insomnia during climacteric.

High-Intensity Exercise

Several studies evaluated the effect of exercise on chronic insomnia among peri-menopausal women. In general, all of them showed positive results, leading to significant benefits in several sleep-related variables. However, the studies were heterogeneous in several aspects such as experimental design, definition of exercise, and outcome measures [36]. Thus, despite the fact that high-intensity physical exercise can be recommended as a useful tool for chronic insomnia in climacteric women, we still cannot draw conclusions about which practices, durations, and other exercise-related variables should be applied.

It is important to bear in mind that the postmenopause period encompasses several other relevant comorbidities in relation to physical exercise practice, such as hypertension and cardiovascular diseases, osteoporosis, and diabetes, among others. In this respect, exercise prescription should be adapted and contextualized to each individual. The prescription, evaluation, and follow-up of the exercise by a qualified professional are advised.

Hypnosis

Hypnosis is a method that changes the state of human consciousness, reducing peripheral awareness and involving focused attention by simple professional suggestion [66]. There are few studies about its efficacy in postmenopausal insomnia; however, one study did demonstrate improvement in Pittsburgh Sleep Quality Index scores and a reduction of hot flashes frequency after 5 weeks of clinical hypnosis [67]. Its use is suggested with this population [36], but it needs to be conducted by an expert professional to ensure that it is used safely and without side effects.

Yoga

Yoga is a concept from India that combines mind (meditation) and body practices (*asanas*, postures, breathing). In the West, yoga is often used solely as a physical exercise. Four months of Yoga was able to decrease the score of Insomnia Severity Index in perimenopausal women with chronic insomnia [68], demonstrating that this practice should be considered for climacteric women [36].

Massage

Massage therapy is another resource that is known to be safe. It acts on arterial and venous blood flow, and the lymphatic system [69]. Randomized clinical trials have demonstrated that massage improves subjective sleep in women in menopausal transition and in postmenopause [70, 71]; thus this method may be considered as another tool for the treatment of insomnia in women [36].

Acupuncture

Acupuncture is a therapeutic technique from traditional eastern medicine. Acupuncture is based on the belief that diseases are caused by an imbalance in energies which can be remedied by stimulating specific points on the skin.

A review of all the clinical trials in the current literature indicates that acupuncture does not seem to be an effective treatment for insomnia in postmenopause [36]. However, the high level of heterogeneity of these studies prevents us definitively from concluding that acupuncture has no therapeutic value. Although more evidence of its efficacy is required, it could be used with this population as a complementary treatment because it may have some positive effect and there are few side effects [72].

Final Considerations

Insomnia is commonly observed in women, especially in menopausal transition and postmenopause. Together with other symptoms from this period of life, this disorder negatively impacts their quality of life.

There is a lack of consistency among many studies which use similar therapeutic interventions (e.g., HT, exercise, and massage). The studies use very heterogeneous groups of women—some with chronic insomnia, some without chronic insomnia, some who are going through menopause, and some who are postmenopausal. This deficiency in standardized methods makes it difficult to identify the best therapeutic option for insomnia after menopause. Nevertheless, this does not seem a problem to choose the best intervention for these women. Although it is not clear which of these specific treatments is the most effective, we believe that the best intervention should be based on care being delivered by a multidisciplinary team that can provide an individualized and personal evaluation of the patient as a whole, and which looks at the body and mind from a hormonal to a biopsychological context in order to promote better health and a better quality of life.

Acknowledgements   The valuable assistance of Gabriel Pires and Lais Berro is appreciated.

References

1. World Health Organization. Research on the menopause in the 1990s. Geneva: World Health Organization; 1994.
2. International Menopause Society. Menopause terminology. http://www.imsociety.org/menopause_terminology.php
3. Soules MR, Sherman S, Parrott E, Rebar R, Santoro N, Utian W, et al. Executive summary: stages of reproductive aging workshop (STRAW). Climacteric. 2001;4(4):267–72.
4. Girão MJBC, Lima GR, Baracat EC. Ginecologia—Série Ginecologia UNIFESP. Brazil: Manole; 2009. 980 p.
5. American Psychiatric Association. Diagnostic and statistic manual of mental disorders. 5th ed. Arlington County, VA: American Psychiatric Publishing; 2013.

6. Castro LS, Poyares D, Leger D, Bittencourt L, Tufik S. Objective prevalence of insomnia in the São Paulo, Brazil epidemiologic sleep study. Ann Neurol. 2013;74(4):537–46.
7. Bittencourt LR, Santos-Silva R, Taddei JA, Andersen ML, de Mello MT, Tufik S. Sleep complaints in the adult Brazilian population: a national survey based on screening questions. J Clin Sleep Med. 2009;5(5):459–63.
8. Foley DJ, Monjan AA, Brown SL, Simonsick EM, Wallace RB, Blazer DG. Sleep complaints among elderly persons: an epidemiologic study of three communities. Sleep. 1995;18(6):425–32.
9. Hachul H, Frange C, Bezerra AG, Hirotsu C, Pires GN, Andersen ML, et al. The effect of menopause on objective sleep parameters: data from an epidemiologic study in São Paulo, Brazil. Maturitas. 2015;80(2):170–8.
10. Vigeta SM, Hachul H, Tufik S, de Oliveira EM. Sleep in postmenopausal women. Qual Health Res. 2012;22(4):466–75.
11. von Mühlen DG, Kritz-Silverstein D, Barrett-Connor E. A community-based study of menopause symptoms and estrogen replacement in older women. Maturitas. 1995;22(2):71–8.
12. Campos HH, Bittencourt LRA, Haidar MA, Tufik S, Baracat EC. Sleep disturbance prevalence in postmenopausal women. Rev Bras Ginecol Obstet. 2005;27(12):6.
13. Young T, Rabago D, Zgierska A, Austin D, Laurel F. Objective and subjective sleep quality in premenopausal, perimenopausal, and postmenopausal women in the Wisconsin Sleep Cohort Study. Sleep. 2003;26(6):667–72.
14. Okun ML, Kravitz HM, Sowers MF, Moul DE, Buysse DJ, Hall M. Psychometric evaluation of the Insomnia Symptom Questionnaire: a self-report measure to identify chronic insomnia. J Clin Sleep Med. 2009;5(1):41–51.
15. Hachul H, Bittencourt LR, Soares JM, Tufik S, Baracat EC. Sleep in post-menopausal women: differences between early and late post-menopause. Eur J Obstet Gynecol Reprod Biol. 2009;145(1):81–4.
16. Calleja-Agius J, Brincat MP. The urogenital system and the menopause. Climacteric. 2015;18 Suppl 1:18–22.
17. Furtado D, Hachul H, Andersen ML, Castro RA, Girão MB, Tufik S. Nocturia×disturbed sleep: a review. Int Urogynecol J. 2012;23(3):255–67.
18. World Health Organization. Life expectancy—data by WHO region. http://apps.who.int/gho/data/view.main.690?lang=en
19. Ensrud KE, Stone KL, Blackwell TL, Sawaya GF, Tagliaferri M, Diem SJ, et al. Frequency and severity of hot flashes and sleep disturbance in postmenopausal women with hot flashes. Menopause. 2009;16(2):286–92.
20. Da Fonseca AM, Bagnoli VR, Souza MA, Azevedo RS, Couto EB, Soares JM, et al. Impact of age and body mass on the intensity of menopausal symptoms in 5968 Brazilian women. Gynecol Endocrinol. 2013;29(2):116–8.
21. Cray L, Woods NF, Mitchell ES. Symptom clusters during the late menopausal transition stage: observations from the Seattle Midlife Women's Health Study. Menopause. 2010;17(5):972–7.
22. Brown JP, Gallicchio L, Flaws JA, Tracy JK. Relations among menopausal symptoms, sleep disturbance and depressive symptoms in midlife. Maturitas. 2009;62(2):184–9.
23. Sandilyan MB, Dening T. Mental health around and after the menopause. Menopause Int. 2011;17(4):142–7.
24. Wesstrom J, Nilsson S, Sundstrom-Poromaa I, Ulfberg J. Restless legs syndrome among women: prevalence, co-morbidity and possible relationship to menopause. Climacteric. 2008;11(5):422–8.
25. Guilleminault C, Palombini L, Poyares D, Chowdhuri S. Chronic insomnia, postmenopausal women, and sleep disordered breathing: part 1. Frequency of sleep disordered breathing in a cohort. J Psychosom Res. 2002;53(1):611–5.
26. Guilleminault C, Palombini L, Poyares D, Chowdhuri S. Chronic insomnia, premenopausal women and sleep disordered breathing: part 2. Comparison of nondrug treatment trials in normal breathing and UARS post menopausal women complaining of chronic insomnia. J Psychosom Res. 2002;53(1):617–23.

27. Bixler EO, Vgontzas AN, Lin HM, Ten Have T, Rein J, Vela-Bueno A, et al. Prevalence of sleep-disordered breathing in women: effects of gender. Am J Respir Crit Care Med. 2001;163(3 Pt 1):608–13.

28. Andersen ML, Bittencourt LR, Antunes IB, Tufik S. Effects of progesterone on sleep: a possible pharmacological treatment for sleep-breathing disorders? Curr Med Chem. 2006;13(29):3575–82.

29. Hachul de Campos H, Brandão LC, D'Almeida V, Grego BH, Bittencourt LR, Tufik S, et al. Sleep disturbances, oxidative stress and cardiovascular risk parameters in postmenopausal women complaining of insomnia. Climacteric. 2006;9(4):312–9.

30. Parish JM. Sleep-related problems in common medical conditions. Chest. 2009;135(2): 563–72.

31. Martínez-Jauand M, Sitges C, Femenia J, Cifre I, González S, Chialvo D, et al. Age-of-onset of menopause is associated with enhanced painful and non-painful sensitivity in fibromyalgia. Clin Rheumatol. 2013;32(7):975–81.

32. Lizcano F, Guzmán G. Estrogen deficiency and the origin of obesity during menopause. Biomed Res Int. 2014;2014:757461.

33. Zargarian N, Lindquist R, Gross CR, Treat-Jacobson D. Outcome measures of behavioral weight loss programs in perimenopause. South Med J. 2014;107(8):486–96.

34. Terauchi M, Hiramitsu S, Akiyoshi M, Owa Y, Kato K, Obayashi S, et al. Associations between anxiety, depression and insomnia in peri- and post-menopausal women. Maturitas. 2012;72(1):61–5.

35. Stuenkel CA. Menopausal hormone therapy: current considerations. Endocrinol Metab Clin North Am. 2015;44(3):565–85.

36. Attarian H, Hachul H, Guttuso T, Phillips B. Treatment of chronic insomnia disorder in menopause: evaluation of literature. Menopause. 2015;22(6):674–84.

37. Marjoribanks J, Farquhar C, Roberts H, Lethaby A. Trial does not change the conclusions of Cochrane review of long term hormone therapy for perimenopausal and postmenopausal women. BMJ. 2012;345:e8141. author reply e64.

38. Kripke DF, Langer RD, Kline LE. Hypnotics' association with mortality or cancer: a matched cohort study. BMJ Open. 2012;2(1):e000850.

39. Kao CH, Sun LM, Liang JA, Chang SN, Sung FC, Muo CH. Relationship of zolpidem and cancer risk: a Taiwanese population-based cohort study. Mayo Clin Proc. 2012;87(5):430–6.

40. Farkas RH, Unger EF, Temple R. Zolpidem and driving impairment—identifying persons at risk. N Engl J Med. 2013;369(8):689–91.

41. Joffe H, Petrillo L, Viguera A, Koukopoulos A, Silver-Heilman K, Farrell A, et al. Eszopiclone improves insomnia and depressive and anxious symptoms in perimenopausal and postmenopausal women with hot flashes: a randomized, double-blinded, placebo-controlled crossover trial. Am J Obstet Gynecol. 2010;202(2):171.e1–11.

42. Greenblatt DJ, Harmatz JS, Roth T, Singh NN, Moline ML, Harris SC, et al. Comparison of pharmacokinetic profiles of zolpidem buffered sublingual tablet and zolpidem oral immediate-release tablet: results from a single-center, single-dose, randomized, open-label crossover study in healthy adults. Clin Ther. 2013;35(5):604–11.

43. Dobkin RD, Menza M, Bienfait KL, Allen LA, Marin H, Gara MA. Ramelteon for the treatment of insomnia in menopausal women. Menopause Int. 2009;15(1):13–8.

44. Ensrud KE, Joffe H, Guthrie KA, Larson JC, Reed SD, Newton KM, et al. Effect of escitalopram on insomnia symptoms and subjective sleep quality in healthy perimenopausal and postmenopausal women with hot flashes: a randomized controlled trial. Menopause. 2012;19(8):848–55.

45. Soares CN, Arsenio H, Joffe H, Bankier B, Cassano P, Petrillo LF, et al. Escitalopram versus ethinyl estradiol and norethindrone acetate for symptomatic peri- and postmenopausal women: impact on depression, vasomotor symptoms, sleep, and quality of life. Menopause. 2006;13(5):780–6.

46. Defronzo Dobkin R, Menza M, Allen LA, Marin H, Bienfait KL, Tiu J, et al. Escitalopram reduces hot flashes in nondepressed menopausal women: a pilot study. Ann Clin Psychiatry. 2009;21(2):70–6.

47. Suvanto-Luukkonen E, Koivunen R, Sundström H, Bloigu R, Karjalainen E, Häivä-Mällinen L, et al. Citalopram and fluoxetine in the treatment of postmenopausal symptoms: a prospective, randomized, 9-month, placebo-controlled, double-blind study. Menopause. 2005;12(1):18–26.
48. Frey BN, Haber E, Mendes GC, Steiner M, Soares CN. Effects of quetiapine extended release on sleep and quality of life in midlife women with major depressive disorder. Arch Womens Ment Health. 2013;16(1):83–5.
49. Dolev Z. Case series of perimenopausal women with insomnia treated with mirtazapine followed by prolonged-release melatonin add-on and monotherapy. Arch Womens Ment Health. 2011;14(3):269–73.
50. Yurcheshen ME, Guttuso T, McDermott M, Holloway RG, Perlis M. Effects of gabapentin on sleep in menopausal women with hot flashes as measured by a Pittsburgh Sleep Quality Index factor scoring model. J Womens Health (Larchmt). 2009;18(9):1355–60.
51. Guttuso T. Nighttime awakenings responding to gabapentin therapy in late premenopausal women: a case series. J Clin Sleep Med. 2012;8(2):187–9.
52. Mucci M, Carraro C, Mancino P, Monti M, Papadia LS, Volpini G, et al. Soy isoflavones, lactobacilli, Magnolia bark extract, vitamin D3 and calcium. Controlled clinical study in menopause. Minerva Ginecol. 2006;58(4):323–34.
53. Hachul H, Brandão LC, D'Almeida V, Bittencourt LR, Baracat EC, Tufik S. Isoflavones decrease insomnia in postmenopause. Menopause. 2011;18(2):178–84.
54. Holzl J, Godau P. Receptor bindings studies with Valeriana officinalis on the benzodiazepine receptor. Planta Med. 1989;55(6):642.
55. Bent S, Padula A, Moore D, Patterson M, Mehling W. Valerian for sleep: a systematic review and meta-analysis. Am J Med. 2006;119(12):1005–12.
56. Sarris J, Byrne GJ. A systematic review of insomnia and complementary medicine. Sleep Med Rev. 2011;15(2):99–106.
57. Taavoni S, Ekbatani N, Kashaniyan M, Haghani H. Effect of valerian on sleep quality in postmenopausal women: a randomized placebo-controlled clinical trial. Menopause. 2011;18(9):951–5.
58. Kohama T, Negami M. Effect of low-dose French maritime pine bark extract on climacteric syndrome in 170 perimenopausal women: a randomized, double-blind, placebo-controlled trial. J Reprod Med. 2013;58(1–2):39–46.
59. Rotem C, Kaplan B. Phyto-Female Complex for the relief of hot flushes, night sweats and quality of sleep: randomized, controlled, double-blind pilot study. Gynecol Endocrinol. 2007;23(2):117–22.
60. Green SM, Haber E, McCabe RE, Soares CN. Cognitive-behavioral group treatment for menopausal symptoms: a pilot study. Arch Womens Ment Health. 2013;16(4):325–32.
61. Alder J, Eymann Besken K, Armbruster U, Decio R, Gairing A, Kang A, et al. Cognitive-behavioural group intervention for climacteric syndrome. Psychother Psychosom. 2006;75(5):298–303.
62. Hunter MS, Liao KL. Determinants of treatment choice for menopausal hot flushes: hormonal versus psychological versus no treatment. J Psychosom Obstet Gynaecol. 1995;16(2):101–8.
63. Morgenthaler T, Kramer M, Alessi C, Friedman L, Boehlecke B, Brown T, et al. Practice parameters for the psychological and behavioral treatment of insomnia: an update. An American Academy of Sleep Medicine report. Sleep. 2006;29(11):1415–9.
64. Smith MT, Perlis ML, Park A, Smith MS, Pennington J, Giles DE, et al. Comparative meta-analysis of pharmacotherapy and behavior therapy for persistent insomnia. Am J Psychiatry. 2002;159(1):5–11.
65. Morin CM, Vallières A, Guay B, Ivers H, Savard J, Mérette C, et al. Cognitive behavioral therapy, singly and combined with medication, for persistent insomnia: a randomized controlled trial. JAMA. 2009;301(19):2005–15.
66. Becker PM. Hypnosis in the management of sleep disorders. Sleep Med Clin. 2015;10(1):85–92.
67. Elkins GR, Fisher WI, Johnson AK, Carpenter JS, Keith TZ. Clinical hypnosis in the treatment of postmenopausal hot flashes: a randomized controlled trial. Menopause. 2013;20(3):291–8.

68. Afonso RF, Hachul H, Kozasa EH, Oliveira DS, Goto V, Rodrigues D, et al. Yoga decreases insomnia in postmenopausal women: a randomized clinical trial. Menopause. 2012;19(2): 186–93.
69. Weinrich SP, Haddock S, Robinson K. Therapeutic massage in older persons: research issues. Br J Nurs. 1999;8(3):159–64.
70. Oliveira D, Hachul H, Tufik S, Bittencourt L. Effect of massage in postmenopausal women with insomnia: a pilot study. Clinics (Sao Paulo). 2011;66(2):343–6.
71. Oliveira DS, Hachul H, Goto V, Tufik S, Bittencourt LR. Effect of therapeutic massage on insomnia and climacteric symptoms in postmenopausal women. Climacteric. 2012;15(1):21–9.
72. Bezerra AG, Pires GN, Andersen ML, Tufik S, Hachul H. Acupuncture to treat sleep disorders in postmenopausal women: a systematic review. Evid Based Complement Alternat Med. 2015;2015:563236.

Chapter 11
Insomnia in Patients with Comorbid Medical Problems

Rachel Paul and Ron C. Anafi

Abstract Almost every medical disease can be associated with insomnia. Insomnia may result directly from the pathophysiology of the illness, as a consequence of pain or other disease symptoms, as an unintended side effect of treatment, or as a manifestation of the anxiety and uncertainty attached to the diagnosis. Improving sleep quality often requires optimally managing other disease symptoms and selecting medications that minimize adverse side effects. Importantly, many medical conditions and medications alter the risks and symptoms of intrinsic sleep disorders that can present as insomnia and sleep fragmentation. Conversely some hypnotics can affect medical conditions. As patients with medical comorbidities tend to be older and take multiple medications, they are also at an increased risk for adverse drug reactions. Non-pharmacologic treatments for insomnia should be given special consideration in this population.

Keywords Insomnia • Sleep • Health • Medical conditions • Frailty syndrome • Poly-pharmacy • Comorbidities • Intrinsic sleep disorders • Risk factors

Introduction

Patients with medical comorbidities commonly experience disrupted and non-restorative sleep. Clinical experience and a growing body of epidemiologic data suggest that almost every medical disorder can be associated with insomnia.

Depending on the comorbidity, insomnia may result from the pathophysiology of the illness itself, as a consequence of pain or other disease symptoms, as an unintended side effect of treatment, or as a manifestation of the anxiety and

R. Paul, M.D.
Department of Sleep Medicine, University of Pennsylvania, Philadelphia, PA 19104, USA
e-mail: Rachel.paul@mwhc.com

R.C. Anafi, M.D., Ph.D. (✉)
Division of Sleep Medicine and Center for Sleep and Circadian Neurobiology, University of Pennsylvania, TRL, 125 South 31st Street, Suite 2100, Philadelphia, PA 19104, USA
e-mail: ron.anafi@uphs.upenn.edu

© Springer International Publishing Switzerland 2017
H.P. Attarian (ed.), *Clinical Handbook of Insomnia*, Current Clinical Neurology,
DOI 10.1007/978-3-319-41400-3_11

199

uncertainty attached to the diagnosis. Treating comorbid insomnia often requires a comprehensive plan and the collaboration of primary care physicians and specialists. Improving sleep quality may rely, in part, on the optimal management of other disease symptoms and the selection of medications that minimize adverse side effects. Patients with medical comorbidities present a unique challenge to the sleep specialist.

A history and clinical evaluation for evidence of intrinsic sleep disorders should be performed in all patients complaining of difficulties with sleep or poor sleep quality. In patients with medical comorbidities, this evaluation needs to be adjusted as the risks and symptoms of intrinsic sleep disorders are altered. Patients with congestive heart failure (CHF) and obstructive sleep apnea (OSA) are less likely to describe excessive daytime sleepiness and more likely to have sleep fragmentation and reduced sleep time. Similarly several commonly prescribed medications increase the risk of restless leg syndrome (RLS), periodic limb movements (PLM), circadian disruption, OSA, and other intrinsic sleep disorders that may present as insomnia.

Patients with medical comorbidities frequently take multiple medications. They are often older and, due to their illnesses, frail [1, 2]. Concerns over poly-pharmacy and the increased risk of falls associated with hypnotic use take on special importance in this population [3–6]. Current guidelines emphasize the role of non-pharmacologic insomnia treatments as first-line therapy [7]. In patients with medical comorbidities this recommendation has added weight. Most studies on the efficacy of biofeedback, mindfulness, cognitive behavioral therapy for insomnia (CBTi), and other non-pharmacologic treatments have focused on otherwise healthy subjects. A growing body of evidence suggests that these therapies are also effective in patients with medical comorbidities [8, 9].

In this chapter we review the epidemiologic data linking insomnia with various medical conditions. We aim to emphasize medical conditions and treatments that alter the likelihood or presentation of intrinsic sleep disorders. We also highlight studies evaluating the efficacy of either pharmacologic or non-pharmacologic insomnia treatments in these specific populations.

Cardiovascular Disease and Insomnia

Cardiovascular disease remains the leading cause of mortality in the USA [10, 11] and is well associated with poor sleep quality and insomnia [12]. In a cross-sectional study ($n = 772$) people with heart disease reported chronic insomnia symptoms at nearly twice the rate of those without heart disease (44.1% versus 22.8%) [13].

Nocturnal angina can lead to sudden awakenings and sleep fragmentation. An observational study of 1588 adults evaluating insomnia risk factors found that angina was independently associated with sleep disturbance [14]. Autonomic tone fluctuates with sleep stage. Increasing heart rate and blood pressure associated with REM lead to an increase in cardiac metabolic demand. The demand placed on stenotic coronary arteries may precipitate angina. Polysomnographic studies of patients have shown that ischemic events are more likely to occur during REM [15]. Arousal inducing arrhythmias may also be unmasked during sleep. Objective changes in sleep architecture were reported to occur after an acute ischemic event although these changes normalized at a 6-month follow-up [16]. Earlier data suggested that poor subjective sleep quality is associated with recurrent cardiac events and conveys a poorer prognosis in women with coronary artery disease [17].

Among patients with congestive heart failure, paroxysmal nocturnal dyspnea (PND) and orthopnea can interfere with sleep [12, 18]. Heart failure patients are also at greater risk for both OSA and central sleep apnea (CSA) [19, 20]. Indeed the distinction between PND and CSA is sometimes unclear. Moreover in this population, sleep apnea is poorly associated with excessive daytime sleepiness [19, 21]. Rather patients with CHF and sleep-disordered breathing showed reduced sleep time and increased sleep fragmentation [19, 21]. Smaller studies suggest that the patients with CHF are at increased risk for periodic limb movements [22, 23]. However in at least one study, PLMs did not result in a marked reduction in sleep quality [23]. CSA and Cheyne-Stokes respirations make this patient population particularly vulnerable to sleep fragmentation and poor sleep quality [19, 20]. Sleep-disordered breathing can also exacerbate heart failure, with frequent apnea-induced arousals increasing sympathetic, blood pressure, and heart rate [24].

There is suggestion that the relationship between insomnia and cardiovascular disease may be bidirectional. A population-based study of 52, 610 men and women in Norway concluded that difficulties initiating and maintaining sleep, along with non-restorative sleep, were associated with a moderately increased risk of acute myocardial infarction [25]. The Nord-Trondelag Health Studies (HUNT 2 and HUNT 3) were extensive population-based studies that followed 25,715 Norwegians over an 11-year period. The studies found that insomnia was a statistically significant risk factor for the incidence of multiple medical conditions, including myocardial infarction [26]. Although these and other studies suggest a correlation between chronic insomnia and the subsequent development of heart disease, the data falls far short of proving causation. It is also unclear if early insomnia management prevents heart disease.

Medications used in the treatment of cardiovascular disease may manifest in insomnia. In hypervolemic patients, diuretics can improve cardiac output and central sleep apnea [27]. However when taken late in the day, diuretics also cause nocturia and frequent awakenings. Beta-specific adrenergic blocking agents reduce sympathetic tone to the pineal gland and have been shown to suppress nighttime melatonin [28–30] and worsen sleep quality [30]. However non-selective beta blockers like carvedilol (alpha-1 blocking) and nebivolol do not appear to suppress melatonin synthesis [29]. Indeed nightly melatonin supplementation improves polysomnographic measures of sleep in hypertensive patients taking beta-1-specific blockers [31]. However it is not clear if subjective sleep measures are similarly improved [31]. There is also some evidence that melatonin decreases blood pressure [32]. Hmg-CoA reductase inhibitors used in the treatment of hypercholesterolemia have been linked to nightmares and sleep disturbance [33]. Larger studies are required to confirm this observation and provide a mechanistic understanding.

Special consideration is needed when selecting hypnotics for a patient with cardiovascular disease. Tricyclic antidepressants (TCAs) including doxepin and trazodone can reduce heart rate variability, slow intraventricular conduction, and induce tachyarrhythmias. Patients with underlying cardiac conduction disease who take TCAs are at an increased risk for cardiac events [34]. CBTi may thus have a particularly favorable risk/benefit profile in this population [35]. In patients with cardiac disease and OSA, positive airway pressure improves hypoxemia, reduces sympathetic tone, and decreases cardiac afterload. PAP therapy can also improve sleep quality and daytime sleepiness in patients with OSA [36]. However recent data suggests that the treatment of CSA with positive pressure therapy may actually be harmful in patients with heart failure and reduced ejection fraction [37, 38].

Pulmonary Disease and Insomnia

Insomnia has been associated with a host of pulmonary conditions including interstitial lung disease, bronchitis, cystic fibrosis, and lung cancer [39–41]. The prevalence of self-reported insomnia among patients with chronic obstructive pulmonary disease (COPD) is nearly twice that observed in controls [42–44]. Patients with insomnia and COPD have less sleep as assessed by actigraphy [42]. Asthmatics are more likely to experience insomnia than healthy controls, and those with poorly controlled asthma report more sleep disturbance [45]. Indeed circadian and sleep-related changes in inflammation, vagal tone, and smooth muscle physiology result in worsening of asthma symptoms during sleep [46, 47]. Several hypotheses have been advanced to explain the association between COPD and insomnia: nocturnal dyspnea and cough, comorbid nicotine use, increased work of breathing, medication use, and hypoxia- or hypercapnia-mediated arousal [48, 49]. Among patients with COPD, current smokers have more sleep complaints than former smokers [42, 44]. Hypercapnic states may be a stronger trigger for arousal than eucapnic states [50, 51]. Patients with asthma and COPD are also more likely to complain of anxiety, depression, and nightmares, all of which may contribute to sleep disturbance [52].

Standard treatments for COPD and asthma can affect sleep quality. However, relevant studies are small and report somewhat conflicting results. In general, the positive effects of a medication in reducing nocturnal respiratory symptoms must be balanced against potential wake-promoting side effects. Systemic corticosteroids are commonly used in the treatment of pulmonary and rheumatic diseases. Self-reported sleep problems increase with corticosteroid use in a dose-dependent fashion [53, 54]. Yet in a small study involving patients with nocturnal asthma, a time-delayed steroid formulation improved sleep in conjunction with asthma symptoms [55]. Theophylline is also well linked to insomnia. Using theophylline earlier in the day may lessen the effect on sleep quality, and if dyspnea improves, there may be no net adverse effect on sleep [56]. Similarly, while adrenergic beta agonists are stimulants, inhaler use was not found to be a significant factor in a regression model describing insomnia symptoms in a small COPD cohort [42]. Tiotropium, a short-acting anticholinergic bronchodilator, was not found to adversely effect sleep quality and long-acting ipratropium may actually improve sleep quality [57, 58]. Oxygen use was associated with improved sleep quality in a few small studies but others have not shown benefit.

Patients with intrinsic lung disease and insomnia should be screened for other sleep disorders. Recent data suggests that patients with COPD have a higher incidence of RLS [59–61]. COPD and other lung diseases may also increase the clinical severity of OSA by reducing pulmonary reserve. In these patients with the so-called overlap syndrome, PAP therapy can improve mortality.

The use of hypnotics in patients with pulmonary disease requires caution. Both short-acting and long-acting benzodiazepines have been shown to depress objective measures of respiratory function in patients with COPD, even in patients with chronic, stable disease [62, 63]. Conflicting data suggests that low doses of the short-acting benzodiazepine temazepam did not alter respiratory measures and improved sleep in patients with severe COPD and insomnia [64]. Non-benzodiazepine receptor agonists, such as zolpidem and zopiclone, have less of an effect on ventilatory drive [65, 66]. Nonetheless the potential for concern remains. Melatonin and ramelteon, a selective melatonin M1/2 agonist, appear to be safe and effective in treating insomnia in patients with COPD [67–69]. Melatonin may even reduce dyspnea and lung oxidative stress in patients with COPD [70]. Finally, patients with COPD have been included as part of a larger evaluation of CBTi that revealed a significant benefit [8, 9]. A small study focused on the use of CBTi in patients with COPD also found a positive effect [71].

Renal Disease and Insomnia

Patients with chronic kidney disease (CKD) are vulnerable to multiple sleep disorders, including RLS, PLM disorder, circadian disruption, CSA, and OSA, all of which can contribute to sleep fragmentation, poor sleep quality, and insomnia [72]. A study of 124 patients with newly diagnosed renal disease showed that sleep disorders occur early in the course of chronic kidney disease. About 59.7% of patients studied reported insomnia symptoms (including frequent awakenings, early morning awakenings, increased sleep latency, and non-refreshing sleep) and 29.8% of patients endorsed the use of hypnotic drugs [73]. Insomnia symptoms may also result as nocturnal melatonin secretion decreases with the progression of renal dysfunction [74].

Patients on hemodialysis have a similar, if not higher, prevalence of insomnia. One study of 694 patients found that 45% complained of either delayed sleep onset or difficulty with sleep maintenance. The study also found that there was a significantly higher risk of insomnia among patients who had been on dialysis for greater than 12 months, in patients who were dialyzed in the morning, and in patients with higher parathyroid hormone levels [75]. Fifty-two percent of patients who complained of insomnia also complained of RLS [75]. Other studies have estimated the incidence of insomnia and sleep complaints (including excessive daytime sleepiness) as high as ~70 % among patients undergoing dialysis [76]. Poor sleep quality has a negative impact on health-related quality of life for patients with chronic kidney disease [77]. Kidney transplant may improve insomnia in renal patients. One study found that the prevalence of insomnia was nearly halved post-transplant [78].

It is important to screen for and manage possible comorbid sleep disorders in patients with insomnia and comorbid CKD. As noted, RLS is very common among patients undergoing dialysis [79], although some data suggests that the risk is more modest among those with more mild kidney disease [80]. The pathophysiology of RLS remains unclear. However iron deficiency and neuropathy are well-identified risk factors for RLS and both are common among patients with ESRD. Iron dextran transiently improves RLS symptoms in dialysis patients [81]. In addition to standard therapies, short daily dialysis [82] and regular aerobic exercise [83] have been shown to improve RLS in patients with ESRD.

When someone lays supine interstitial fluid redistributes to the upper airway, increases tissue volume, and may contribute to upper airway obstruction [84]. Volume status and fluid redistribution may be partly responsible for the higher risk of sleep-disordered breathing among patients with CKD and ESRD [85, 86]. This suggests that, in patients undergoing intermittent dialysis, sleep-disordered breathing may be unmasked or become more severe as the time from the most recent dialysis session increases. In small studies, nightly peritoneal dialysis improved apnea and sleep disruption [87, 88]. Larger clinical studies evaluating the effect of more aggressive fluid management are still lacking, as are trials comparing polysomnographic results at different stages of the dialysis cycle.

CKD leads to uremia and electrolyte disturbance that have been linked to insomnia [89]. CKD is also associated with a blunting of the normal circadian pattern in serum melatonin concentration [74]. Melatonin rhythms are further disrupted in patients undergoing intermittent daily dialysis [90, 91]. Smaller studies have shown a partial improvement in melatonin rhythms and sleep quality with nocturnal hemodialysis and nocturnal peritoneal dialysis [90, 91].

When using hypnotics or medications for RLS, dosing must often be adjusted for glomerular filtration rate. Zaleplon, a non-benzodiazepine hypnotic, has been shown to improve sleep latency and effective sleep quality in patients with chronic kidney disease with few side effects [92]. Melatonin also appears to be effective in this population [93]. Non-pharmacological therapies should be considered. In a small, pilot study CBTi improved sleep quality and reduced fatigue in patients with chronic kidney disease undergoing peritoneal dialysis [94].

Gastrointestinal Disorders and Insomnia

GERD is a well-known cause of sleep disturbance and secondary insomnia. GERD is also associated with other known causes of sleep disruption including nocturnal wheezing and cough. A nationwide American Gastroenterological Association telephone survey of 1000 patients experiencing weekly heartburn symptoms revealed that 79% of respondents report nocturnal symptoms [95]. Among those, 75% reported poor sleep quality related to acid reflux symptoms and 40% believed that their nighttime symptoms impacted their ability to function the next day. Gastric acid secretion follows a circadian rhythm which causes acid secretion to peak at night [96]. One study found that even asymptomatic patients and patients with minimal GERD symptoms have abnormal acid production, as well as sleep disturbance [97]. The same study showed that asymptomatic GERD patients had improvement in sleep efficiency after treatment with rabeprazole, a proton pump inhibitor. Esomeprazole and dexlansoprazole have also been shown to improve heartburn and subjective sleep quality in patients with GERD [98, 99]. There prevalence of GERD in patients with OSA has been estimated to be as high as 76% [100]. While GERD and OSA share common risk factors including obesity, it has also been theorized that the drops in intrathoracic pressure characterizing apneic episodes induce reflux of gastric contents into the thoracic cavity [101]. Alternatively inflammation and changes in the sensory innervation of the upper airway that result from GERD may provoke apnea [101]. Indeed PAP therapy has been shown to improve GERD symptoms in patients with comorbid OSA [102]. Conversely, treatment with PPIs has been shown to decrease the number of obstructive events in patients with GERD and OSA [103].

Any gastrointestinal disorder that causes pain, including esophagitis, peptic and duodenal ulcers, and irritable bowel syndrome, can contribute to sleep disturbance. One prospective study found that IBS patients had a significant reduction in slow-wave sleep, higher Epworth scores, and increased sleep fragmentation compared to age-matched controls [104]. A small randomized, placebo-controlled study concluded that melatonin 3 mg at bedtime improved abdominal pain in patients with IBS who complain of sleep disturbance; however there was no actual improvement in sleep quality at this dose [105].

It is well known that sleep disturbance, including delayed sleep onset and reduced sleep duration, is associated with hepatic encephalopathy. Cirrhotic patients with normal cognition and without evidence of hepatic encephalopathy also complain of poor sleep quality [106, 107]. This may be related to alterations in circadian timing. Patients with chronic liver failure have a delayed peak in serum melatonin, an increased daytime serum melatonin concentration, and a reduced peak-trough differential [108, 109]. The reduction in serum melatonin amplitude correlated with disease severity [108].

Secondary insomnia in patients with gastrointestinal disorders may improve with treatment of the underlying condition. If hypnotics are used, it is important to note that benzodiazepines and non-benzodiazepine receptor agonists may worsen GERD by decreasing gut motility and lowering esophageal sphincter tone [110–112]. Reduced hepatic clearance of benzodiazepines may result in increased daytime sleepiness and adversely affect cognition. Alternatively melatonin has been shown to improve GERD symptoms [113, 114] and in a small pilot study, ramelteon improved both GERD symptoms and sleep disturbance [115]. However, reduced hepatic melatonin clearance remains a concern [108, 116]. Dopamine receptor antagonists like prochlorperazine or metoclopramide are often used as anti-emetics or pro-motility agents and may precipitate RLS.

Genitourinary Conditions and Insomnia

Nocturia becomes more common in both men and women with age. It is also an under-appreciated cause of sleep disturbance in the elderly. A 2003 National Sleep Foundation survey of 1424 older patients, aged 55–84, found that 53 % of subjects reported sleep disturbance related to "nightly or almost nightly" nocturia. Nocturia was also found to be an independent risk factor for self-reported insomnia (75 % increased risk) and reduced sleep quality (71 % increased risk) [117].

One of the most common causes of nocturia-related sleep disturbance in men is benign prostatic hyperplasia (BPH). A cross-sectional study of 2179 men with BPH found that 60.9 % of those studied complained of insomnia. The number of episodes of nocturia per night were correlated with wake after sleep onset and Epworth sleepiness scale, but not total sleep time and sleep onset [118]. Another study comparing medical versus surgical management of BPH found that transurethral resection of the prostate (TURP) resulted in significant improvement in the number of nocturnal awakenings compared to tamsulosin [119]. Overactive bladder is another common genitourinary condition with a significant impact on sleep quality that contributes to poor quality of life and depression among both men and women [120]. It's important to counsel patients to avoid liquids, especially caffeinated beverages close to bedtime. Although medications for overactive bladder can improve nocturia-related awakenings, they can also alter sleep structure by suppressing REM [121, 122]. Finally, it is important to remember that untreated OSA is also a common cause of both nocturia and increased daytime urinary frequency [123]. The diagnosis of OSA should be considered in patients with sleep maintenance insomnia and nocturia.

Medications, such as diuretics, can also contribute to nocturia. Timing diuretics earlier in the afternoon may significantly reduce nighttime awakenings due to nocturia. Desmopressin has been shown to be an effective treatment for nocturia in men and women with a decrease in the total number of voids and an increase in the duration of sleep time before the first void [124, 125].

Endocrine Conditions and Insomnia

Basic science, case reports, and clinical teaching connect various endocrine disorders with insomnia and other sleep disorders. In particular, several endocrine disorders have been associated with an increased risk for sleep-disordered breathing [126]. However, clinical studies testing and validating these connections are sometimes lacking [126]. Moreover the secretion of several hormones is tied to either sleep/wake state or circadian time [127]. Associations between sleep disorders and hormonal changes are likely bidirectional, complicating the interpretation of simple observational data.

Hyperthyroidism is classically associated with palpitations, weight loss, anxiety, and insomnia [128]. Exogenous administration of thyroid hormone into the sleep-promoting pre-optic nucleus promotes wakefulness in mice [129]. In a study of patients with thyrotoxicosis, hyperkinetic symptoms were associated with difficulty falling asleep [130]. However the prevalence of insomnia in this population was not compared to a control. Indeed, a small study found only an increased frequency of PLMs in women with Grave's disease and no other significant changes in sleep quality indexes when compared to control [131]. Supratherapeutic administration of thyroid hormone did not alter sleep architecture in normal subjects [132]. Using data from a larger study, Akatsu and colleagues investigated the relationship between thyroid function and sleep quality in 682 men [133]. Only small numbers of men with subclinical hyperthyroidism and hypothyroidism were followed. However, neither was significantly associated with subjective sleep complaint or objective differences in actigraphic sleep measures [133]. Hypothyroidism is associated with sleepiness and fatigue and has been linked to the development of obstructive sleep apnea in several studies. In some studies thyroid supplementation improves apnea but this has not been observed universally.

Acromegaly, caused by excess growth hormone production, results in soft tissue changes believed to precipitate OSA [134–136]. In addition patients with acromegaly are at an increased risk of CSA [136]. Hormonally induced changes in the chemo-sensitivity of respiratory control centers is hypothesized to mediate this risk [137]. Octreotide treatment improves, but does not fully correct, apnea in many of these patients [138].

Adrenal insufficiency is associated with fatigue and poor sleep quality [139, 140]. Cortisol replacement therapy that better replicated the normal circadian cortisol rhythm improved insomnia in a case report [141]. A small controlled trial found that timed cortisol admiration increased the amount of REM sleep but not subjective sleep measures of sleep quality [142]. Data describing the effect off Cushing's syndrome on sleep are sparse. Nonetheless, exogenous steroids to induce insomnia in a dose-dependent manner [53, 54] and Cushing's and elevated plasma cortisol have been associated both with insomnia [143] and OSA [144].

Men with low serum testosterone often note increased daytime fatigue, and this association remains significant in patients with OSA [145]. On the other hand exogenous testosterone supplementation is believed to precipitate or worsen OSA, and it has been recommended that testosterone supplementation be avoided in the setting of untreated apnea [146]. Again however, the data is sparse. In a study of obese men with severe OSA and low plasma testosterone levels, testosterone supplementation acutely worsened the oxygen desaturation index and nocturnal hypoxemia, but this effect disappeared after 12 weeks [147]. Perhaps due to variations in dose and timing, a collection of small studies yielded conflicting results [146]. Menopause and the associated changes in serum estrogen and progesterone can also have a marked effect on sleep. Hot flashes, insomnia, non-restorative sleep, and an increased prevalence of OSA have all been described [148]. Hormone replacement therapy, selective serotonin reuptake inhibitors, hypnotics, and non-pharmacologic therapies have all shown some therapeutic benefit in studies. These findings are reviewed in Chap. 10.

Ocular Disorders and Insomnia

Visual and non-visual light perception play a key role in regulation of the sleep-wake cycle. The paired suprachiasmatic nuclei (SCN) of the hypothalamus act as a "master circadian pacemaker" [149]. The SCN receives input from melanopsin-containing retinal ganglion cells sensitive to blue light. The SCN also receives from classical photoreceptor cells via accessory pathways or via their influence on the melanopsin-containing ganglion cells [150, 151]. The important role of light perception in coordinating sleep timing likely contributes to the high prevalence of sleep disturbance among the visually impaired. One study found that out of 403 subjects, 48.7 % reported disturbed sleep, including prolonged sleep latency, reduced sleep duration, and daytime naps. There was a higher prevalence of sleep disturbance among those with a complete loss of light perception than among those with more moderate visual loss [152].

Age-related changes to the eye can also contribute to sleep disturbance. Over time, the lens of the eye acquires a yellow discoloration that preferentially blocks blue light [153]. Although this may not affect visual acuity, it may induce sleep disturbance. In a cross-sectional, population-based study of 970 participants who had yellowing of the lens, there was an inverse relationship between blue light lens transmission and the risk of sleep disturbance [154]. Of those who endorsed sleep disturbances, 82.6 % endorsed both insomnia and the use of hypnotics [154]. Both self-reported sleep symptoms and the circadian modulation of serum melatonin appear to improve after cataract surgery [155–159]. It remains controversial if the use of artificial lenses that block a narrow portion of the blue-light spectrum, developed for retinal UV protection, might attenuate the improvement after cataract surgery [155, 160, 161].

Non-24-h sleep-wake disorder, also known as "free-running circadian" disorder, may account for significant sleep disturbance in those who are completely blind. The typical presenting symptoms include periodic insomnia and daytime sleepiness. The totally blind are also susceptible to free-running temperature, cortisol, and melatonin levels despite the presence of non-photic behavioral and environmental time cues [162]. Both melatonin and the melatonin agonist, tasimelteon, have been shown to entrain the circadian rhythm in blind individuals and improve nocturnal sleep parameters [163, 164].

Dermatologic Disorders and Insomnia

The skin is the body's largest organ and is innervated by a dense collection of somatic afferent nerve fibers and receptors. Damage, pressure, or irritation of the dermis act through dermal nerve endings to cause pain and itching. Both pruritus and pain are commonly cited insomnia triggers and infectious, allergic, or inflammatory skin conditions are all associated with disturbed sleep [165, 166].

Patients with herpes zoster report insomnia as one of the most significant symptoms [167]. Nearly 65% of children with eczema report insomnia and that number jumps to over 85% among patients with active disease [168]. Adults with eczema are also likely to have insomnia and describe either short or long sleep time [169]. Interestingly in patients with atopic dermatitis subjective itchiness does not appear to correlate with scratching observed during a PSG-monitored study [170]. Arousals from sleep related to scratching occurred primarily in stage N1 and N2 sleep and correlated with disease severity [170]. Indeed a structural modeling study concluded that the increase in depression and attention-deficit hyperactivity observed in children with eczema is wholly explained via eczema's deleterious effect on sleep [168].

Circadian modulation of fibroblast molecular physiology, serum cortisol, and pro-inflammatory cytokines along with sleep-related changes in dermal temperature is theorized to increase the symptoms of eczema and other immune-mediated skin disorders at night [165, 166]. Itching during sleep may also worsen the underlying skin condition the following day.

Non-pharmacologic treatments for insomnia related to dermatologic disease often focus on the skin condition. The use of occlusive dressings and bandages can improve skin hydration and reduce pruritus but may also restrict movement during sleep. Watching humorous films before sleep reduced nighttime awakenings in patients with atopic dermatitis as compared to watching nonhumorous films [171].

Oral corticosteroids can improve dermatologic symptoms and thus sleep, but might also induce insomnia at higher doses [172]. Antihistamines are often considered first-line agents as they may reduce itching and have hypnotic properties. However, tolerance to these sedative effects can develop quickly [173]. The tricyclic antidepressant doxepin has been shown to be effective over several months [174] and has selective antihistaminergic properties at low dose [175]. Thus doxepin is a reasonable choice for patients with insomnia and pruritus; however it has not been specifically studied in this population.

Cancer and Insomnia

A review of 15 studies on insomnia and cancer concluded that approximately 30–50% of cancer patients report insomnia [176]. In a sample of 121 patients with cancer, more patients reported insomnia than pain, anorexia, fatigue, or nausea [177].

The etiology of insomnia and sleep disturbance among cancer patients is often multifactorial. Patients with lung cancer or tumors affecting the upper airway may develop nocturnal hypoxemia or OSA. Patients with cancers compromising endocrine or neurologic function may also have disrupted sleep as a result. It is likely that anxiety, depression, and pain from invasive tumors and surgery all contribute to poor sleep quality. Studies have also shown that there is a significant association between radiation and chemotherapy with insomnia [178, 179]. Radiation therapy, in particular, affects sleep quality. Radiation activates cellular pathways that increase the sleep-modulating cytokines, IL-6 and TNF-a [180, 181]. Increases in these cytokines are associated with fever, pain, and insomnia. In one study, patients undergoing radiation therapy experienced declines in sleep efficiency. Patients who had undergone more radiation treatments complained of more sleep disturbance [182]. Adjunctive treatments, such as hormonal therapy or surgical oophorectomy used in the treatment of breast and reproductive cancers, cause hormonal changes and impact sleep. Similarly the treatment of thyroid cancers with exogenous thyroid hormone to suppress endogenous TSH may worsen insomnia. Corticosteroids and opiates, used in the management of cancer symptoms or medication side effects, also contribute to insomnia. Frequent sleep interruptions experienced during hospitalizations may trigger insomnia that may persistent when patients return home [183]. A significant number of patients can experience symptoms of insomnia for several years after their cancer diagnosis [184, 185].

Several investigators have evaluated non-pharmacologic therapies for cancer-related insomnia. CBTi has been found to be effective in multiple studies [186, 187]. One study evaluating the efficacy of CBTi among breast cancer survivors found that CBTi improved the Insomnia Severity Index (ISI), decreased in the use of sleep aids, lowered levels of depression and anxiety, and increased a measure of quality of life at post-treatment compared to controls [188]. The positive therapeutic effects of CBTi were maintained 1 year after treatment [188]. Patients treated with CBTi alone or with CBTi and temazepam were more likely to have improvements in sleep efficiency compared to control or medication alone (47%) and placebo (22%) [189]. A recent study evaluating the long-term efficacy of a video-based CBTi platform in breast cancer survivors showed improvement over control but did not demonstrate equivalence with in-person CBTi [190]. The addition of the stimulant armodafinil to combat cancer-related fatigue did not appear to augment the effect of CBTi in a small study [191]. Several studies evaluating mindfulness-based interventions for insomnia [192–194], including a recent meta-analysis [195], have shown benefit. However there have been some exceptions and at least one study found that improvements were not long lasting [196]. A recent non-inferiority study comparing mindfulness therapy with CBTi found CBTi to be superior [197]. Finally a recent small study found that biofeedback was effective in improving subjective sleep quality measures among breast cancer survivors [198].

References

1. Cesari M, Prince M, Thiyagarajan JA, De Carvalho IA, Bernabei R, Chan P, et al. Frailty: an emerging public health priority. J Am Med Dir Assoc. 2016;17(3):188–92.
2. Fried LP, Tangen CM, Walston J, Newman AB, Hirsch C, Gottdiener J, et al. Frailty in older adults: evidence for a phenotype. J Gerontol A Biol Sci Med Sci. 2001;56(3):M146–56.
3. Willson MN, Greer CL, Weeks DL. Medication regimen complexity and hospital readmission for an adverse drug event. Ann Pharmacother. 2014;48(1):26–32.
4. Wimmer BC, Bell JS, Fastbom J, Wiese MD, Johnell K. Medication regimen complexity and polypharmacy as factors associated with all-cause mortality in older people: a population-based cohort study. Ann Pharmacother. 2016;50(2):89–95.

5. Charlesworth CJ, Smit E, Lee DSH, Alramadhan F, Odden MC. Polypharmacy among adults aged 65 years and older in the United States: 1988–2010. J Gerontol A Biol Sci Med Sci. 2015;70(8):989–95.
6. Maher RL, Hanlon J, Hajjar ER. Clinical consequences of polypharmacy in elderly. Expert Opin Drug Saf. 2013;13(1):57–65.
7. Schutte-Rodin S, Broch L, Buysse D, Dorsey C, Sateia M. Clinical guideline for the evaluation and management of chronic insomnia in adults. J Clin Sleep Med. 2008;4(5):487–504.
8. Geiger-Brown JM, Rogers VE, Liu W, Ludeman EM, Downton KD, Diaz-Abad M. Cognitive behavioral therapy in persons with comorbid insomnia: meta-analysis. Sleep Med Rev. 2015;23:54–67.
9. Wu JQ, Appleman ER, Salazar RD, Ong JC. Cognitive behavioral therapy for insomnia comorbid with psychiatric and medical conditions: a meta-analysis. JAMA Intern Med. 2015;175(9):1461–72.
10. Murphy SL, Xu J, Kochanek KD. National vital statistics reports. National Vital Statistics Reports 61.4; 2013. http://www.nber.org/mortality/2007/nvsr58_19.pdf.
11. Mozaffarian D, Benjamin EJ, Go AS, Arnett DK, Blaha MJ, Cushman M, et al. Heart disease and stroke statistics-2016 update: a report from the American Heart Association. Circulation. 2015;133(4):e38–360.
12. Malhotra A, Loscalzo J. Sleep and cardiovascular disease: an overview. Prog Cardiovasc Dis. 2009;51(4):279–84.
13. Taylor DJ, Mallory LJ, Lichstein KL, Durrence HH, Riedel B, Bush AJ. Comorbidity of chronic insomnia with medical problems. Sleep. 2007;30(2):5–10.
14. Hartz AJ, Daly JM, Kohatsu ND, Stromquist AM, Jogerst GJ, Kukoyi OA. Risk factors for insomnia in a rural population. Ann Epidemiol. 2007;17(12):940–7.
15. Kales J, Kales A. Evaluation, diagnosis, and treatment of clinical condtions related to sleep. JAMA. 1970;213(13):2229–35.
16. Schiza SE, Simantirakis E, Bouloukaki I, Mermigkis C, Arfanakis D, Chrysostomakis S, et al. Sleep patterns in patients with acute coronary syndromes. Sleep Med. 2010;11(2):149–53.
17. Leineweber C, Kecklund G, Janszky I, Åkerstedt T, Orth-Gomér K. Poor sleep increases the prospective risk for recurrent events in middle-aged women with coronary disease. J Psychosom Res. 2003;54(2):121–7.
18. Nagai M, Hoshide S, Kario K. Sleep duration as a risk factor for cardiovascular disease—a review of the recent literature. Curr Cardiol Rev. 2010;6(1):54–61.
19. MacDonald M, Fang J, Pittman SD, White DP, Malhotra A. The current prevalence of sleep disordered breathing in congestive heart failure patients treated with beta-blockers. J Clin Sleep Med. 2008;4(1):38–42.
20. Butt M, Dwivedi G, Khair O, Lip GYH. Obstructive sleep apnea and cardiovascular disease. Int J Cardiol. 2010;139(1):7–16.
21. Arzt M, Young T, Finn L, Skatrud JB, Ryan CM, Newton GE, et al. Sleepiness and sleep in patients with both systolic heart failure and obstructive sleep apnea. Arch Intern Med. 2006;166(16):1716–22.
22. Hanly PJ, Zuberi-Khokhar N. Periodic limb movements during sleep in patients with congestive heart failure. Chest. 1996;109(6):1497–502.
23. Skomro R, Silva R, Alves R, Figueiredo A, Lorenzi-Filho G. The prevalence and significance of periodic leg movements during sleep in patients with congestive heart failure. Sleep Breath. 2009;13(1):43–7.
24. Rosen D, Roux FJ, Shah N. Sleep and breathing in congestive heart failure. Clin Chest Med. 2014;35:521–34.
25. Laugsand LE, Vatten LJ, Platou C, Janszky I. Insomnia and the risk of acute myocardial infarction: a population study. Circulation. 2011;124(19):2073–81.
26. Sivertsen B, Lallukka T, Salo P, Pallesen S, Hysing M, Krokstad S, et al. Insomnia as a risk factor for ill health: results from the large population-based prospective HUNT Study in Norway. J Sleep Res. 2014;23(2):124–32.

27. Javaheri S. Acetazolamide improves central sleep apnea in heart failure: a double-blind, prospective study. Am J Respir Crit Care Med. 2006;173(2):234–7.
28. Van Den Heuvel CJ, Reid KJ, Dawson D. Effect of atenolol on nocturnal sleep and temperature in young men: reversal by pharmacological doses of melatonin. Physiol Behav. 1997;61(6):795–802.
29. Stoschitzky K, Stoschitzky G, Brussee H, Bonell C, Dobnig H. Comparing beta-blocking effects of bisoprolol, carvedilol and nebivolol. Cardiology. 2006;106:199–206.
30. Brismar K, Hylander B, Eliasson K, Rössner S, Wetterberg L. Melatonin secretion related to side-effects of beta-blockers from the central nervous system. Acta Med Scand. 1988;223(6):525–30.
31. Scheer FAJL, Morris CJ, Garcia JI, Smales C, Kelly EE, Marks J, et al. Repeated melatonin supplementation improves sleep in hypertensive patients treated with beta-blockers: a randomized controlled trial. Sleep. 2012;35(10):1395–402.
32. Reiter RJ, Tan D-X, Paredes SD, Fuentes-Broto L. Beneficial effects of melatonin in cardiovascular disease. Ann Med. 2010;42(4):276–85.
33. Tuccori M, Montagnani S, Mantarro S, Capogrosso-Sansone A, Ruggiero E, Saporiti A, et al. Neuropsychiatric adverse events associated with statins: epidemiology, pathophysiology, prevention and management. CNS Drugs. 2014;28(3):249–72.
34. Hamer M, David Batty G, Seldenrijk A, Kivimaki M. Antidepressant medication use and future risk of cardiovascular disease: the Scottish Health Survey. Eur Heart J. 2011;32(4): 437–42.
35. Redeker NS, Jeon S, Andrews L, Cline J, Jacoby D, Mohsenin V. Feasibility and efficacy of a self-management intervention for insomnia in stable heart failure. J Clin Sleep Med. 2015;11(10):1109–19. http://www.aasmnet.org/jcsm/ViewAbstract.aspx?pid=30210.
36. Bradley TD, Floras JS. Sleep apnea and heart failure: part I: obstructive sleep apnea. Circulation. 2003;107(12):1671–8.
37. Bradley TD, Logan AG, Kimoff RJ, Sériès F, Morrison D, Ferguson K, et al. Continuous positive airway pressure for central sleep apnea and heart failure. N Engl J Med. 2005;353(19):2025–33.
38. Cowie M, Woehrle H. Adaptive servo-ventilation for central sleep apnea in systolic heart failure. N Engl J Med. 2015;373(12):1095–105. http://www.nejm.org/doi/full/10.1056/NEJMoa1506459.
39. Milioli G, Bosi M, Poletti V, Tomassetti S, Grassi A, Riccardi S, et al. Sleep and respiratory sleep disorders in idiopathic pulmonary fibrosis. Sleep Med Rev. 2016;26:57–63. doi:10.1016/j.smrv.2015.03.005.
40. Caverley PM. The effect of oxygenation on sleep quality in chronic bronchitis and emphysema. Am Rev Respir Dis. 1982;126(2):206–10.
41. Fauroux B, Pepin J-L, Boelle P-Y, Cracowski C, Murris-Espin M, Nove-Josserand R, et al. Sleep quality and nocturnal hypoxaemia and hypercapnia in children and young adults with cystic fibrosis. Arch Dis Child. 2012;97(11):960–6.
42. Budhiraja R, Parthasarathy S, Budhiraja P, Habib MP, Wendel C, Quan SF. Insomnia in patients with COPD. Sleep. 2012;35(3):369–75.
43. Ohayon MM. Chronic Obstructive Pulmonary Disease and its association with sleep and mental disorders in the general population. J Psychiatr Res. 2014;54:79–84.
44. Valipour A, Lavie P, Lothaller H, Mikulic I, Burghuber OC. Sleep profile and symptoms of sleep disorders in patients with stable mild to moderate chronic obstructive pulmonary disease. Sleep Med. 2011;12(4):367–72.
45. Wertz DA, Pollack M, Rodgers K, Bohn RL, Sacco P, Sullivan SD. Impact of asthma control on sleep, attendance at work, normal activities, and disease burden. Ann Allergy Asthma Immunol. 2010;105(2):118–23.
46. Durrington HJ, Farrow SN, Loudon AS, Ray DW. The circadian clock and asthma. Thorax. 2014;69(1):90–2.
47. Mehra R. Understanding nocturnal asthma. The plot thickens. Am J Respir Crit Care Med. 2014;190(3):243–4.

48. Budhiraja R, Siddiqi TA, Quan SF. Sleep disorders in chronic obstructive pulmonary disease: etiology, impact, and management. J Clin Sleep Med. 2015;11(3):259–70.
49. Roth T. Hypnotic use for insomnia management in chronic obstructive pulmonary disease. Sleep Med. 2009;10(1):19–25.
50. Berthon-Jones M, Sullivan CE. Ventilatory and arousal responses to hypoxia in sleeping humans. Am Rev Respir Dis. 1982;125:632–9.
51. Berthon-Jones M, Sullivan CE. Ventilation and arousal responses to hypercapnia in normal sleeping humans. J Appl Physiol Respir Environ Exerc Physiol. 1984;57:59–67.
52. Wood JM. Prevalence of nightmares among patients with asthma and chronic obstructive airways disease. Am Phys Assoc. 1993;3(4):231–41.
53. Ciriaco M, Ventrice P, Russo G, Scicchitano M, Mazzitello G, Scicchitano F, et al. Corticosteroid-related central nervous system side effects. J Pharmacol Pharmacother. 2013;4 Suppl 1:S94–8.
54. Curtis JR, Westfall AO, Allison J, Bijlsma JW, Freeman A, George V, et al. Population-based assessment of adverse events associated with long-term glucocorticoid use. Arthritis Rheum. 2006 Jun 15;55(3):420–6.
55. Alavoine L, Taillé C, Ball J, Knauer C, Witte S, Kent J, et al. Nocturnal asthma: proof-of-concept open-label study with delayed-release prednisone. Pulm Ther. 2015;1(1):43–52.
56. Berry RB, Desa MM, Branum JP, Light RW. Effect of theophylline on sleep and sleep-disordered breathing in patients with chronic obstructive pulmonary disease. Am Rev Respir Dis. 1991;143(2):245–50.
57. McNicholas WT, Calverley PMA, Lee A, Edwards JC, Williams A, Rees J, et al. Long-acting inhaled anticholinergic therapy improves sleeping oxygen saturation in COPD. Eur Respir J. 2004;23(6):825–31.
58. Martin RJ, Bucki Bartelson BL, Smith P, Hudgel DW, Lewis D, Pohl G, et al. Effect of ipratropium bromide treatment on oxygen saturation and sleep quality in COPD. Chest. 1999;115(5):1338–45.
59. Lo Coco D, Mattaliano A, Lo Coco A, Randisi B. Increased frequency of restless legs syndrome in chronic obstructive pulmonary disease patients. Sleep Med. 2009;10(5):572–6.
60. Aras G, Kadakal F, Purisa S, Kanmaz D, Aynaci A, Isik E. Are we aware of restless legs syndrome in COPD patients who are in an exacerbation period? Frequency and probable factors related to underlying mechanism. COPD. 2011;8(6):437–43.
61. Cavalcante AGM, de Bruin PFC, de Bruin VMS, Pereira EDB, Cavalcante MM, Nunes DM, et al. Restless legs syndrome, sleep impairment, and fatigue in chronic obstructive pulmonary disease. Sleep Med. 2012;13(7):842–7.
62. Jolly E, Aguirre L, Jorge E, Luna C. Acute effect of lorazepam on respiratory muscles in stable patients with chronic obstructive pulmonary disease. Medicina (B Aires). 1996;56 (5 Pt 1):472–8.
63. Cohn MA, Morris DD, Juan D. Effects of estazolam and flurazepam on cardiopulmonary function in patients with chronic obstructive pulmonary disease. Drug Saf. 1992;7(2):152–8.
64. Stege G, Heijdra YF, van den Elshout FJJ, van de Ven MJT, de Bruijn PJ, van Sorge AA, et al. Temazepam 10 mg does not affect breathing and gas exchange in patients with severe normocapnic COPD. Respir Med. 2010;104(4):518–24.
65. Berry RB, Patel PB. Effect of zolpidem on the efficacy of continuous positive airway pressure as treatment for obstructive sleep apnea. Sleep. 2006;29(8):1052–6.
66. Beaupré A, Soucy R, Phillips R, Bourgouin J. Respiratory center output following zopiclone or diazepam administration in patients with pulmonary disease. Respiration. 1988;54:235–40.
67. Shilo L, Dagan Y, Smorjik Y, Weinberg U, Dolev S, Komptel B, et al. Effect of melatonin on sleep quality of COPD intensive care patients: a pilot study. Chronobiol Int. 2000;17:71–6.
68. Nunes DM, Mota RMS, Mochado MO, Pereira EDB, deBruin VMS, deBruin PFC. Effect of melatonin administration on subjective sleep quality in chronic obstructive pulmonary disease. Braz J Med Biol Res. 2008;41(10):926–31.
69. Kryger M, Wang-Weigand S, Zhang J, Roth T. Effect of Ramelteon, a selective MT1/MT2-receptor agonist, on respiration during sleep in mild to moderate COPD. Sleep Breath. 2008;12:243–50.

70. Matos Cavalcante AG, Bruin PFC, Bruin VMS, Nunes DM, Pereira EDB, Cavalcante MM. Melatonin reduces lung oxidative stress in patients with chronic obstructive pulmonary disease: a randomized, double-blind, placebo-controlled study. J Pineal Res. 2012;53:238–44.
71. Kapella MC, Herdegen JJ, Perlis ML, Shaver JL, Larson JL, Law JA, et al. Cognitive behavioral therapy for insomnia comorbid with COPD is feasible with preliminary evidence of positive sleep and fatigue effects. Int J Chron Obstruct Pulmon Dis. 2011;6:625–35.
72. Koch BCP, Nagtegaal JE, Kerkhof GA, ter Wee PM. Circadian sleep-wake rhythm disturbances in end-stage renal disease. Nat Rev Nephrol. 2009;5(7):407–16.
73. De Santo RM, Bartiromo M, Cesare CM, Cirillo M. Sleep disorders occur very early in chronic kidney disease. J Nephrol. 2008;21 Suppl 13:S59–65.
74. Koch BCP, Van Der Putten K, Van Someren EJW, Wielders JPM, Ter Wee PM, Nagtegaal JE, et al. Impairment of endogenous melatonin rhythm is related to the degree of chronic kidney disease (CREAM study). Nephrol Dial Transplant. 2010;52:513–9.
75. Sabbatini M, Minale B, Crispo A, Pisani A, Ragosta A, Esposito R, et al. Insomnia in maintenance haemodialysis patients. Nephrol Dial Transplant. 2002;17(5):852–6.
76. Eryavuz N, Yuksel S, Acarturk G, Uslan I, Demir S, Demir M, et al. Comparison of sleep quality between hemodialysis and peritoneal dialysis patients. Int Urol Nephrol. 2008;40(3):785–91.
77. Iliescu EA, Coo H, McMurray MH, Meers CL, Quinn MM, Singer MA, et al. Quality of sleep and health-related quality of life in haemodialysis patients. Nephrol Dial Transplant. 2003;18(1):126–32.
78. Novak M, Molnar MZ, Ambrus C, Kovacs AZ, Koczy A, Remport A, et al. Chronic insomnia in kidney transplant recipients. Am J Kidney Dis. 2006;74:655–65.
79. Chavoshi F, Einollahi B, Sadeghniat Haghighi K, Saraei M, Izadianmehr N. Prevalence and sleep related disorders of restless leg syndrome in hemodialysis patients. Nephrourol Mon. 2015;7(2):e24611.
80. Calviño J, Cigarrán S, Lopez LM, Martinez A, Sobrido M-J. Restless legs syndrome in non-dialysis renal patients: is it really that common? J Clin Sleep Med. 2015;11(1):57–60.
81. Sloand JA, Shelly MA, Feigin A, Bernstein P, Monk RD. A double-blind, placebo-controlled trial of intravenous iron dextran therapy in patients with ESRD and restless legs syndrome. Am J Kidney Dis. 2004;43(4):663–70.
82. Jaber BL, Schiller B, Burkart JM, Daoui R, Kraus MA, Lee Y, et al. Impact of short daily hemodialysis on restless legs symptoms and sleep disturbances. Clin J Am Soc Nephrol. 2011;6(5):1049–56.
83. Giannaki CD, Hadjigeorgiou GM, Karatzaferi C, Maridaki MD, Koutedakis Y, Founta P, et al. A single-blind randomized controlled trial to evaluate the effect of 6 months of progressive aerobic exercise training in patients with uraemic restless legs syndrome. Nephrol Dial Transplant. 2013;28(11):2834–40.
84. Redolfi S, Yumino D, Ruttanaumpawan P, Yau B, Su M-C, Lam J, et al. Relationship between overnight rostral fluid shift and Obstructive Sleep Apnea in nonobese men. Am J Respir Crit Care Med. 2009;179(3):241–6.
85. Elias RM, Bradley TD, Kasai T, Motwani SS, Chan CT. Rostral overnight fluid shift in end-stage renal disease: relationship with obstructive sleep apnea. Nephrol Dial Transplant. 2012;27(4):1569–73.
86. Elias RM, Chan CT, Paul N, Motwani SS, Kasai T, Gabriel JM, et al. Relationship of pharyngeal water content and jugular volume with severity of obstructive sleep apnea in renal failure. Nephrol Dial Transplant. 2013;28(4):937–44.
87. Lyons OD, Chan CT, Yadollahi A, Bradley TD. Effect of ultrafiltration on sleep apnea and sleep structure in patients with end-stage renal disease. Am J Respir Crit Care Med. 2015;191(11):1287–94.
88. Tang SCW, Lam B, Lai ASH, Pang CBY, Tso WK, Khong PL, et al. Improvement in sleep apnea during nocturnal peritoneal dialysis is associated with reduced airway congestion and better uremic clearance. Clin J Am Soc Nephrol. 2009;4(2):410–8.
89. Virga G, Stanic L, Mastrosimone S, Gastaldon F, da Porto A, Bonadonna A. Hypercalcemia and insomnia in hemodialysis patients. Nephron. 2000;85(1):94–5.

90. Koch BCP, Hagen EC, Nagtegaal JE, Boringa JBS, Kerkhof GA, Ter Wee PM. Effects of nocturnal hemodialysis on melatonin rhythm and sleep-wake behavior: an uncontrolled trial. Am J Kidney Dis. 2009;53(4):658–64.
91. Koch BCP, Nagtegaal JE, Hagen EC, ter Wee PM, Kerkhof GA. Different melatonin rhythms and sleep-wake rhythms in patients on peritoneal dialysis, daytime hemodialysis and nocturnal hemodialysis. Sleep Med. 2010;11(3):242–6.
92. Sabbatini M, Crispo A, Pisani A, Ragosta A, Cesaro A, Mirenghi F, Cianciaruso B, Federico S. Zaleplon improves sleep quality in maintenance hemodialysis patients. Nephron Clin Pract. 2003;94(4):c99–103.
93. Edalat-Nejad M, Haqhverdi F, Hossein-Tabar T, Ahmadian M. Melatonin improves sleep quality in hemodialysis patients. Indian J Nephrol. 2013;23(4):264–9.
94. Chen HY, Chiang CK, Wang HH, Hung KY, Lee YJ, Peng YS, et al. Cognitive-behavioral therapy for sleep disturbance in patients undergoing peritoneal dialysis: a pilot randomized controlled trial. Am J Kidney Dis. 2008;52:314–23.
95. Shaker R, Castell DO, Schoenfeld PS, Spechler SJ. Nighttime heartburn is an under-appreciated clinical problem that impacts sleep and daytime function: the results of a Gallup survey conducted on behalf of the American Gastroenterological Association. Am J Gastroenterol. 2003;98:1487–93.
96. Moore JG, Englert E. Circadian rhythm of gastric acid secretion in man. Nature. 1970;226:1261–2.
97. Shaheen NJ, Madanick RD, Alattar M, Morgan DR, Davis PH, Galanko JA, et al. Gastroesophageal reflux disease as an etiology of sleep disturbance in subjects with insomnia and minimal reflux symptoms: a pilot study of prevalence and response to therapy. Dig Dis Sci. 2008;53:1493–9.
98. Johnson DA, Orr WC, Crawley JA, Traxler B, McCullough J, Brown KA, et al. Effect of esomeprazole on nighttime heartburn and sleep quality in patients with GERD: a randomized, placebo-controlled trial. Am J Gastroenterol. 2005;11:1914–22.
99. Fass R, Johnson DA, Orr WC, Han C, Mody R, Stern KN, et al. The effect of dexlansoprazole MR on nocturnal heartburn and GERD-related sleep disturbances in patients with symptomatic GERD. Am J Gastroenterol. 2011;106:421–31.
100. Heinemann S, Graf KI, Karaus M, Dorow P. Occurrence of obstructive sleep related respiratory disorder in conjunction with gastroesophageal reflux. Pneumologie. 1995;49:139–41.
101. Eskiizmir G, Kezirian E. Is there a vicious cycle between obstructive sleep apnea and laryngopharyngeal reflux disease? Med Hypotheses. 2009;73(5):706–8.
102. Green BT, Broughton WA, O'Connor JB. Marked improvement in nocturnal gastroesophageal reflux in a large cohort of patients with obstructive sleep apnea treated with continuous positive airway pressure. Arch Intern Med. 2003;163:41–5.
103. Senior BA et al. Gastroesophageal reflux and obstructive sleep apnea. Laryngoscope. 2001;111(12):2144–6.
104. Rotem AY, Sperber AD, Krugliak P, Freidman B, Tal A, Tarasiuk A. Polysomnographic and actigraphic evidence of sleep fragmentation in patients with irritable bowel syndrome. Sleep. 2003;26:747–52.
105. Song GH, Leng PH, Gwee KA, Moochhala SM, Ho KY. Melatonin improves abdominal pain in irritable bowel syndrome patients who have sleep disturbances: a randomised, double blind, placebo controlled study. Gut. 2005;54:1402–7.
106. Córdoba J, Cabrera J, Lataif L, Penev P, Zee P, Blei AT. High prevalence of sleep disturbance in cirrhosis. Hepatology. 1998;27(2):339–45.
107. Groeneweg M, Quero JC, De Bruijn I, Hartmann IJC, Essink-Bot ML, Hop WCJ, et al. Subclinical hepatic encephalopathy impairs daily functioning. Hepatology. 1998;28(1):45–9.
108. Chojnacki C, Wachowska-Kelly P, Błasiak J, Reiter RJ, Chojnacki J. Melatonin secretion and metabolism in patients with hepatic encephalopathy. J Gastroenterol Hepatol. 2013;28(2):342–7.
109. Velissaris D, Karamouzos V, Polychronopoulos P, Karanikolas M. Chronotypology and melatonin alterations in minimal hepatic encephalopathy. J Circadian Rhythms. 2009;7:6.
110. Fass R, Quan SF, O'Connor GT, Ervin A, Iber C. Predictors of heartburn during sleep in a large prospective cohort study. Chest. 2005;127(5):1658–66.

111. Hall AW, Moossa AR, Clark J, Cooley GR, Skinner DB. The effects of premedication drugs on the lower oesophageal high pressure zone and reflux status of rhesus monkeys and man. Gut. 1975 May;16(5):347–52.

112. Gagliardi GS, Shah AP, Goldstein M, Denua-Rivera S, Doghramji K, Cohen S, et al. Effect of zolpidem on the sleep arousal response to nocturnal esophageal acid exposure. Clin Gastroenterol Hepatol. 2009;7(9):948–52.

113. Kandil TS, Mousa AA, El-Gendy AA, Abbas AM. The potential therapeutic effect of melatonin in Gastro-Esophageal Reflux Disease. BMC Gastroenterol. 2010;10:7.

114. de Oliveira Torres JDF, de Souza Pereira R. Which is the best choice for gastroesophageal disorders: Melatonin or proton pump inhibitors? World J Gastrointest Pharmacol Ther. 2010;1(5):102–6.

115. Jha LK, Fass R, Gadam R, Maradey-Romero C, Nasrollah L, Hershcovici T, Quan SF, Dickman R. The Effect of Ramelteon on Heartburn Symptoms of Patients With Gastroesophageal Reflux Disease and Chronic Insomnia: A Pilot Study. J Clin Gastroenterol. 2016;50(2):e19–24.

116. Lane EA, Moss HB. Pharmacokinetics of melatonin in man: first pass hepatic metabolism. J Clin Endocrinol Metab. 1985;61(6):1214–6.

117. Bliwise DL, Foley DJ, Vitiello MV, Ansari FP, Ancoli-Israel S, Walsh JK. Nocturia and disturbed sleep in the elderly. Sleep Med. 2009;10:540–8.

118. Leger D, Comet D, Haab F, Ohayon MM. Prostatic hyperplasia is highly associated with nocturia and excessive sleepiness: a cross-sectional study Emmanuel Chartier-Kastler. BMJ Open. 2012;2:e000505.

119. Simaioforidis V, Papatsoris AG, Chrisofos M, Chrisafis M, Koritsiadis S, Deliveliotis C. Tamsulosin versus transurethral resection of the prostate: effect on nocturia as a result of benign prostatic hyperplasia. Int J Urol. 2011;18(3):243–8.

120. Stewart WF, Van Rooyen JB, Cundiff GW, Abrams P, Herzog AR, Corey R, et al. Prevalence and burden of overactive bladder in the United States. World J Urol. 2003;20:327–36.

121. Rackley R, Weiss JP, Rovner ES, Wang JT, Guan Z, 037 STUDY GROUP. Nighttime dosing with tolterodine reduces overactive bladder-related nocturnal micturitions in patients with overactive bladder and nocturia. Urology. 2006;67(4):731–6.

122. Diefenbach K, Donath F, Maurer A, Quispe Bravo S, Wernecke KD, Schwantes U, et al. Randomised, double-blind study of the effects of oxybutynin, tolterodine, trospium chloride and placebo on sleep in healthy young volunteers. Clin Drug Investig. 2003;23:395–404.

123. Kemmer H, Mathes AM, Dilk O, Gröschel A, Grass C, Stöckle M. Obstructive sleep apnea syndrome is associated with overactive bladder and urgency incontinence in men. Sleep. 2009;32(2):271–5.

124. Lose G, Lalos O, Freeman RM, Van Kerrebroeck P. Efficacy of desmopressin (Minirin) in the treatment of nocturia: a double-blind placebo-controlled study in women. Am J Obstet Gynecol. 2003;189:1106–13.

125. Hospital S. Efficacy of desmopressin in the treatment of nocturia: a double-blind placebo-controlled study in men. BJU Int. 2002;89:855–62.

126. Morgan D, Tsai SC. Sleep and the endocrine system. Crit Care Clin. 2015;31(3):403–18.

127. Spiegel K, Leproult R, Van Cauter E. Impact of sleep debt on metabolic and endocrine function. Lancet. 1999;354(9188):1435–9.

128. Lu CL, Lee YC, Tsai SJ, Hu PG, Sim CB. Psychiatric disturbances associated with hyperthyroidism: an analysis report of 30 cases. Zhonghua Yi Xue Za Zhi (Taipei). 1995;56(6):393–8.

129. Moffett SX, Giannopoulos PF, James TD, Martin JV. Effects of acute microinjections of thyroid hormone to the preoptic region of hypothyroid adult male rats on sleep, motor activity and body temperature. Brain Res. 2013;1516:55–65.

130. Sridhar GR, Putcha V, Lakshmi G. Sleep in thyrotoxicosis. Indian J Endocrinol Metab. 2011;15(1):23–6.

131. Tobaldini E, Porta A, Bulgheroni M, Pecis M, Muratori M, Bevilacqua M, et al. Increased complexity of short-term heart rate variability in hyperthyroid patients during orthostatic

challenge. Conf Proc IEEE Eng Med Biol Soc. 2008;2008:1988–91. doi:10.1109/IEMBS.2008.4649579.

132. Kraemer S, Danker-Hopfe H, Pilhatsch M, Bes F, Bauer M. Effects of supraphysiological doses of levothyroxine on sleep in healthy subjects: a prospective polysomnography study. J Thyroid Res. 2011;2011:420580.

133. Akatsu H, Ewing SK, Stefanick ML, Fink HA, Stone KL, Barrett-Connor E, et al. Association between thyroid function and objective and subjective sleep quality in older men: the osteoporotic fractures in men (MrOS) study. Endocr Pract. 2014;20(6):576–86.

134. Colao A, Ferone D, Marzullo P, Lombardi G. Systemic complications of acromegaly: epidemiology, pathogenesis, and management. Endocr Rev. 2004;25(1):102–52.

135. Grunstein RR. Sleep apnea in acromegaly. Ann Intern Med. 1991;115(7):527.

136. Roemmler J, Gutt B, Fischer R, Vay S, Wiesmeth A, Bidlingmaier M, et al. Elevated incidence of sleep apnoea in acromegaly-correlation to disease activity. Sleep Breath. 2012;16(4):1247–53.

137. Grunstein RR, Ho KY, Berthon-Jones M, Stewart D, Sullivan CE. Central sleep apnea is associated with increased ventilatory response to carbon dioxide and hypersecretion of growth hormone in patients with acromegaly. Am J Respir Crit Care Med. 1994;150(2):496–502.

138. Grunstein RR. Effect of octreotide, a somatostatin analog, on sleep apnea in patients with acromegaly. Ann Intern Med. 1994;121(7):478.

139. Aulinas A, Webb SM. Health-related quality of life in primary and secondary adrenal insufficiency. Expert Rev Pharmacoecon Outcomes Res. 2014 Dec;14(6):873–88.

140. Løvås K, Husebye ES, Holsten F, Bjorvatn B. Sleep disturbances in patients with Addison's disease. Eur J Endocrinol. 2003;148(4):449–56.

141. Voss U, Tuin I, Krakow K. Sleep improvement in an insomniac patient with global pituitary insufficiency after change from triple to quadruple cortisol replacement therapy. Sleep Med. 2007;8(5):517–9.

142. García-Borreguero D, Wehr TA, Larrosa O, Granizo JJ, Hardwick D, Chrousos GP, et al. Glucocorticoid replacement is permissive for rapid eye movement sleep and sleep consolidation in patients with adrenal insufficiency. J Clin Endocrinol Metab. 2000;85(11):4201–6.

143. Shipley JE, Schteingart DE, Tandon R, Starkman MN. Sleep architecture and sleep apnea in patients with Cushing's disease. Sleep. 1992;15(6):514–8.

144. Berger G, Hardak E, Shaham B, Avitan E, Yigla M. Preliminary prospective explanatory observation on the impact of 3-month steroid therapy on the objective measures of sleep-disordered breathing. Sleep Breath. 2012;16(2):549–53.

145. Bercea RM, Mihaescu T, Cojocaru C, Bjorvatn B. Fatigue and serum testosterone in obstructive sleep apnea patients. Clin Respir J. 2015;9(3):342–9.

146. Hanafy HM. Testosterone therapy and obstructive sleep apnea: is there a real connection? J Sex Med. 2007;4(5):1241–6.

147. Hoyos CM, Killick R, Yee BJ, Grunstein RR, Liu PY. Effects of testosterone therapy on sleep and breathing in obese men with severe obstructive sleep apnoea: a randomized placebo-controlled trial. Clin Endocrinol (Oxf). 2012;77(4):599–607.

148. Xu Q, Lang C. Examining the relationship between subjective sleep disturbance and menopause: a systematic review and meta-analysis. Menopause. 2014;21(12):1301–18.

149. Takahashi JS, Hong H-K, Ko CH, McDearmon EL. The genetics of mammalian circadian order and disorder: implications for physiology and disease. Nat Rev Genet. 2008;9(10):764–75.

150. Paul KN, Saafir TB, Tosini G. The role of retinal photoreceptors in the regulation of circadian rhythms. Rev Endocr Metab Disord. 2009;10(4):271–8.

151. Ho Mien I, Chua EC-P, Lau P, Tan L-C, Lee IT-G, Yeo S-C, et al. Effects of exposure to intermittent versus continuous red light on human circadian rhythms, melatonin suppression, and pupillary constriction. PLoS One. 2014;9(5):e96532.

152. Tabandeh H, Lockley SW, Buttery R, Skene DJ, Defrance R, Arendt J, et al. Disturbance of sleep in blindness. Am J Ophthalmol. 1998;126:707–12.

153. Kessel L, Lundeman JH, Herbst K, Andersen TV, Larsen M. Age-related changes in the transmission properties of the human lens and their relevance to circadian entrainment. J Cataract Refract Surg. 2010;36:308–12.

154. Kessel L, Siganos G, Jørgensen T, Larsen M. Sleep disturbances are related to decreased transmission of blue light to the retina caused by lens yellowing. Sleep. 2011;34(9):1215–9.
155. Turner PL, Van Someren EJW, Mainster MA. The role of environmental light in sleep and health: effects of ocular aging and cataract surgery. Sleep Med Rev. 2010;14:269–80.
156. Tanaka M, Hosoe K, Hamada T, Morita T. Change in sleep state of the elderly before and after cataract surgery. J Physiol Anthropol. 2010;29(6):219–24.
157. Asplund R, Lindblad BE. Sleep and sleepiness 1 and 9 months after cataract surgery. Arch Gerontol Geriatr. 2004;38(1):69–75.
158. Asplund R, Ejdervik LB. The development of sleep in persons undergoing cataract surgery. Arch Gerontol Geriatr. 2002;35(2):179–87.
159. Ayaki M, Muramatsu M, Negishi K, Tsubota K. Improvements in sleep quality and gait speed after cataract surgery. Rejuvenation Res. 2013;16(1):35–42.
160. Mainster MA, Turner PL. Blue-blocking IOLs decrease photoreception without providing significant photoprotection. Surv Ophthalmol. 2010;55:272–83.
161. Landers JA, Tamblyn D, Perriam D. Effect of a blue-light-blocking intraocular lens on the quality of sleep. J Cataract Refract Surg. 2009;35:83–8.
162. Sack RL, Lewy AJ, Blood ML, Keith LD, Nakagawa H. Circadian rhythm abnormalities in totally blind people: incidence and clinical significance. J Clin Endocrinol Metab. 1992;75:127–34.
163. Sack RL, Brandes RW, Kendall AR, Lewy AJ. Entrainment of free-running circadian rhythms by melatonin in blind people. N Engl J Med. 2000;343(15):1070–7.
164. Lockley S, Dressman M, Torres R, Lavedan C, Licamele L, Polymeropoulos M. Tasimelteon treatment entrains the circadian clock and demonstrates significant benefit on sleep and wake parameters in totally blind individuals with non-24 hour circadian rhythms. Sleep Med. 2013;14(Supplement 1):e178.
165. Fishbein AB, Vitaterna O, Haugh IM, Bavishi AA, Zee PC, Turek FW, et al. Nocturnal eczema: review of sleep and circadian rhythms in children with atopic dermatitis and future research directions. J Allergy Clin Immunol. 2015;136(5):1170–7.
166. Gupta MA, Gupta AK. Sleep-wake disorders and dermatology. Clin Dermatol. 2013;31(1):118–26.
167. Goh C-L, Khoo L. A retrospective study of the clinical presentation and outcome of herpes zoster in a tertiary dermatology outpatient referral clinic. Int J Dermatol. 1997;36(9):667–72.
168. Camfferman D, Kennedy JD, Gold M, Martin AJ, Winwood P, Lushington K. Eczema, sleep, and behavior in children. J Clin Sleep Med. 2010;6(6):581–8.
169. Silverberg J, Garg N, Paller A. Sleep disturbances in adults with eczema are associated with impaired overall health: a US population-based study. J Invest Dermatol. 2015;135(1):56–66.
170. Bender BG, Ballard R, Canono B, Murphy JR, Leung DYM. Disease severity, scratching, and sleep quality in patients with atopic dermatitis. J Am Acad Dermatol. 2008;58(3):415–20.
171. Kimata H. Viewing humorous film improves night-time wakening in children with atopic dermatitis. Indian Pediatr. 2007;44(4):281–5.
172. Kenna HA, Poon AW, de los Angeles CP, Koran LM. Psychiatric complications of treatment with corticosteroids: review with case report. Psychiatry Clin Neurosci. 2011;65(6):549–60.
173. Richardson GS, Roehrs TA, Rosenthal L, Koshorek G, Roth T. Tolerance to daytime sedative effects of H1 antihistamines. J Clin Psychopharmacol. 2002;22(5):511–5.
174. Krystal AD, Durrence HH, Scharf M, Jochelson P, Rogowski R, Ludington E, et al. Efficacy and safety of doxepin 1 mg and 3 mg in a 12-week sleep laboratory and outpatient trial of elderly subjects with chronic primary insomnia. Sleep. 2010;33(11):1553–61.
175. Yeung W-F, Chung K-F, Yung K-P, Ng TH-Y. Doxepin for insomnia: a systematic review of randomized placebo-controlled trials. Sleep Med Rev. 2015;19:75–83.
176. Savard J, Morin CM. Insomnia in the context of cancer: a review of a neglected problem. J Clin Oncol. 2001;19:895–908.
177. Chen M-L, Chang H-K. Physical symptom profiles of depressed and nondepressed patients with cancer. Palliat Med. 2004;18:712–8.
178. Palesh OG, Roscoe JA, Mustian KM, Roth T, Savard J, Ancoli-Israel S, et al. Prevalence, demographics, and psychological associations of sleep disruption in patients with cancer: University of Rochester Cancer Center-Community Clinical Oncology Program. J Clin Oncol. 2010;28:292–8.

179. Hickok JT, Morrow GR, Roscoe JA, Mustian K, Okunieff P. Occurrence, severity, and longitudinal course of twelve common symptoms in 1129 consecutive patients during radiotherapy for cancer. J Pain Symptom Manage. 2005;30(5):433–42.
180. Vgontzas AN, Zoumakis M, Papanicolaou DA, Bixler EO, Prolo P, Lin H-M, et al. Chronic insomnia is associated with a shift of interleukin-6 and tumor necrosis factor secretion from nighttime to daytime. Metabolism. 2002;51:887–92.
181. Sprod L, Palesh O, Janelsins M, Peppone L, Heckler C, Adams M, et al. Exercise, sleep quality, and mediators of sleep in breast and prostate cancer patients receiving radiation therapy. Commun Oncol. 2010;7:463–71.
182. Miaskowski C, Lee KA. Pain, fatigue, and sleep disturbances in oncology outpatients receiving radiation therapy for bone metastasis: a pilot study. J Pain Symptom Manage. 1999;17:320–32.
183. Nelson JE, Meier DE, Oei EJ, Nierman DM, Senzel RS, Manfredi PL, et al. Self-reported symptom experience of critically ill cancer patients receiving intensive care. Crit Care Med. 2001;29(2):277–82.
184. Savard J, Simard S, Blanchet J, Ivers H, Morin CM. Prevalence, clinical characteristics, and risk factors for insomnia in the context of breast cancer. Sleep. 2001;24(5):583–90.
185. Savard J, Ivers H, Villa J, Caplette-Gingras A, Morin CM. Natural course of insomnia comorbid with cancer: an 18-month longitudinal study. J Clin Oncol. 2011;29:3580–6.
186. Fleming L, MacMahon K. CBT-I in cancer: we know it works, so why are we waiting? Curr Sleep Med Rep. 2015;1(3):177–83.
187. Garland SN, Johnson JA, Savard J, Gehrman P, Perlis M, Carlson L, et al. Sleeping well with cancer: a systematic review of cognitive behavioral therapy for insomnia in cancer patients. Neuropsychiatr Dis Treat. 2014;10:1113–24.
188. Espie CA, Fleming L, Cassidy J, Samuel L, Taylor LM, White CA, et al. Randomized controlled clinical effectiveness trial of cognitive behavior therapy compared with treatment as usual for persistent insomnia in patients with cancer. J Clin Oncol. 2008;26:4651–8.
189. Morin CM, Bootzin RR, Buysse DJ, Edinger JD, Espie CA, Lichstein KL. Psychological and behavioral treatment of insomnia: update of the recent evidence (1998–2004). Sleep. 2006;29(11):1398–414.
190. Savard J, Ivers H, Savard M-H, Morin CM. Long-term effects of two formats of cognitive behavioral therapy for insomnia comorbid with breast cancer. Sleep. 2015;39(4):813–23.
191. Heckler CE, Garland SN, Peoples AR, Perlis ML, Shayne M, Morrow GR, et al. Cognitive behavioral therapy for insomnia, but not armodafinil, improves fatigue in cancer survivors with insomnia: a randomized placebo-controlled trial. Support Care Cancer. 2015;24(5):2059–66.
192. Lengacher CA, Johnson-Mallard V, Post-White J, Moscoso MS, Jacobsen PB, Klein TW, et al. Randomized controlled trial of mindfulness-based stress reduction (MBSR) for survivors of breast cancer. Psychooncology. 2009;18(12):1261–72.
193. Lengacher CA, Reich RR, Paterson CL, Jim HS, Ramesar S, Alinat CB, et al. The effects of mindfulness-based stress reduction on objective and subjective sleep parameters in women with breast cancer: a randomized controlled trial. Psychooncology. 2015;24(4):424–32.
194. Johns SA, Brown LF, Beck-Coon K, Monahan PO, Tong Y, Kroenke K. Randomized controlled pilot study of mindfulness-based stress reduction for persistently fatigued cancer survivors. Psychooncology. 2015;24(8):885–93.
195. Ledesma D, Kumano H. Mindfulness-based stress reduction and cancer: a meta-analysis. Psychooncology. 2009;18(6):571–9.
196. Andersen SR, Würtzen H, Steding-Jessen M, Christensen J, Andersen KK, Flyger H, et al. Effect of mindfulness-based stress reduction on sleep quality: results of a randomized trial among Danish breast cancer patients. Acta Oncol. 2013;52(2):336–44.
197. Garland SN, Carlson LE, Stephens AJ, Antle MC, Samuels C, Campbell TS. Mindfulness-based stress reduction compared with cognitive behavioral therapy for the treatment of insomnia comorbid with cancer: a randomized, partially blinded, noninferiority trial. J Clin Oncol. 2014;32(5):449–57.
198. Alvarez J, Meyer FL, Granoff DL, Lundy A. The effect of EEG biofeedback on reducing postcancer cognitive impairment. Integr Cancer Ther. 2013;12(6):475–87.

Chapter 12
Sleep Disturbance in Cancer Survivors

Heather L. McGinty, Allison J. Carroll, and Stacy D. Sanford

Abstract Sleep disturbance is highly prevalent among survivors of cancer across the continuum of care. There are numerous unique factors among survivors that may precipitate and/or perpetuate sleep disturbance, including, but not limited to, cancer diagnosis and treatment. Similar to the general population, sleep disturbance is negatively associated with multiple domains of quality of life, including the emotional and physical well-being of cancer survivors. Moreover, sleep disturbance often co-occurs with other common behavioral symptoms such as fatigue, pain, depression, and cognitive impairment. Routine screening for sleep disturbance is recommended, especially at key transitions in care (e.g., a change in treatment or transition off of treatment). Guidelines for thorough assessment and treatment of sleep disturbance exist; however, research examining sleep in cancer survivors is a growing area of inquiry. The best empirical support to date is for treating insomnia among cancer survivors using cognitive behavioral therapy for insomnia. Additional clinical research is warranted to establish the efficacy of treatment modalities, including pharmacotherapy, for sleep disturbance among cancer survivors.

Keywords Cancer • Sleep disturbance • Insomnia • Assessment • Treatment • Quality of life

H.L. McGinty, Ph.D.
Department of Medical Social Sciences, Northwestern University Feinberg School of Medicine, 633 N. St. Clair St., Suite 19-052, Chicago, IL 60611, USA
e-mail: heather.mcginty@northwestern.edu

A.J. Carroll, M.S.
Department of Preventive Medicine, Northwestern University Feinberg School of Medicine, 680 N Lake Shore Drive Ste 1400, Chicago, IL 60657, USA
e-mail: allisoncarroll2016@u.northwestern.edu

S.D. Sanford, Ph.D. (✉)
Department of Medical Social Sciences, Northwestern University Feinberg School of Medicine, 633 N. St. Clair St., Suite 19-052, Chicago, IL 60611, USA

Department of Psychiatry and Behavioral Sciences, Northwestern University Feinberg School of Medicine, 675 N. Saint Clair, Suite 21-100, Chicago, IL 60611, USA
e-mail: ssanfor1@nm.org

© Springer International Publishing Switzerland 2017
H.P. Attarian (ed.), *Clinical Handbook of Insomnia*, Current Clinical Neurology,
DOI 10.1007/978-3-319-41400-3_12

Introduction

Cancer survivorship spans the time from when a person is first diagnosed with cancer through to end of life, encompassing both those with active disease and on treatment as well as those enjoying several disease-free years [1]. In 2014, the American Cancer Society estimated there to be nearly 14.5 million cancer survivors and projected that this number will grow to nearly 19 million cancer survivors by the year 2024 as cancer detection and treatments continue to improve [1]. This growing population of cancer survivors carries unique healthcare concerns and symptom profiles with which all healthcare providers should become familiar. Increasing interest in patient-reported outcomes in cancer has revealed that insomnia and other symptoms of disturbed sleep are some of the most common problems endorsed by patients across the cancer survivorship continuum [2]. However, patients may not discuss sleep complaints with their oncology treatment team [3], which highlights the importance of screening and assessing these concerns, but also makes it difficult to ascertain the full extent of the problem in this population [2]. In this chapter, we provide the latest information about the prevalence, presentation, impact, assessment, and available treatments of sleep disturbance in cancer survivors.

Sleep Disturbance over the Cancer Care Continuum

Sleep complaints can occur at any time in the cancer continuum from pre-diagnosis through long-term cancer survivorship. Common symptoms are increased daytime sleepiness, nighttime awakenings, sleep latency, and/or time in bed awake (e.g., poor sleep efficiency), as well as decreased daytime activity and/or disruption in diurnal sleeping patterns [2]. Note sleep disturbances experienced in the context of cancer may not always meet full criteria for a sleep disorder. Even so, rates of sleep disturbance among patients with cancer are estimated to be three times the rate observed in the general population; an estimated 10–15 % of the general population has sleep disturbance compared to 30–50 % of cancer survivors [4]. Depending on how and when sleep disturbance is assessed, approximately 20–75 % of patients with cancer report at least one form of sleep complaint during their initial cancer diagnosis, while on treatment, following completion of successful treatment, or at the end of life [4–6].

Although few studies have directly compared the rates of insomnia and sleep disturbance between cancer sites, one study of a variety of cancer types during chemotherapy revealed clinical insomnia rates that were highest among patients with genitourinary tract cancer (54 %), lung cancer (51 %), and breast cancer (46 %) [5]. When assessing subjective sleep complaints, the available studies indicate that women with breast cancer tend to have the highest rates of overall sleep complaints at over 80 % during chemotherapy [5] and report greater subjective sleep impairment than comparison groups of cancer survivors [7, 8]. However, patients with lung cancer have demonstrated higher rates of objective sleep disruption compared to patients with breast cancer [9].

Unfortunately, there are a range of negative consequences associated with sleep disturbance among cancer survivors. Survivors with sleep disturbance are more likely to report impairments in daytime functioning, including fatigue, depression, anxiety, and impaired cognition (e.g., "chemo brain") [5, 10, 11]. A number of studies have evaluated the impact of sleep disturbance on health-related quality of life in cancer survivors before, during, and after treatment completion. In general, sleep disruption is related to poorer quality of life for patients with a history of cancer. For example, patients with breast cancer at various points in their treatment trajectory reported poorer physical functioning, bodily pain, vitality, emotional well-being, and mental health if they had poorer sleep quality than those reporting good sleep [12]. In a large sample with mixed cancer types, greater sleep impairment at any point in cancer care was associated with poorer physical, social, economic, psychological/spiritual, or familial well-being even after controlling for factors such as age and treatment history [13]. The prevalence and impact of sleep disturbance on quality of life across the different time points in cancer survivorship are further outlined below from the point of diagnosis to treatment to post-treatment and long-term survivorship or end of life.

Pre-treatment

The time period immediately following diagnosis is particularly distressing for most cancer survivors and presents challenges to both sleep and overall well-being. In one study, distress was higher in those patients with insomnia symptoms who were closer to cancer diagnosis than for those whose insomnia had persisted for several months after diagnosis, which highlights the impact of recent cancer diagnosis on both sleep disturbance and emotional distress [14]. Few studies have assessed sleep or insomnia rates prior to the start of any cancer treatment and those which have often combined these rates with patients either on or post-treatment. However, approximately 43 % of patients with mixed cancer types surveyed prior to starting chemotherapy met clinical criteria for an insomnia syndrome [5]. Among women who are diagnosed with breast cancer and scheduled to begin chemotherapy, both objective and subjective measures of sleep indicate that these women experience significant sleep disturbance (e.g., awake for 25 % of time in bed) and poor quality of sleep [15, 16]. Among women with breast cancer who met criteria for clinical insomnia, approximately a third reported that sleep became problematic only following their cancer diagnosis and the majority reported that cancer exacerbated an existing sleep problem [17]. Qualitative studies also indicate that a cancer diagnosis itself can exacerbate existing sleep problems or contribute to a new onset of insomnia, which may then persist for years following the termination of cancer treatment [18].

On Treatment (Surgery, Chemotherapy, Radiation Therapy, Endocrine Therapies)

The varying forms of treatment for cancer can further impact sleep over the continuum of cancer care. Of note, many of the patients in the "pre-treatment" studies above, while naive to chemotherapy, may have undergone surgery or biopsies prior to assessment that have the potential to impact sleep. For example, over 30 % of men who underwent radical prostatectomy for prostate cancer reported impaired sleep, and nearly 20 % of these patients met the criteria for insomnia syndrome [19]. Among women with breast cancer who had undergone surgery, over 50 % of the patients reported elevated sleep disturbance with the most common problem being sleep maintenance difficulty [16]. Sleep disturbance following cancer surgery tends to persist even after the expected recovery period has elapsed [20].

Not surprisingly, patients who undergo intensive treatments such as hospitalizations for cancer or stem cell transplants also suffer quality of life impairment that is associated with sleep disturbances. For instance, greater problems with overall physical symptoms or physical functioning, bodily pain, and emotional distress were associated with poorer sleep (i.e., longer time to sleep onset and shorter sleep duration) among adults hospitalized for cancer [21]. The first year following bone marrow transplant is associated with a number of physical symptoms, including difficulty sleeping for approximately 20 % of patients [22]. Another study of longer term stem cell transplant survivors (mean of 43.5 months post-transplant) observed that 51 % of patients reported some sleep difficulties, with nearly 16 % reporting moderate to severe sleep problems [23].

During chemotherapy, regardless of the number of treatments or cycles, between 60 and 80 % of patients report experiencing at least some symptoms of insomnia, and approximately half of those patients meet the criteria for insomnia syndrome [5, 11]. A prospective evaluation of sleep problems in patients receiving chemotherapy found that sleep disturbance worsens over time as the patient progresses through treatment cycles [24]. A more recent longitudinal study suggests that sleep disturbance during chemotherapy for breast cancer is strongly mediated by chemotherapy side effects [8]. Others have reported consistent impairments in subjective and objective sleep quality (e.g., total night sleep time, wake time at night) in women with breast cancer before and during chemotherapy, and also observed increases in daytime napping during chemotherapy [25]. In a large study evaluating patients with mixed cancer sites, insomnia during chemotherapy was associated with greater depression and fatigue than those who did not report insomnia syndromes [5]. Patients receiving chemotherapy for lung cancer who reported sleep disturbances had significantly poorer perceived cognitive functioning and worse performance statuses when statistically controlling for the influence of other symptoms (e.g., shortness of breath, pain, or depressive symptom severity) on quality of life [11].

Radiation therapy may also impact sleep disturbance, though perhaps to a lesser degree than other treatments for cancer. For example, over 50 % of breast cancer survivors reported sleep disturbance while they were undergoing radiation therapy [17].

Again, a more recent study suggests that sleep disturbance is exacerbated by radiation therapy for women with breast cancer. Data showed insomnia symptom severity increasing over the course of treatment [8]. However, in longitudinal studies of patients with breast or prostate cancer with no history of chemotherapy, sleep disturbance appears to be most severe prior to initiating radiation therapy and in the early weeks of treatment, but improves over time and after completion of treatment [7, 26]. Therefore, although many patients report sleep disturbance prior to and during radiation therapy, there is insufficient evidence that radiation therapy alone results in chronic sleep problems.

The hormonal changes that often result from cancer and/or cancer treatment can have a significant impact on sleep. Whether resulting from chemotherapy-induced menopause or androgen deprivation therapy-induced andropause, hot flashes and night sweats in particular are associated with greater sleep impairment in cancer patients [8, 27]. Hot flashes are related to greater reported time spent awake during the night, as well as objective changes in sleep structure indicating less efficient and more disrupted sleep in women with breast cancer [28]. In prostate cancer, nocturnal awakenings and/or daytime sleepiness, nocturia, and hot flashes were symptoms found to cluster together for those patients undergoing androgen deprivation therapy [29]. When specifically assessing for insomnia syndrome, severe insomnia symptoms are reported by men undergoing androgen deprivation therapy for prostate cancer; however, receipt of hormone therapy was not related to insomnia syndrome among women with breast cancer [8].

Post-treatment and Long-Term Survivorship

For many survivors, sleep disturbance continues after completion of treatment and into long-term survivorship. For example, sleep disturbances persist for 40–65 % of breast cancer survivors after treatment, and these disturbances are not solely related to the use of adjuvant endocrine therapies [30–32]. Several studies demonstrate that these sleep complaints can persist several weeks or months following completion of chemotherapy treatment [10, 33]. Over half of long-term lung cancer survivors (>5 years post-diagnosis) report poor sleep quality; in fact, poor sleep quality is nearly twice as common in long-term lung cancer survivors compared to non-cancer controls [34]. These survivors with sleep impairments also reported poorer overall quality of life than non-cancer controls even after controlling for the impact of dyspnea [34]. Similar impairments in sleep and quality of life are found in pediatric cancer survivors, even decades later as adult survivors, although the percentage of adult survivors of childhood cancers who self-report poor sleep quality is somewhat lower than survivors of adult cancers (17 % report poor sleep quality, 14 % report excessive daytime sleepiness) [35]. Regardless, evidence indicates that poor sleep quality is associated with poorer quality of life in this population, especially related to neurocognitive impairment even after controlling for the influences of cranial radiation, steroids, antimetabolite chemotherapy, sex, and current age [36].

Advanced Disease

No known studies have directly compared insomnia rates between cancer stages (e.g., early stage vs. metastatic disease). However, several studies have evaluated sleep in patients with metastatic cancer or those receiving palliative care, thereby giving us important information about sleep impairment in advanced cancer. One study measuring sleep disturbance among women with a diagnosis of metastatic breast cancer revealed that 64 % of these women reported one or more types of sleep disturbance, including problems getting to sleep, maintaining sleep, early-morning awakenings, and daytime sleepiness [37]. Seventy-five percent of patients receiving radiation therapy for various types of metastatic cancer reported poor sleep efficiency and demonstrated several objective and subjective sleep impairments that were associated with poorer functional status [38]. Furthermore, patients with advanced cancer in an inpatient setting report poor sleep (i.e., diurnal sleep, non-restorative sleep, difficulties falling or staying asleep, and nightmares), with 30 % of patients reporting an average sleep duration of less than 5 h per night. Moreover, these sleep problems are associated with poorer performance statuses, anxiety, depression, and confusion [39]. A more recent study of 820 patients with advanced cancers being treated in palliative care settings found that 60 % of patients report sleep disturbance, and multiple factors were associated with poor sleep, including depression and anxiety symptoms, Karnofsky score, and certain medications (e.g., corticosteroids and opioids) [40].

Risk Factors for Sleep Disturbance in Cancer

Speilman's three-factor model of insomnia serves as a good framework for discussing risk factors for sleep disturbance in cancer [41]. The "3 P" model, as highlighted in Table 12.1, denotes three etiologic factors associated with insomnia in cancer: predisposing, precipitating, and perpetuating factors. Predisposing factors include enduring personal traits that are known to increase susceptibility to sleep disturbance such as aging, personal or family history of insomnia, gender, race, arousability, or decreased homeostatic sleep drive [42, 43]. Of note, contrary to studies in the general population, a large cohort study found that younger cancer survivors are more likely to present with insomnia symptoms or insomnia syndrome compared to older survivors [5].

Precipitating factors are situations or events that can trigger sleep disturbance; these may be either acute or chronic events. For cancer survivors, this includes stressful points in cancer care such as diagnosis, hospitalizations, or recurrence. These also include psychological factors such as anxiety, depression, or increased levels of stress that may interfere with sleep, as well as physiological effects of disease or treatment, including late effects and symptoms such as pain, nausea/vomiting, hot flashes, cortisol disruption, or variations in cytokine production [43].

Table 12.1 Summary of potential etiologic factors of insomnia in the context of cancer

Predisposing factors
Hyperarousability trait
Decreased homeostatic sleep drive
Female gender
Age
Familial history of insomnia
Personal history of insomnia
Pre-existing psychiatric disorder
Precipitating factors
Cancer diagnosis
Surgery
Chemotherapy
Radiotherapy
Hormonal therapy
Hospitalization
Bone marrow transplantation
Psychological factors (e.g., new-onset mood or anxiety disorder)
Palliative medications (e.g., corticosteroids, antiemetics, stimulants, opioids)
Disease and/or treatment effects
Nausea/vomiting
Pain
Frequent urination
Hot flashes
Perpetuating factors
Maladaptive sleep behaviors
Excessive amount of time spent in bed
Irregular sleep-wake schedule
Napping
Engaging in sleep-interfering activities in the bedroom
Faulty beliefs and attitudes about sleep
Unrealistic sleep requirement expectations
Faulty appraisals of sleep difficulties
Misattributions of daytime impairments
Misconceptions about the causes of insomnia

Note: Adapted with permission from Morin, C.M. and Savard, J. (2001) Insomnia in the Context of Cancer: A Review of a Neglected Problem. *Journal of Clinical Oncology,* 19;895–908

Finally, perpetuating factors maintain sleep disturbance even after the precipitating factors have resolved. These include maladaptive behaviors and cognitions about sleep, including excessive time in bed, irregular sleep-wake scheduling, napping, conditioning non-sleep activities in the bed, poor sleep hygiene, unrealistic expectations about sleep requirements, and biased appraisals of sleep difficulties or daytime impairments [2, 42]. These perpetuating factors are similar for cancer survivors as well as non-cancer populations and may prolong sleep disturbance for years if not intervened upon.

Impact of Poor Sleep on Cancer and Its Treatment

It is commonly accepted knowledge that melatonin production plays an integral role in regulating circadian rhythms and promoting sleep, but laboratory studies also demonstrate its role in increasing immune functioning and inhibiting tumor cell growth [44]. Further, some literature suggests that disruptions in sleep and/or circadian rhythms can predispose people to cancer. This theory is largely supported by cohort studies and case–control trials that demonstrate an increased risk of developing cancer among shift workers as well as studies that demonstrate an association between circadian clock, endoplasmic reticulum stress signaling, and oncogenesis ([for a review, please see: [44, 45]). In fact, the International Agency for Research on Cancer has stated that shift work is "probably" a carcinogen based on animal studies and epidemiological evidence [46]. Interestingly, epidemiological studies have demonstrated elevations in various inflammatory markers and increased risk of cancer in association with shortened sleep duration, or paradoxically, with prolonged sleep duration [45]. However, to date, there are no prospective studies to demonstrate that treating disordered sleep or circadian rhythm disruptions prevents cancer or positively impacts cancer outcomes such as recurrences [45]. Additionally, variability across existing studies in design and methodology makes it difficult to draw conclusions as results have been mixed [45].

Symptom Clusters

It is clear that sleep disruption is often tied to other physical or psychological symptoms in cancer survivors, just as observed in those with no history of cancer. Many have postulated that the tight association between cancer-related sleep disturbance and other symptoms (e.g., fatigue, pain, depressed mood, or cognitive complaints) represents a "symptom cluster" which is defined as three or more concurrent symptoms that are related to each other regardless of their underlying etiology [47]. Recognizing the interrelationships between symptoms improves the symptom management by targeting symptom clusters rather than solely focusing on the most troubling symptom and discouraging the use of interventions which may aggravate one or more of the related symptoms. Therefore, identifying those symptoms which cluster with sleep disruption is an important consideration for healthcare providers who treat cancer survivors. The most often recognized behavioral symptom cluster in cancer populations includes any combination of sleep disturbance, fatigue, pain, and depressed mood [33, 48, 49]. These symptoms are also the most commonly

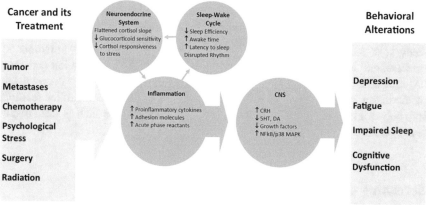

Fig. 12.1 Neuroendocrine-immune mechanisms and mediators of behavioral comorbidities in patients with cancer. Various aspects of being diagnosed with and treated for cancer activate inflammation through tissue damage/destruction and/or psychological stress. Cytokines of the innate immune response along with lifestyle changes, pain, and other consequences of cancer and its treatment alter the sleep-wake cycle, which in turn contributes to disruption of the neuroendocrine system, in particular, the hypothalamic-pituitary-adrenal (HPA) axis. Given the role of the HPA axis and glucocorticoids in regulating inflammatory responses, altered HPA axis function may disrupt glucocorticoid-mediated negative regulation of inflammation. Unrestrained inflammation and the associated increased release of proinflammatory cytokines, in turn, interact with central nervous system (CNS) pathways that regulate behavior, leading to pathophysiologic changes that underlie depression, fatigue, impaired sleep, and cognitive dysfunction. Figure adapted with permission from Miller AH, Ancoli-Israel SA, Bower JE, Capuron L, Irwin MR. Neuroendocrine-immune mechanisms of behavioral comorbidities in patiens with cancer. J Clin Oncol 2008; 26(6):971–82

reported in cancer survivors and, in the case of depression, sleep disturbance and fatigue may represent symptoms of the same problem (i.e., clinical depression with vegetative symptoms) [49]. More recently, subjective cognitive impairment has also been discussed in this context and was correlated longitudinally with sleep disturbance, fatigue, and depression in women with breast cancer [50].

Furthermore, shared associations between symptoms on a longitudinal basis suggest a shared underlying pathophysiological mechanism, indicating that efforts to document the mechanism for one symptom of interest may have broader applicability to all symptoms in the cluster. The role of pro-inflammatory cytokines has been increasingly implicated as a common neuroendocrine-immune mechanism underlying the behavioral symptoms of sleep disturbance, fatigue, depression, and cognitive dysfunction in individuals with cancer (see Fig. 12.1) [51, 52]. Observational and experimental data indicate that cancer survivors experience inflammation and support a relationship between sleep disturbance and innate immune cytokines [53]. However, to date, the relationship between sleep and inflammatory markers in cancer survivors has not been rigorously examined and results from existing studies have been mixed. For example, one breast cancer study found some inflammatory markers to be associated with fatigue in women treated with chemotherapy, but no such association was found for patient-reported sleep disturbance and depression, or for patients who did not receive chemotherapy [54]. However, the authors also note limitations of the study such as the cross-sectional design, their focus on only three inflammatory markers, and lack of clarity about the clinical significance of depression and sleep disturbance scores in their sample. Ultimately, variability across studies in design and methodology makes it difficult to draw conclusions. The exact nature of the relationship between immunologic processes and behavioral symptoms such as sleep disturbance remains speculative and additional research is required.

Screening and Assessing Sleep in Cancer Survivors

The high prevalence of sleep disturbance in cancer survivors paired with the complexity of factors that may contribute to such disturbance over the continuum of care merits routine screening for sleep disturbance followed by comprehensive assessment of contributing factors for positive screens. Both the Pan-Canadian practice guidelines [55] and the National Comprehensive Cancer Network (NCCN) survivorship guidelines [56] recommend routine screening and assessment at key transitions in care or changes in clinical status (e.g., at diagnosis, initiating new treatment, at completion of treatment).

Patient-reported outcome measures are most commonly used to screen for sleep disturbance. An example includes the 7-item Insomnia Severity Index [57] as suggested by the National Cancer Institute: PDQ® Sleep Disorders [4]. The Pan-Canadian guidelines suggest screening with the Edmonton Symptom Assessment Scale (ESAS; "other" item) [58] followed by two additional questions that screen for impairments in daytime functioning and frequency of disturbance: (1) *Do you have problems with your sleep or sleep disturbance on average (routinely, in the past month, etc.) for three or more nights a week?* (2) *If yes, does the problem with your sleep negatively affect your daytime function or quality of life?* Unfortunately, the ESAS does not specifically ask about sleep disturbance. Alternatively, they suggest using the eight-item PROMIS® "sleep thermometer tool" [59]. The NCCN Guidelines for Supportive Care Survivorship provide a detailed algorithm for screening for insomnia and other sleep disorders as well as assessment of contributing factors, treatment of contributing factors, and referral and/or treatment of sleep disorders. These guidelines are available online for clinicians to review and are summarized in Table 12.2 [56].

Table 12.2 Summary of 2015 NCCN survivorship guidelines for sleep screening, assessment, and treatment recommendations

Screening and assessment questions to be asked at regular intervals, especially when there is a change in clinical status or treatment:

- **Insomnia**
  - Are you currently taking medication to help you sleep?
  - Do you have difficulty falling or staying asleep?
  - How long does it take to fall asleep?
  - How many times do you wake up every night?
  - How long have you had difficulty falling or staying asleep?

Meets the criteria if difficulty falling asleep and/or maintaining sleep:

- Occurs at least three times per week
- Has a duration >4 weeks
  - Short-term insomnia if <3 months
  - Chronic insomnia if ≥3 months
- **Hypersomnia**
  - Do you fall asleep while reading, watching television, talking to friends, or driving?
  - Are you excessively sleepy during the day?
- **Obstructive sleep apnea (OSA)**
  - Do you snore, gasp for breath, or stop breathing during sleep? OR have you been told that you do so?
- **Restless leg syndrome (RLS)**
  - Do you have the urge to move the legs, usually accompanied by an uncomfortable, deep-seeded sensation that is brought on by rest? IF SO, are these symptoms more frequent or severe in the evening?

History and presentation (skip if no concerns for sleep disorder/disturbance):

- Assessment of treatable contributing factors:
  - Comorbidities:
    - Alcohol and/or substance abuse
    - Obesity
    - Cardiac dysfunction
    - Endocrine dysfunction (e.g., hypothyroidism)
    - Anemia: Examine iron and ferritin levels
    - Emotional distress: Screen for anxiety and depression
    - Neurologic disorders
    - Psychiatric disorders
  - Medications—Consider persistent use of:
    - Sleep aids (including over-the-counter)
    - Pain medications
    - Antiemetics
    - Stimulants
    - Antidepressants
    - Anti-psychotics
    - Sedative/hypnotics

(continued)

Table 12.2 (continued)

• Antihistamines
– Review caffeine intake
– Review history of chemotherapy
– Pain
– Fatigue
– Shift work
– Current coping strategies (relaxation techniques, meditation, etc.)
Insomnia disorder screening criteria met
• Obtain details about course of insomnia
– Insomnia problematic, causing decreased daytime functioning, poor quality of life, or distress to patient
• Address comorbid conditions if:
Medical, neurologic, or psychiatric condition(s), recurrence of cancer, pain, or if symptoms are associated with shift work
• Address medications that may cause insomnia
• Provide treatment for problematic insomnia:
Sleep hygiene education
Cognitive behavioral therapy
Pharmacologic intervention, if safe, for difficulty falling asleep, maintaining sleep, or nonrestorative sleep
Refer to sleep specialist for chronic or refractory symptoms
– If insomnia not problematic:
• Sleep hygiene education
• Reassess as needed
Sleep disturbance and/or excessive sleepiness (hypersomnias, OSA, RLS, or circadian rhythm sleep disorders) criteria met
• Further assessment to determine type and severity of problem:
– Associated with insufficient sleep time:
• Testing: Sleep log or diary
• Diagnosis: Insufficient sleep syndrome
• Treatment:
Increase time for sleep
Sleep hygiene education
– Associated with observed apneas, snoring:
• Testing:
Polysomnography (PSG)
Refer to sleep specialist for further evaluation
• Diagnosis: Obstructive sleep apnea (OSA)
• Treatment:
Weight loss
Exercise
Refer to sleep specialist
– Associated with uncomfortable sensation:

(continued)

Table 12.2 (continued)

• Testing:
Ferritin level <45–50 ng per mL
Refer to sleep specialist for further evaluation
• Diagnosis: Restless leg syndrome (RLS)
• Treatment management options:
Dopamine agonists
Benzodiazepines (BZD)
Gabapentin (enacarbil)
Opioids
Iron replacement as clinically indicated
Refer to sleep specialist
– Refer to sleep specialist if any of the following:
• Prolonged wakefulness or awakenings
• Prolonged nocturnal sleep (i.e., >9 h for adults)
• Cataplexy, frequent short naps, vivid dreams, disrupted sleep, or sleep paralysis
• Excessive daytime sleepiness not associated with other symptoms

Treating Sleep Disturbances and Contributing Factors

The first step in treatment for insomnia is to intervene on any possible contributing factors. Choosing a treatment direction can be challenging, as the treatment for one symptom may exacerbate another. Therefore, assessing for symptoms that commonly cluster together (sleep disturbance, fatigue, depression, pain, or cognitive impairment) may assist treatment planning. Many medications can lead to insomnia or hypersomnia, and when possible, it may be helpful to alter or change the patient's medications. The following medication types are examples of drugs associated with various forms of sleep impairment: analgesics (opioids and nonsteroidal anti-inflammatory drugs), antidepressants (tricyclic drugs and selective serotonin reuptake inhibitors [SSRIs]), antiemetics (dopamine antagonists, anticholinergic agents, 5-HT$_3$ antagonists), and corticosteroids (prednisone and dexamethasone) [43]. Even so, adequate treatment of symptoms such as pain, fatigue, or emotional distress is crucial. For example, it may be necessary to help the patient engage in adequate pain management strategies including appropriate pharmacotherapy or physical therapy, while also being mindful over time that some pain medications like opioids may exacerbate sleep difficulties (e.g., sleep apnea). If a patient is experiencing significant cancer-related fatigue, then this can exacerbate or trigger difficulties with sleep as patients attempt to compensate with less daytime activity and more daytime naps. Several psychological or behavioral interventions can reduce cancer-related fatigue, including pharmacological treatments, incorporating physical activity, and reducing maladaptive thoughts about fatigue [60, 61]. Stimulant medications are sometimes prescribed to help manage fatigue, but can exacerbate sleep disturbance. Addressing these factors may be the only intervention required for a subset of patients with sleep complaints.

Patients who exhibit risk factors for sleep disorders other than insomnia such as sleep apnea, narcolepsy, periodic limb movement disorder, or a circadian rhythm disorder warrant referrals to a sleep specialist for a more formal evaluation via objective measures such as actigraphy or polysomnography. Briefly, the following are risk factors for sleep apnea: loud snoring, older age, male gender, obesity, large neck circumference, and comorbid health conditions such as hypertension, diabetes mellitus, congestive heart failure, or stroke [62]. The STOP Questionnaire [63] is commonly used to screen for sleep apnea. Risk factors for restless leg syndrome include periodic limb movements during sleep, female gender, and highly soluble transferrin receptor [64]. Patients with several risk factors for these sleep disorders or those who exhibit symptoms of circadian rhythm sleep disorders should receive additional objective sleep monitoring prior to engaging in interventions designed primarily to treat insomnia. Additional guidelines for assessment and treatment of sleep disorders as provided by the NCCN are listed in Table 12.2.

If symptoms of insomnia persist once the above contributing factors are addressed, it may become necessary to refer patients out to a behavioral sleep specialist (The American Board of Sleep Medicine maintains an online list of certified behavioral sleep medicine specialists: http://www.absm.org/BSMSpecialists.aspx). Clinicians who specialize in behavioral sleep medicine are commonly mental health professionals, and can offer psychological and behavioral therapies and/or pharmacotherapy. Psychological and/or behavioral interventions for insomnia are recommended as an initial approach to treatment, when possible [65]. Because psychological distress, including depression and anxiety, is highly comorbid in cancer survivors, assessing for these factors and their potential contribution to sleep disturbance is especially relevant for these patients in order to make an informed referral to a mental health professional.

A recent meta-analysis provides strong support for the efficacy of cognitive behavioral therapy for insomnia (CBTi) in cancer survivors, demonstrating medium to large effect sizes compared to control groups [66]. In cancer survivors, both individual and group-delivered CBTi has also been shown to improve subjective sleep outcomes (e.g., patient-reported sleep quality, greater sleep duration, and fewer nights with hypnotic medication) as well as mood, cancer-related fatigue, and quality of life [67]. Some studies tailored CBTi to include components of fatigue management (e.g., appropriate napping during the day, expectations regarding fatigue) that may be of special significance to persons with cancer [68].

To address the limitations of face-to-face treatment delivery in cancer survivors, different modalities of CBTi delivery have been evaluated and found to be both effective and feasible for reaching a broader population of patients. One study observed that video-delivered CBTi was clinically effective for treating insomnia in breast cancer survivors, though those who received face-to-face CBTi evidenced greater insomnia remission rates [69]. An Internet-based CBTi program delivered to a small group of patients with cancer evidenced greater reductions in sleep problems compared to a wait-list control group [70]. It should be noted that these CBTi studies have been conducted in patients with early-stage cancers and therefore the efficacy of CBTi for patients with advanced cancer is unknown [67].

Targeting dysfunctional beliefs about sleep and reducing daytime napping have been identified as key predictors of CBTi treatment response [71]. Trials evaluating behavioral therapy alone have demonstrated improvements in subjective, but not objective, measures of sleep; furthermore, improvements are not maintained over time in this form of treatment [72]. Finally, individual or group-based mindfulness-based stress reduction (MBSR) for oncology populations can significantly improve sleep and decrease stress in cancer survivors. Although MBSR had similar outcomes compared to CBTi, CBTi produced more rapid and durable improvements in sleep [73].

Physical activity has also been evaluated as a possible treatment for sleep disturbance in cancer survivors. In systematic reviews and meta-analyses of exercise interventions for health-related quality of life among patients on or post-cancer treatment, results indicate that even mild exercise such as walking can reduce sleep disturbance in heterogeneous populations with various tumor sites, stages, and treatment histories, although it should be noted that individuals who were terminally ill or in palliative care were excluded [74–76]. Among women with ovarian cancer, those who met public health physical activity guidelines of the Centers for Disease Control and Prevention (30% of the sample) self-reported significantly shorter sleep latency, higher sleep quality, greater sleep efficiency, and less sleep aid use compared to the women who did not meet the physical activity guidelines [77].

Some studies have observed that yoga practice is related to improvements in both subjective and objective measures (e.g., inflammation) of sleep and health, with a direct correlation between greater intensity of yoga practice with better sleep outcomes [78, 79]. Whereas those studies comprised primarily breast cancer survivors, benefits to sleep were also found in one small study ($N=39$) of lymphoma survivors comparing Tibetan yoga practice to standard care [80]. It should be noted, however, that there is not sufficient evidence to indicate that yoga can improve sleep in patients with hematological malignancies according to a recent Cochrane review [81].

Bright light and melatonin treatments are commonly employed for circadian rhythm disorders in the general population, but these treatments have not been thoroughly evaluated in cancer survivors. Preliminary research of women receiving chemotherapy for breast cancer has shown that women who received bright light therapy every morning for 30 min report less sleep dysregulation, use less sleep medication, and rate daytime dysfunction as less severe compared to a dim light control group [82, 83]. Regarding melatonin, there is no existing literature, to our knowledge, indicating benefits to subjective or objective measures of sleep in cancer survivors. Most of the literature examining melatonin in oncology populations is related to the hypothesized link between inappropriate melatonin timing and risk for cancer and/or the potential benefit of melatonin supplements for slowing the progression of malignant tumor growth (e.g., [84, 85]), as opposed to using melatonin to treat circadian rhythm problems in patients with cancer [86]. Therefore, although bright light therapy and melatonin have been shown to be effective in the general population for improving sleep related to circadian rhythm desynchronization, the efficacy of these interventions in cancer survivors remains to be seen.

Pharmacological treatments are effective for treating insomnia in the general population, but they are only recommended for short-term use for best results and to reduce the likelihood of dependence [87]. Reported use of hypnotic medication among patients with cancer differs by tumor site, ranging from as little as 15–20 % among patients with prostate, colon, or gastrointestinal cancer to 20–30 % among patients with breast cancer, and up to 40 % among patients with lung cancer [88–91]. The rates of current sleep aid prescription use were reportedly similar among cancer survivors (≥5 years post-diagnosis) and healthy non-cancer controls in a nationally representative sample [92].

To date, no randomized controlled trials have evaluated hypnotic medications for improving sleep disturbance in cancer survivors. However, the efficacy of antidepressants in cancer survivors with comorbid sleep disturbance and depression has been evaluated. For example, mirtazapine showed some preliminary benefit for insomnia symptoms in a small sample of patients with various tumor sites and comorbid mood disorder when compared to imipramine and placebo [93]. Paroxetine demonstrated some improvements in sleep during a trial investigating its efficacy for treating depression in patients with various tumor sites; however, the rates of sleep problems remained quite high [94].

In summary, because there are a number of possible contributing factors to poor sleep in cancer survivors, these should all be addressed before engaging in further treatment in order to reduce patient burden. CBTi, as in the general population, remains the most effective and well-studied treatment for insomnia in cancer populations. Exercise, bright light therapy, melatonin, and hypnotic medications have not been sufficiently evaluated in cancer survivors, though preliminary results for exercise (walking and yoga, in particular) show promise for aiding in the treatment of insomnia in this population.

Summary

Research examining sleep in cancer survivors is a growing area of inquiry. The current literature indicates higher prevalence of both sleep disturbance and insomnia syndrome among cancer survivors than what is observed in the general population. There is a high prevalence of sleep disturbance across the continuum of care from point of diagnosis and for many, persists after completion of treatment. The nature of cancer and its treatment exposes survivors to many potential precipitating and/or perpetuating factors that are atypical for the general population. Further, sleep disturbance rarely presents as a single symptom, but more often co-occurs with symptoms such as fatigue, pain, depression, and/or cognitive impairment. This adds a level of complexity to assessment and often requires individualized treatment plans. As a result, treatment of disturbed sleep among patients with a history of cancer must take all these factors into consideration to appropriately adapt successful interventions to their unique needs.

Qualitative interviews with survivors with mixed cancer types revealed several aspects of quality of life that were impaired when patients reported comorbid chronic insomnia, including fatigue, impaired daytime functioning such as reduced social activities, changes in temperament, catastrophizing about the possibility of cancer recurrence, and a sense of pressure to return to "normal" following cancer treatment [18]. To our knowledge, the impact of this added pressure to return to a healthy baseline or fear of recurrence on recovery or maintenance of sleep disturbance in cancer survivors has not been examined. Much of what we have learned suggests that the impact of sleep disturbance on quality of life is similar to what is observed among healthy controls or individuals with other health conditions and disturbed sleep [34, 95].

Finally, because research in this area is relatively new compared to other populations with sleep complaints, there is a need for additional research. The available literature evaluating the prevalence and degree of sleep disturbance in cancer survivors primarily relies on convenience samples and brief screening tools for measurement of sleep disturbance (as opposed to diagnostic criteria for insomnia), and the populations studied have either focused on a few specific cancer types (e.g., breast or lung cancer most commonly) or have used samples that are too heterogeneous to compare sleep disturbance across cancer sites [53]. Hence, the methodological shortcomings of the available research make it difficult to characterize sleep and sleep problems in cancer survivors. There is a need for more prospective research evaluating patients from the time of diagnosis through long-term survivorship. To date, CBTi has been the most thoroughly investigated intervention for sleep disturbance in cancer care. Thus, randomized controlled trials studying the safety and efficacy of other commonly used treatments for sleep disturbance such as hypnotic medications, bright light therapy, and/or melatonin within cancer survivors is warranted given the high prevalence and notable impact sleep disturbance has on the quality of life of survivors.

References

1. American Cancer Society. Cancer treatment and survivorship facts & figures 2014–2015. Atlanta: American Cancer Society; 2014.
2. Savard J, Morin CM. Insomnia in the context of cancer: a review of a neglected problem. J Clin Oncol. 2001;19(3):895–908.
3. Davidson JR, Feldman-Stewart D, Brennenstuhl S, Ram S. How to provide insomnia interventions to people with cancer: insights from patients. Psychooncology. 2007;16(11):1028–38. doi:10.1002/pon.1183.
4. National Cancer Institute. Sleep Disorders—For Health Professionals (PDQ®). Bethesda, MD: National Cancer Institute; 2015 [updated April 23, 2014; cited May 7, 2015]; Available from: http://cancer.gov/cancertopics/pdq/supportivecare/sleepdisorders/HealthProfessional.
5. Palesh OG, Roscoe JA, Mustian KM, Roth T, Savard J, Ancoli-Israel S, Heckler C, Purnell JQ, Janelsins MC, Morrow GR. Prevalence, demographics, and psychological associations of

sleep disruption in patients with cancer: University of Rochester Cancer Center-Community Clinical Oncology Program. J Clin Oncol. 2010;28(2):292–8. doi:10.1200/jco.2009.22.5011.

6. Hugel H, Ellershaw JE, Cook L, Skinner J, Irvine C. The prevalence, key causes and management of insomnia in palliative care patients. J Pain Symptom Manage. 2004;27(4):316–21. doi:10.1016/j.jpainsymman.2003.09.010.

7. Thomas KS, Bower J, Hoyt MA, Sepah S. Disrupted sleep in breast and prostate cancer patients undergoing radiation therapy: the role of coping processes. Psychooncology. 2010;19(7):767–76. doi:10.1002/pon.1639.

8. Savard J, Ivers H, Savard MH, Morin CM. Cancer treatments and their side effects are associated with aggravation of insomnia: results of a longitudinal study. Cancer. 2015;121(10):1703–11. doi:10.1002/cncr.29244.

9. Silberfarb PM, Hauri PJ, Oxman TE, Schnurr P. Assessment of sleep in patients with lung cancer and breast cancer. J Clin Oncol. 1993;11(5):997–1004.

10. Sanford SD, Wagner LI, Beaumont JL, Butt Z, Sweet JJ, Cella D. Longitudinal prospective assessment of sleep quality: before, during, and after adjuvant chemotherapy for breast cancer. Support Care Cancer. 2013;21(4):959–67. doi:10.1007/s00520-012-1612-7.

11. Chen ML, Yu CT, Yang CH. Sleep disturbances and quality of life in lung cancer patients undergoing chemotherapy. Lung Cancer. 2008;62(3):391–400. doi:10.1016/j.lungcan.2008.03.016.

12. Fortner BV, Stepanski EJ, Wang SC, Kasprowicz S, Durrence HH. Sleep and quality of life in breast cancer patients. J Pain Symptom Manage. 2002;24(5):471–80. doi:10.1016/S0885-3924(02)00500-6.

13. Lis C, Gupta D, Grutsch J. The relationship between insomnia and patient satisfaction with quality of life in cancer. Support Care Cancer. 2008;16(3):261–6. doi:10.1007/s00520-007-0314-z.

14. Taylor LM, Espie CA, White CA. Attentional bias in people with acute versus persistent insomnia secondary to cancer. Behav Sleep Med. 2003;1(4):200–12. doi:10.1207/S15402010BSM0104_3.

15. Ancoli-Israel S, Liu L, Marler MR, Parker BA, Jones V, Sadler GR, Dimsdale J, Cohen-Zion M, Fiorentino L. Fatigue, sleep, and circadian rhythms prior to chemotherapy for breast cancer. Support Care Cancer. 2006;14(3):201–9. doi:10.1007/s00520-005-0861-0.

16. Berger AM, Farr LA, Kuhn BR, Fischer P, Agrawal S. Values of sleep/wake, activity/rest, circadian rhythms, and fatigue prior to adjuvant breast cancer chemotherapy. J Pain Symptom Manage. 2007;33(4):398–409. doi:10.1016/j.jpainsymman.2006.09.022.

17. Savard J, Simard S, Blanchet J, Ivers H, Morin CM. Prevalence, clinical characteristics, and risk factors for insomnia in the context of breast cancer. Sleep. 2001;24(5):583–90.

18. Fleming L, Gillespie S, Espie CA. The development and impact of insomnia on cancer survivors: a qualitative analysis. Psychooncology. 2010;19(9):991–6. doi:10.1002/pon.1652.

19. Savard J, Simard S, Hervouet S, Ivers H, Lacombe L, Fradet Y. Insomnia in men treated with radical prostatectomy for prostate cancer. Psychooncology. 2005;14(2):147–56. doi:10.1002/pon.830.

20. Van Onselen C, Paul SM, Lee K, Dunn L, Aouizerat BE, West C, Dodd M, Cooper B, Miaskowski C. Trajectories of sleep disturbance and daytime sleepiness in women before and after surgery for breast cancer. J Pain Symptom Manage. 2013;45(2):244–60. doi:10.1016/j.jpainsymman.2012.02.020.

21. Eyigor S, Eyigor C, Uslu R. Assessment of pain, fatigue, sleep and quality of life (QoL) in elderly hospitalized cancer patients. Arch Gerontol Geriatr. 2010;51(3):e57–61. doi:10.1016/j.archger.2009.11.018.

22. Heinonen H, Volin L, Uutela A, Zevon M, Barrick C, Ruutu T. Quality of life and factors related to perceived satisfaction with quality of life after allogeneic bone marrow transplantation. Ann Hematol. 2001;80(3):137–43.

23. Andrykowski MA, Carpenter JS, Greiner CB, Altmaier EM, Burish TG, Antin JH, Gingrich R, Cordova MJ, Henslee-Downey PJ. Energy level and sleep quality following bone marrow transplantation. Bone Marrow Transplant. 1997;20(8):669–79. doi:10.1038/sj.bmt.1700949.

24. Savard J, Liu L, Natarajan L, Rissling MB, Neikrug AB, He F, Dimsdale JE, Mills PJ, Parker BA, Sadler GR, Ancoli-Israel S. Breast cancer patients have progressively impaired sleep-wake activity rhythms during chemotherapy. Sleep. 2009;32(9):1155–60.
25. Liu L, Mills PJ, Rissling M, Fiorentino L, Natarajan L, Dimsdale JE, Sadler GR, Parker BA, Ancoli-Israel S. Fatigue and sleep quality are associated with changes in inflammatory markers in breast cancer patients undergoing chemotherapy. Brain Behav Immun. 2012;26(5):706–13. doi:10.1016/j.bbi.2012.02.001.
26. Dhruva A, Paul SM, Cooper BA, Lee K, West C, Aouizerat BE, Dunn LB, Swift PS, Wara W, Miaskowski C. A longitudinal study of measures of objective and subjective sleep disturbance in patients with breast cancer before, during, and after radiation therapy. J Pain Symptom Manage. 2012;44(2):215–28. doi:10.1016/j.jpainsymman.2011.08.010.
27. Kumar RJ, Barqawi A, Crawford ED. Adverse events associated with hormonal therapy for prostate cancer. Rev Urol. 2005;7 Suppl 5:S37–43.
28. Savard J, Davidson JR, Ivers H, Quesnel C, Rioux D, Dupéré V, Lasnier M, Simard S, Morin CM. The association between nocturnal hot flashes and sleep in breast cancer survivors. J Pain Symptom Manage. 2004;27(6):513–22. doi:10.1016/j.jpainsymman.2003.10.013.
29. Hanisch LJ, Gehrman PR. Circadian rhythm of hot flashes and activity levels among prostate cancer patients on androgen deprivation therapy. Aging Male. 2011;14(4):243–8. doi:10.3109/13685538.2011.582528.
30. Bardwell WA, Profant J, Casden DR, Dimsdale JE, Ancoli-Israel S, Natarajan L, Rock CL, Pierce JP. The relative importance of specific risk factors for insomnia in women treated for early-stage breast cancer. Psychooncology. 2008;17(1):9–18.
31. Janz NK, Mujahid M, Chung LK, Lantz PM, Hawley ST, Morrow M, Schwartz K, Katz SJ. Symptom experience and quality of life of women following breast cancer treatment. J Womens Health. 2007;16(9):1348–61.
32. Otte JL, Carpenter JS, Russell KM, Bigatti S, Champion VL. Prevalence, severity, and correlates of sleep-wake disturbances in long-term breast cancer survivors. J Pain Symptom Manage. 2010;39(3):535–47.
33. Hoffman AJ, Given BA, von Eye A, Gift AG, Given CW. Relationships among pain, fatigue, insomnia, and gender in persons with lung cancer. Oncol Nurs Forum. 2007;34(4):785–92. doi:10.1188/07.onf.785-792.
34. Gooneratne NS, Dean GE, Rogers AE, Nkwuo JE, Coyne JC, Kaiser LR. Sleep and quality of life in long-term lung cancer survivors. Lung Cancer. 2007;58(3):403–10. doi:10.1016/j.lungcan.2007.07.011.
35. Mulrooney DA, Ness KK, Neglia JP, Whitton JA, Green DM, Zeltzer LK, Robison LL, Mertens AC. Fatigue and sleep disturbance in adult survivors of childhood cancer: a report from the Childhood Cancer Survivor Study (CCSS). Sleep. 2008;31(2):271–81.
36. Clanton NR, Klosky JL, Li C, Jain N, Srivastava DK, Mulrooney D, Zeltzer L, Stovall M, Robison LL, Krull KR. Fatigue, vitality, sleep, and neurocognitive functioning in adult survivors of childhood cancer: a report from the Childhood Cancer Survivor Study. Cancer. 2011;117(11):2559–68.
37. Palesh OG, Collie K, Batiuchok D, Tilston J, Koopman C, Perlis ML, Butler LD, Carlson R, Spiegel D. A longitudinal study of depression, pain, and stress as predictors of sleep disturbance among women with metastatic breast cancer. Biol Psychol. 2007;75(1):37–44. doi:10.1016/j.biopsycho.2006.11.002.
38. Miaskowski C, Lee KA. Pain, fatigue, and sleep disturbances in oncology outpatients receiving radiation therapy for bone metastasis: a pilot study. J Pain Symptom Manage. 1999;17(5):320–32.
39. Mercadante S, Girelli D, Casuccio A. Sleep disorders in advanced cancer patients: prevalence and factors associated. Support Care Cancer. 2004;12(5):355–9. doi:10.1007/s00520-004-0623-4.
40. Mercadante S, Aielli F, Adile C, Ferrera P, Valle A, Cartoni C, Pizzuto M, Caruselli A, Parsi R, Cortegiani A, Masedu F, Valenti M, Ficorella C, Porzio G. Sleep disturbances in patients with advanced cancer in different palliative care settings. J Pain Symptom Manage. 2015;23(15):410–8.

41. Spielman AJ, Caruso LS, Glovinsky PB. A behavioral perspective on insomnia treatment. Psychiatr Clin North Am. 1987;10(4):541–53.
42. Fiorentino L, Ancoli-Israel S. Insomnia and its treatment in women with breast cancer. Sleep Med Rev. 2006;10(6):419–29. doi:10.1016/j.smrv.2006.03.005.
43. Vena C, Parker K, Cunningham M, Clark J, McMillan S. Sleep-wake disturbances in people with cancer part I: an overview of sleep, sleep regulation, and effects of disease and treatment. Oncol Nurs Forum. 2004;31(4):735–46. doi:10.1188/04.onf.735-746.
44. Blask DE. Melatonin, sleep disturbance, and cancer risk. Sleep Med Rev. 2009;13(4):257–64. doi:10.1016/j.smrv.2008.07.007.
45. Davis MP, Goforth HW. Long-term and short-term effects of insomnia in cancer and effective interventions. Cancer J. 2014;20(5):330–44. doi:10.1097/ppo.0000000000000071.
46. Straif K, Baan R, Grosse Y, Secretan B, El Ghissassi F, Bouvard V, Altieri A, Benbrahim-Tallaa L, Cogliano V. Carcinogenicity of shift-work, painting, and fire-fighting. Lancet Oncol. 2007;8(12):1065–6.
47. Dodd M, Janson S, Facione N, Faucett J, Froelicher ES, Humphreys J, Lee K, Miaskowski C, Puntillo K, Rankin S, Taylor D. Advancing the science of symptom management. J Adv Nurs. 2001;33(5):668–76.
48. Barsevick AM. The concept of symptom cluster. Semin Oncol Nurs. 2007;23(2):89–98. doi:10.1016/j.soncn.2007.01.009.
49. Donovan KA, Jacobsen PB. Fatigue, depression, and insomnia: evidence for a symptom cluster in cancer. Semin Oncol Nurs. 2007;23(2):127–35. doi:10.1016/j.soncn.2007.01.004.
50. Sanford SD, Beaumont JL, Butt Z, Sweet JJ, Cella D, Wagner LI. Prospective longitudinal evaluation of a symptom cluster in breast cancer. J Pain Symptom Manage. 2014;47(4):721–30. doi:10.1016/j.jpainsymman.2013.05.010.
51. Miller AH, Ancoli-Israel S, Bower JE, Capuron L, Irwin MR. Neuroendocrine-immune mechanisms of behavioral comorbidities in patients with cancer. J Clin Oncol. 2008;26(6):971–82. doi:10.1200/jco.2007.10.7805.
52. Thornton LM, Andersen BL, Blakely WP. The pain, depression, and fatigue symptom cluster in advanced breast cancer: covariation with the hypothalamic-pituitary-adrenal axis and the sympathetic nervous system. Health Psychol. 2010;29(3):333–7.
53. Irwin MR. Depression and insomnia in cancer: prevalence, risk factors, and effects on cancer outcomes. Curr Psychiatry Rep. 2013;15(11):404. doi:10.1007/s11920-013-0404-1.
54. Bower JE, Ganz PA, Irwin MR, Kwan L, Breen EC, Cole SW. Inflammation and behavioral symptoms after breast cancer treatment: do fatigue, depression, and sleep disturbance share a common underlying mechanism? J Clin Oncol. 2011;29(26):3517–22.
55. Howell D, Oliver TK, Keller-Olaman S, Davidson J, Garland S, Samuels C, Savard J, Harris C, Aubin M, Olson K, Sussman J, Macfarlane J, Taylor C. A Pan-Canadian practice guideline: prevention, screening, assessment, and treatment of sleep disturbances in adults with cancer. Support Care Cancer. 2013;21(10):2695–706. doi:10.1007/s00520-013-1823-6.
56. NCCN. Survivorship. National Comprehensive Cancer Network; 2015 [updated 2015; cited May 7, 2015]; Version 1.2015: Available from: http://www.nccn.org/professionals/physician_gls/f_guidelines.asp#supportive.
57. Savard MH, Savard J, Simard S, Ivers H. Empirical validation of the Insomnia Severity Index in cancer patients. Psychooncology. 2005;14(6):429–41. doi:10.1002/pon.860.
58. Chang VT, Hwang SS, Feuerman M. Validation of the Edmonton Symptom Assessment Scale. Cancer. 2000;88(9):2164–71.
59. Buysse DJ, Yu L, Moul DE, Germain A, Stover A, Dodds NE, Johnston KL, Shablesky-Cade MA, Pilkonis PA. Development and validation of patient-reported outcome measures for sleep disturbance and sleep-related impairments. Sleep. 2010;33(6):781–92.
60. Minton O, Richardson A, Sharpe M, Hotopf M, Stone P. A systematic review and meta-analysis of the pharmacological treatment of cancer-related fatigue. J Natl Cancer Inst. 2008;100(16):1155–66. doi:10.1093/jnci/djn250.
61. NCCN. Cancer-related fatigue: clinical practice guidelines in oncology. J Natl Compr Canc Netw. 2003;1(3):308–31.

62. Young T, Skatrud J, Peppard PE. Risk factors for obstructive sleep apnea in adults. JAMA. 2004;291(16):2013–6.
63. Chung F, Yegneswaran B, Liao P, Chung SA, Vairavanathan S, Islam S, Khajehdehi A, Shapiro CM. STOP questionnaire: a tool to screen patients for obstructive sleep apnea. Anesthesiology. 2008;108(5):812–21. doi:10.1097/ALN.0b013e31816d83e4.
64. Hogl B, Kiechl S, Willeit J, Saletu M, Frauscher B, Seppi K, Muller J, Rungger G, Gasperi A, Wenning G, Poewe W. Restless legs syndrome: a community-based study of prevalence, severity, and risk factors. Neurology. 2005;64(11):1920–4.
65. Schutte-Rodin S, Broch L, Buysse D, Dorsey C, Sateia M. Clinical guideline for the evaluation and management of chronic insomnia in adults. J Clin Sleep Med. 2008;4(5):487–504.
66. Johnson JA, Rash JA, Campbell TS, Savard J, Gehrman PR, Perlis M, Carlson LE, Garland SN. A systematic review and meta-analysis of randomized controlled trials of cognitive behavior therapy for insomnia (CBT-I) in cancer survivors. Sleep Med Rev. 2016;27:20–28. doi:10.1016/j.smrv.2015.07.001.
67. Garland SN, Johnson JA, Savard J, Gehrman P, Perlis M, Carlson L, Campbell T. Sleeping well with cancer: a systematic review of cognitive behavioral therapy for insomnia in cancer patients. Neuropsychiatr Dis Treat. 2014;10:1113–24. doi:10.2147/ndt.s47790.
68. Savard J, Simard S, Ivers H, Morin CM. Randomized study on the efficacy of cognitive-behavioral therapy for insomnia secondary to breast cancer, part I: sleep and psychological effects. J Clin Oncol. 2005;23(25):6083–96. doi:10.1200/jco.2005.09.548.
69. Savard J, Ivers H, Savard MH, Morin CM. Is a video-based cognitive behavioral therapy for insomnia as efficacious as a professionally administered treatment in breast cancer? Results of a randomized controlled trial. Sleep. 2014;37(8):1305–14. doi:10.5665/sleep.3918.
70. Ritterband LM, Bailey ET, Thorndike FP, Lord HR, Farrell-Carnahan L, Baum LD. Initial evaluation of an Internet intervention to improve the sleep of cancer survivors with insomnia. Psychooncology. 2012;21(7):695–705. doi:10.1002/pon.1969.
71. Tremblay V, Savard J, Ivers H. Predictors of the effect of cognitive behavioral therapy for chronic insomnia comorbid with breast cancer. J Consult Clin Psychol. 2009;77(4):742–50. doi:10.1037/a0015492.
72. Berger AM, Kuhn BR, Farr LA, Von Essen SG, Chamberlain J, Lynch JC, Agrawal S. One-year outcomes of a behavioral therapy intervention trial on sleep quality and cancer-related fatigue. J Clin Oncol. 2009;27(35):6033–40. doi:10.1200/jco.2008.20.8306.
73. Garland SN, Carlson LE, Stephens AJ, Antle MC, Samuels C, Campbell TS. Mindfulness-based stress reduction compared with cognitive behavioral therapy for the treatment of insomnia comorbid with cancer: a randomized, partially blinded, noninferiority trial. J Clin Oncol. 2014;32(5):449–57. doi:10.1200/jco.2012.47.7265.
74. Mishra SI, Scherer RW, Geigle PM, Berlanstein DR, Topaloglu O, Gotay CC, Snyder C. Exercise interventions on health-related quality of life for cancer survivors. Cochrane Database Syst Rev. 2012;15(8).
75. Mishra SI, Scherer RW, Snyder C, Geigle PM, Berlanstein DR, Topaloglu O. Exercise interventions on health-related quality of life for people with cancer during active treatment. Cochrane Database Syst Rev. 2012;15(8).
76. Chiu HY, Huang HC, Chen PY, Hou WH, Tsai PS. Walking improves sleep in individuals with cancer: a meta-analysis of randomized, controlled trials. Oncol Nurs Forum. 2015;42(2):E54–62. doi:10.1188/15.onf.e54-e62.
77. Stevinson C, Steed H, Faught W, Tonkin K, Vallance JK, Ladha AB, Schepansky A, Capstick V, Courneya KS. Physical activity in ovarian cancer survivors: associations with fatigue, sleep, and psychosocial functioning. Int J Gynecol Cancer. 2009;19(1):73–8. doi:10.1111/IGC.0b013e31819902ec.
78. Mustian KM, Sprod LK, Janelsins M, Peppone LJ, Palesh OG, Chandwani K, Reddy PS, Melnik MK, Heckler C, Morrow GR. Multicenter, randomized controlled trial of yoga for sleep quality among cancer survivors. J Clin Oncol. 2013;31(26):3233–41. doi:10.1200/jco.2012.43.7707.
79. Kiecolt-Glaser JK, Bennett JM, Andridge R, Peng J, Shapiro CL, Malarkey WB, Emery CF, Layman R, Mrozek EE, Glaser R. Yoga's impact on inflammation, mood, and fatigue in breast

cancer survivors: a randomized controlled trial. J Clin Oncol. 2014;32(10):1040–9. doi:10.1200/jco.2013.51.8860.

80. Cohen L, Warneke C, Fouladi RT, Rodriguez MA, Chaoul-Reich A. Psychological adjustment and sleep quality in a randomized trial of the effects of a Tibetan yoga intervention in patients with lymphoma. Cancer. 2004;100(10):2253–60. doi:10.1002/cncr.20236.

81. Felbel S, Meerpohl JJ, Monsef I, Engert A, Skoetz N. Yoga in addition to standard care for patients with haematological malignancies. Cochrane Database Syst Rev. 2014;12(6).

82. Neikrug AB, Rissling M, Trofimenko V, Liu L, Natarajan L, Lawton S, Parker BA, Ancoli-Israel S. Bright light therapy protects women from circadian rhythm desynchronization during chemotherapy for breast cancer. Behav Sleep Med. 2012;10(3):202–16. doi:10.1080/1540200 2.2011.634940.

83. Ancoli-Israel S, Rissling M, Neikrug A, Trofimenko V, Natarajan L, Parker BA, Lawton S, Desan P, Liu L. Light treatment prevents fatigue in women undergoing chemotherapy for breast cancer. Support Care Cancer. 2012;20(6):1211–9. doi:10.1007/s00520-011-1203-z.

84. Lissoni P, Chilelli M, Villa S, Cerizza L, Tancini G. Five years survival in metastatic non-small cell lung cancer patients treated with chemotherapy alone or chemotherapy and melatonin: a randomized trial. J Pineal Res. 2003;35(1):12–5.

85. Sookprasert A, Johns NP, Phunmanee A, Pongthai P, Cheawchanwattana A, Johns J, Konsil J, Plaimee P, Porasuphatana S, Jitpimolmard S. Melatonin in patients with cancer receiving chemotherapy: a randomized, double-blind, placebo-controlled trial. Anticancer Res. 2014;34(12): 7327–37.

86. Jung B, Ahmad N. Melatonin in cancer management: progress and promise. Cancer Res. 2006;66(20):9789–93. doi:10.1158/0008-5472.can-06-1776.

87. National Sleep Foundation. Safe Use of Sleep Aids. 2014 [updated 2014; cited October 2, 2015]; Available from: https://sleepfoundation.org/insomnia/content/safe-use-sleep-aids.

88. Paltiel O, Marzec-Boguslawska A, Soskolne V, Massalha S, Avitzour M, Pfeffer R, Cherny N, Peretz T. Use of tranquilizers and sleeping pills among cancer patients is associated with a poorer quality of life. Qual Life Res. 2004;13(10):1699–706.

89. Casault L, Savard J, Ivers H, Savard MH, Simard S. Utilization of hypnotic medication in the context of cancer: predictors and frequency of use. Support Care Cancer. 2012;20(6):1203–10. doi:10.1007/s00520-011-1199-4.

90. Moore TA, Berger AM, Dizona P. Sleep aid use during and following breast cancer adjuvant chemotherapy. Psychooncology. 2011;20(3):321–5. doi:10.1002/pon.1756.

91. Lee K, Cho M, Miaskowski C, Dodd M. Impaired sleep and rhythms in persons with cancer. Sleep Med Rev. 2004;8(3):199–212. doi:10.1016/j.smrv.2003.10.001.

92. Braun IM, Rao SR, Meyer FL, Fedele G. Patterns of psychiatric medication use among nationally representative long-term cancer survivors and controls. Cancer. 2015;121(1):132–8. doi:10.1002/cncr.29014.

93. Cankurtaran ES, Ozalp E, Soygur H, Akbiyik DI, Turhan L, Alkis N. Mirtazapine improves sleep and lowers anxiety and depression in cancer patients: superiority over imipramine. Support Care Cancer. 2008;16(11):1291–8.

94. Palesh OG, Mustian KM, Peppone LJ, Janelsins M, Sprod LK, Kesler S, Innominato PF, Roth T, Manber R, Heckler C, Fiscella K, Morrow GR. Impact of paroxetine on sleep problems in 426 cancer patients receiving chemotherapy: a trial from the University of Rochester Cancer Center Community Clinical Oncology Program. Sleep Med. 2012;13(9):1184–90. doi:10.1016/j.sleep.2012.06.001.

95. Carpenter JS, Andrykowski MA. Psychometric evaluation of the Pittsburgh Sleep Quality Index. J Psychosom Res. 1998;45(1):5–13.

Chapter 13
Insomnia in Comorbid Neurological Problems

Federica Provini and Carolina Lombardi

Abstract Insomnia is the most common sleep complaint. Insomnia is not a disease but a symptom arising from multiple environmental, medical, and mental disorders. Insomnia can be transient, of short term, or chronic in its presentation. Degenerative and vascular diseases involving the central nervous system (CNS) may impair sleep either as a result of the brain lesion or because of illness-related personal discomfort.

Chronic insomnia can be caused by neurological conditions characterized by movement disorders starting or persisting during sleep that hinder sleep onset and/ or sleep continuity.

Three specific neurological conditions, fatal familial insomnia, a human prion disease; Morvan syndrome, an autoimmune limbic encephalopathy; and Delirium tremens, the well-known alcohol or benzodiazepine withdrawal syndrome, share a common clinical phenotype characterized by an inability to sleep associated with motor and autonomic activation. Agrypnia excitata (AE) is the term, which aptly defines this generalized over-activation syndrome, whose pathogenetic mechanism consists in an intralimbic disconnection releasing the hypothalamus and brainstem reticular formation from corticolimbic control.

F. Provini, M.D., Ph.D. (✉)
Department of Biomedical and Neuromotor Sciences, University of Bologna, Bologna, Italy

IRCCS Institute of Neurological Sciences, Bellaria Hospital,
Via Altura, 3, 40139 Bologna, Italy
e-mail: federica.provini@unibo.it

C. Lombardi, M.D., Ph.D.
Department of Cardiology, Sleep Disorder Center, Instituto Auxologico Italiano IRCCS,
Milan, Italy

© Springer International Publishing Switzerland 2017
H.P. Attarian (ed.), *Clinical Handbook of Insomnia*, Current Clinical Neurology,
DOI 10.1007/978-3-319-41400-3_13

Keywords Insomnia • Degenerative diseases • Movement disorders • Fatal familial insomnia • Morvan syndrome • Delirium tremens • Agrypnia excitata

Poor sleep quality is the most common sleep complaint [1]. Insomnia is when sleep is insufficient, inadequate, or non-restorative resulting in daytime fatigue, irritability, and decreased concentration. Its prevalence varies considerably depending on the definition adopted. Acute insomnia refers to sleep problems lasting from one night to a few weeks, whereas chronic insomnia refers to sleep problems lasting at least three nights weekly for at least 1 month [2]. Epidemiologic evidence concludes that while one-fourth to one-third of the general population report transient or occasional difficulty falling and/or staying asleep, about 10 % of the adult population present chronic complaints and seek help for insomnia [3, 4]. Increasing age, female sex, depressed mood, and physical illness are the most important risk factors for chronic insomnia [3–8].

The inadequate identification and treatment of insomnia have significant medical and public health implications. Chronic insomnia impairs occupational performance and quality of life [9–11].

Objective sleep measures, EEG activity, and physiological findings suggest that insomnia is not a state of sleep loss, but a disorder of hyperarousal present during both night and daytime [9, 12]. Several psychological and physiological factors such as the association with other medical complaints and/or psychological symptoms, particularly anxious-ruminative personality traits, worry and depression can contribute to the onset and perpetuation of insomnia. Stressful life events (difficulties in interpersonal relationships, family discord, problems at work, and financial troubles) may also determine poor sleep quality.

Insomnia is not always a specific illness or disease but can often represent a symptom or consequence of other primary disorders. Positive family history for insomnia is common in patients with a "poor quality of sleep." It is difficult, however, to fathom whether the emotional problems favoring the onset of a sleep disorder in adulthood are due to a genetic predisposition or the result of having lived in a family burdened by affective problems and/or interpersonal conflict [13].

The mechanisms regulating sleep and sleep architecture may be affected by neurological illness, but it should also be borne in mind that neurological disorders and diseases are almost always accompanied by major psychological distress. In addition, the medications used in the treatment of medical and neurological diseases, e.g., β-blockers, some selective serotonin reuptake inhibitors (SSRIs), some neuroleptics, amphetamines, and others, may induce sleep fragmentation, reduce total sleep time, and delay sleep onset. Hence it is difficult to establish whether the onset of chronic insomnia in an individual patient with a neurological illness is due to the disease or to a psychosomatic disorder or an iatrogenic consequence of the neurological impairment.

The neurological diseases most commonly associated with chronic insomnia can be divided into three groups [14, 15]:

(a) Neurological diseases or disorders (degenerative and others) involving the central nervous system (CNS) impairing sleep mainly or exclusively because of illness-related personal discomfort (motor immobility, personal or family life disruption, depression, drugs).
(b) Neurological diseases characterized by movement disorders hindering sleep onset and/or sleep continuity.
(c) CNS lesions (dysfunction) impairing the basic mechanisms of sleep generation (agrypnia or organic insomnia).

Insomnia in Neurological Diseases (Degenerative and Others)

Insomnia and Dementia

Good sleep is an important index of people's quality of life especially in the elderly. An inability to get to sleep, shorter sleep times, and changes in the normal circadian patterns can impact on an individual's overall well-being and can play also a critical role in cognitive functions, alterations being increasingly common as people age. Sleep disturbances were present in 59.2 % of people with dementia and insomnia is reported in 21.8 % of patients [16]. In addition the elderly often present high comorbidity and polytreatment. Many common chronic conditions, such as chronic obstructive pulmonary disease, diabetes, dementia, chronic pain, and cancer, that are more common in the elderly, can also have significant effects on sleep, increasing the prevalence of insomnia compared with the general population.

Moreover aging accompanied by mental deterioration caused by a degenerative (e.g., Alzheimer's) or vascular disease (multi-infarct dementia) may determine more pronounced alterations of the sleep-wake cycle than physiological aging [17]. Comorbid insomnia and other sleep disturbances are common in patients with neurodegenerative disorders, such as Alzheimer's disease (AD) and other dementing disorders [18, 19].

Furthermore, studies of incident dementia suggest that sleep problems increase the risk of dementia [20]. Finally poor sleep results in an increased risk of significant morbidities and even mortality in demented patients [21].

A 24-h actigraphic study performed in institutionalised dementia patients showed four types of abnormal rhythms: a free-running (phase delayed) type, an aperiodic type, an ultradian rhythm type with a cycle lasting 3–4 h, and a flattened amplitude type in which patients were largely bedridden [22].

The factors most strongly associated with night awakenings among patients with AD were male gender, greater memory problems, and decreased functional status [23].

Sundowning defines the tendency of demented people to have nocturnal agitation. Sundowning can be a primary factor leading to the decision to institutionalize a patient. Admission to a nursing home in turn exacerbates the behavioral disorder with mental confusion and hallucinations.

Less severe or better tolerated than nocturnal disruptive behavior are disorders arising during the day. Nursing facilities that routinely put patients to bed during the afternoon for naps had lower rates of agitation than facilities that did not employ this routine [24]. The cause of sundowning in dementia is unknown, but there is some evidence of impaired circadian fluctuations in body temperature and secretion of melatonin and cortisol in patients with dementia compared with an age-matched normal population [25].

However the origin of sleep disorders in dementia is usually multifactorial, including neurodegenerative progression itself and environmental factors; moreover medication used in dementia is often associated with negative effects on sleep [26]. It remains unsettled whether insomnia or sleep disruption in the elderly with dementia is due to an anatomical-functional impairment of the suprachiasmatic nucleus or to a more complex alteration of the neuronal network controlling circadian and homeostatic wake-sleep cycle regulation [25, 27].

The treatment approach to the demented elderly patient with insomnia is difficult and largely based on clinical experience and empiric data rather than a large evidence-based studies. Clinical assessment of secondary causes for sleep disorders, including medical and psychiatric condition and medication side effects, is really important and comorbidities should be treated. After that, using a "less is better" approach in attempting nonpharmacologic interventions before initiating a trial of drug therapy is the optimal first step [28].

Because of environmental and medical conditions, older adults are less likely than younger adults to receive prolonged, high-intensity daily bright light. Keeping patients in well-lit rooms during the day and in the dark and quiet sleeping rooms during the night may help to improve the wake-sleep cycle. Exposure to bright light may help to optimize the sleep-wake cycle in dementia, although optimal timing of such light exposure for older adults (i.e., morning, afternoon, or evening) is uncertain and there is no consensus on the optimum treatment protocol. In addition to sleep improvement, bright light therapy may reduce unwanted behavioral and cognitive symptoms associated with dementia and depression in the elderly [29, 30].

Although potentially effective, benzodiazepines must be used with care. Daytime sedation or worsening of the agitation, two common side effects, may limit the use of benzodiazepines [31]. Clozapine (12.5–25 mg twice a day to be used with care because of potential bone marrow suppression) and risperidone (1.0 mg a day) may be of value and the more recently atypical antipsychotics such as quetiapine (12.5—25 mg) and olanzapine (10—15 mg) showed improvements in nighttime behavior but can also aggravate sometimes sleep-wake cycle disturbances [32].

Administration of 3–5 mg of melatonin 2–3 h before bedtime may also be of some benefit although large-scale studies showing unequivocal efficacy are not available [33, 34].

Ramelteon, a melatonin receptor agonist, seems to have a subjective efficacy in elderly outpatients evaluated in a clinical trial [35].

Insomnia in Neurological Diseases with Motor System Involvement

This group of diseases includes Parkinson disease (PD) and Parkinsonian syndromes or synucleinopathies such as multiple system atrophy (MSA) and dementia with Lewy bodies (DLB) and tauopathies such as progressive supranuclear palsy (PSP) and corticobasal degeneration (CBD), Huntington's disease (HD), progressive dystonia, Tourette's syndrome (TS), and autosomal dominant spinocerebellar ataxia (SCA). Literature reports on insomnia in these diseases are fragmentary, controversial, and mainly anecdotal.

Polysomnographic (PSG) recording is not indicated for the routine evaluation of insomnia in these diseases, but video-PSG may be required in special cases in which motor, [REM sleep behavior disorder (RBD)] or breathing disorders (laryngeal stridor), or excessive daytime sleepiness are prominent. Lacking appropriate therapy, treatment of sleep disturbance is often difficult and is confined to general measures to improve sleep quality (sleep hygiene, etc.) (Table 13.1).

Parkinson's Disease (PD)

Patients with Parkinson's disease (PD) experience major difficulties in maintaining sleep, and present painful nighttime abnormal movements, daytime sleepiness, sleep attacks, and insomnia. According to a recent study insomnia is present in more than one-third of PD patients [36]. Insomnia fluctuates over time in individual patients, and seems to be due to a complex interaction between movement disorders, side effects of dopamine agents, depression, and degeneration of sleep-wake regulating systems. A marked reduction of spindling, sleep fragmentation, and a shorter total sleep time are common in the PSG recordings of PD patients [37].

Dementia with Lewy Bodies (DLB)

Sleep disturbances, in particular hallucinatory episodes and RBD, are very common in diffuse Lewy body disease and are helpful in differentiating DLB from Alzheimer's disease early in the disease course [38–40].

Multiple System Atrophy (MSA)

Sleep disorders are common manifestations in MSA and include reduced and fragmented sleep, motor events (RBD), and/or breathing difficulty (central and obstructive apneas and nocturnal stridor) [41, 42]. RBD and nocturnal stridor may be the first symptoms of the disease. RBD occurs in virtually 100 % of patients, sometimes preceding the onset of waking motor symptoms and autonomic failure by several

Table 13.1 Sleep complains and polysomnographic findings in common and uncommon neurological diseases

Disease	Sleep complain	Polysomnographic findings
Parkinson disease	Difficulties in maintaining sleep, nighttime abnormal movements, daytime sleepiness	Marked reduction of spindling, sleep fragmentation and shorter total sleep time
Dementia with Lewy bodies	Insomnia and RBD	Reduced sleep efficiency; REM sleep without atonia
Multiple system atrophy	Reduced and fragmented sleep. RBD, and nocturnal stridor may be the first symptoms of the disease	Reduced amount of slow-wave sleep and REM sleep, reduced total sleep time, increased sleep latency and recurrent awakenings. Impaired circadian rhythms of temperature and melatonin secretion
Progressive supranuclear palsy	Insomnia and daytime subjective somnolence. RBD seldom occurs	Prolonged sleep latency, decreased total sleep time, decreased sleep efficiency, repeated arousals and awakenings, drastic reduction in the number and amplitude of sleep spindles, and less REM sleep
Corticobasal degeneration	Insomnia	Reduced sleep efficiency
Huntington's disease	Impaired initiation and maintenance of sleep especially in moderate to severe form	Longer sleep latency, lower sleep efficiency, frequent nocturnal awakenings, less slow-wave sleep, increase of periodic limb movements
Progressive dystonia	Insomnia	Increased sleep latency, frequent awakenings, reduced sleep efficiency. REM sleep may be reduced in severely affected patients
Tourette's syndrome	Somnambulism, night terrors, enuresis, increased number of awakenings, and increased motor activity during sleep	Decreased, increased, or unchanged SWS and REM sleep. Tics could appear during sleep recording
Autosomal dominant spinocerebellar ataxia	Impaired sleep, RBD, RLS, stridor, and NREM parasomnias in SCA3 patients	A peculiar EEG pattern characterized by an admixture of different elements of states of being with high-voltage slow waves and increased tonic EMG activity was described in few patients
Restless legs syndrome	Urge to move the limbs, accompanied by uncomfortable and unpleasant sensations in the extremities. The symptoms begin or worsen during periods of inactivity and are worse in the evening	Longer sleep latency, recurrent and prolonged awakenings throughout the night. In 80–100 % of RLS patients, PLMS occur

(continued)

Table 13.1 (continued)

Disease	Sleep complain	Polysomnographic findings
Propriospinal myoclonus	Violent muscle jerks in flexion or extension of the trunk and limbs	The contractions usually arise from the thoraco-abdominal/paraspinal muscles and then spread up and down the spinal cord via slowly conducting pathways
Nocturnal frontal lobe epilepsy	Partial seizures characterized by bizarre motor behaviors or sustained dystonic postures	Ictal and interictal scalp EEG could be normal
REM sleep behavior disorder	Episodes of abnormal and often violent dream-enacting behaviors, especially in the second part of the night	Loss of the physiological muscular atonia during REM sleep
Excessive fragmentary hypnic myoclonus	If severe, excessive fragmentary hypnic myoclonus may disturb sleep onset and continuity, causing insomnia	Arrhythmic, asynchronous, and asymmetric brief twitches involving different body areas and fasciculation potentials during NREM sleep
Facio-mandibular myoclonus	Sudden forceful myoclonus of the masticatory muscles, evident only during sleep, often associated with biting of the tongue and lips	Rhythmic or prolonged tonic contractions of the masticatory muscles
Fatal familial insomnia	Drowsiness, stupor, enacted dreams (gestures mimicking daily life activities with a dream content), autonomic hyperactivation	Complete absence of spindles and delta sleep. Wake or subwakefulness EEG patterns (stage 1 NREM) interspersed by recurrent brief REM sleep episodes without atonia persist throughout the 24 h. Persistent motor activity throughout the 24 h
Morvan syndrome	Severe insomnia associated with autonomic overactivity and enacted dreams	Short clusters of REM sleep emerged from a subwake EEG pattern (stage 1 NREM) during day and night. Enacted dreams mimicking daily life activities coincided with REM sleep episodes
Delirium tremens	Severe insomnia, dream enactment, motor violent agitation, sleeplessness, and sympathetic hyperactivity	Complete sleep-wake disruption with a drastic reduction of spindles and delta sleep. A state between subwakefulness (stage 1) and REM sleep (stage 1+REM) becomes the predominant PSG pattern

years [43]. Nocturnal stridor is a life-threatening condition in MSA due to a sleep-related laryngeal dystonia [44]. PSG recordings in patients with Shy-Drager syndrome show a reduced amount of slow-wave sleep (SWS), reduced REM sleep, reduced total sleep time, increased sleep latency, and recurrent awakenings [45, 46]. The circadian rhythms of temperature and melatonin secretion are also impaired in both MSA and PSP reflecting a severe disruption of the mechanisms regulating autonomic and endocrine homeostasis [47].

Progressive Supranuclear Palsy (PSP) and Corticobasal Degeneration (CBD)

PSP and CBD have overlapping clinical features hampering the clinical distinction between these two entities. Insomnia is a common complaint in these patients [48, 49].

Axial rigidity, dystonia, and postural difficulties may contribute to sleep disruption. PSG recordings in patients with PSP show a prolonged sleep latency, decreased total sleep time, decreased sleep efficiency, repeated arousals and awakenings, a decreased percentage of stage 2 with a drastic reduction in the number and amplitude of sleep spindles, and less REM sleep [48]. REM sleep latency may be reduced in some patients. Isolated cases of RBD associated with PSP have been reported but RBD seldom occurs in PSP and CBD [50–52].

Another characteristic feature of PSP seems to be daytime somnolence. However, subjective sleepiness in these patients may not coincide with objective measurements by Multiple Sleep Latency Test (MSLT).

Huntington's Disease (HD)

Insomnia with impaired initiation and maintenance of sleep is a common complaint, especially in moderate-to-severe HD. Longer sleep latency, lower sleep efficiency, frequent nocturnal awakenings, less slow-wave sleep, and a high prevalence of periodic limb movements are common in patients with HD [53].

Progressive Dystonia

Sleep disturbances occur in many patients with torsion dystonia. Deterioration of sleep parallels disease progression. PSG studies in these patients disclosed increased sleep latency and frequent awakenings with reduced sleep efficiency [54]. REM sleep may be reduced in severely affected patients.

Tourette's Syndrome (TS)

The degree of sleep disturbance and the impact of sleep disturbances on quality of life are correlated with disease severity. Around 40 % of children with TS also have a history of somnambulism, night terrors, or enuresis and are prone to "confusional arousal." An increased number of awakenings and increased motor activity and body movements during sleep have been described in TS irrespective of comorbid attention-deficit hyperactivity disorder [55].

Autosomal Dominant Spinocerebellar Ataxia (SCA)

SCA is a clinically and genetically heterogeneous group of disorders characterized by progressive ataxia, dysarthria, and nystagmus. Sleep disturbances are common features in SCA. In 1978 Osorio and co-workers reported the absence of REM sleep in two patients with spinocerebellar degeneration and described a peculiar EEG pattern characterized by an admixture of different elements of states of being with high-voltage slow waves and increased tonic EMG activity [56]. This non-conventional sleep stage probably represents an example of status dissociatus.

In two small pilot studies, PSG revealed REM sleep without atonia in the majority of patients with spinocerebellar ataxia type 2 (SCA2) [56, 57] and a reduction of REM density [58]. Impaired sleep is a frequent symptom in SCA3 (Machado-Joseph disease) with a very high prevalence of RBD (>50 %) [59, 60], appearing in some cases several years before ataxia [60]. RLS is present in about half of SCA3 patients but is rare in other types of SCA [61]. Stridor and NREM-related parasomnias have also been described in SCA3 patients [60, 62, 63].

Insomnia and Sleep-Related Movement Disorders

The main sleep-related movement disorders hindering sleep onset or interrupting SWS or REM sleep are (1) restless legs syndrome (RLS) and periodic limb movements in sleep (PLMS), (2) propriospinal myoclonus (PSM), (3) nocturnal frontal lobe epilepsy (NFLE), and (4) REM sleep behavior disorder (RBD).

Restless Legs Syndrome (RLS)

RLS is a common sensorimotor disorder clinically characterized by a compelling urge to move the limbs, accompanied by uncomfortable and unpleasant sensations in the extremities [64–66]. Typically, the legs are mostly affected but arm involvement has also been reported [65, 67] (Fig. 13.1). The urge to move the legs or unpleasant sensations begin or worsen during periods of rest or inactivity and are worse in the evening, especially when the patient lies down trying to fall asleep [65, 66]. Any limb movement, such as walking or stretching or rubbing the legs together, making cycling movements, and pacing across the room, partially or totally relieves symptoms, at least as long as the activity continues [64]. In milder forms, the disorder only briefly delays sleep onset and is not a true medical problem. However, more severe forms of RLS may cause severe insomnia by lengthening the time before sleep onset and provoking recurrent and prolonged awakenings throughout the night and impairing quality of life [68]. Idiopathic RLS is often familial with a genetically heterogeneous complex trait [69, 70]. RLS may also occur in acquired forms associated with a variety of neurological disorders (such as Parkinson's disease and Parkinsonian syndromes) and other medical conditions (such as uremia and end-stage renal disease, iron-deficiency anemia, diabetes, and familial amyloidosis). RLS may transiently appear during pregnancy (in most cases, symptoms are mild and they usually resolve after delivery), or intensify during treatment with various drugs (such as typical and atypical neuroleptics, metoclopramide, estrogens, tri- and tetracyclic antidepressants, serotonin reuptake inhibitors) [71].

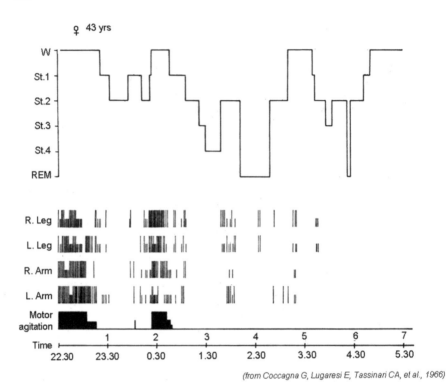

Fig. 13.1 Polysomnographic recording in a patient with restless leg syndrome. Hypnogram (*top*) and schematic representation (*bottom*) of myoclonic jerks, involving legs and arms and motor agitation. Delayed sleep onset and sleep fragmentation result from the motor disturbance (*R* right, *L* left) (reproduced from "Restless Legs", Coccagna G, Lugaresi E, Tassinari CA and Ambrosetto C. Omnia Medica et Therapeutica, 1966 vol.4)

Juvenile onset is the rule in inherited familial forms. Children with RLS commonly report symptoms resembling "growing pains" [72]. RLS was suggested to be highly associated with attention-deficit hyperactivity disorder [73]. Although RLS prevalence is high, only few patients with the condition will be led to consult a physician; severe chronic forms leading patients to seek treatment are present in only about 2–3 % of patients [68, 74]. Older patients tend to complain of more severe RLS symptoms indicating that the frequency and severity of symptoms tend to increase over time together with the progression of the disease. For patients with moderate-to-severe symptoms, drug therapy is required. First-choice treatment relies on low doses of a dopamine agonist; opioids are a second-line option. Clonazepam and gabapentin are alternative treatment possibilities either alone or in combination with dopaminergic therapy [75].

Periodic Limb Movements in Sleep (PLMS)

PLMS occur in 80–100% of patients with RLS [67, 76]. PLMS are characterized by periodic episodes of involuntary, repetitive, and highly stereotyped dorsiflexion of the big toe and/or foot, sometimes associated with flexion of the leg on the thigh and of the thigh on the trunk. Both extremities are usually involved, but as a rule not simultaneously or symmetrically, predominating in one leg or alternating between legs. PLMS appear on falling asleep and continue in light sleep, recurring every 20–40 s. K complexes, increased muscle tone, heart and breathing rates, and raised systemic blood pressure appear simultaneously with PLMS during light sleep, suggesting that PLMS are part of a periodic arousal involving cortical, somatic, and visceral functions [77, 78]. A dual mechanism consisting in an abnormal hyperexcitability of different and unsynchronized primary lumbosacral and, to a lesser extent, cervical spinal generators triggered by sleep-related factors located at a supraspinal but still unresolved level could be the source for PLMS [79].

PLMS occur in a number of sleep disorders such as narcolepsy, sleep apnea syndrome, and RBD. They can also occur as an isolated condition in otherwise healthy subjects, especially in the elderly, and in most cases PLMS are simply a causal PSG observation and are virtually never appreciated by the patient. It is currently controversial whether PLMS themselves cause insomnia or excessive daytime sleepiness. Because the prevalence of PLMS does not differ significantly in people with insomnia and hypersomnia or healthy subjects, except for very peculiar cases in which myoclonic jerks are so frequent and violent as to disrupt nocturnal sleep, PLMS are not the cause of insomnia [67].

Propriospinal Myoclonus (PSM)

PSM is a type of spinal myoclonus in which the myoclonic activity is generated within the spinal cord but does not remain restricted to segmentally innervated muscles and actually spreads up and down the length of the spinal cord along propriospinal pathways intrinsic to the cord [80]. PSM is characterized by violent muscle jerks in flexion or extension of the trunk and abdomen usually arising from the thoraco-abdominal/paraspinal muscles, or cervical muscles such as the sternocleidomastoideus muscle (Fig. 13.2). In some patients and in some instances, jerks may involve only a restricted group of muscles (always including the originator muscle), propagating to more rostral and caudal levels only in the most intense jerks [81]. PSM is usually idiopathic, but is sometimes associated with spinal lesions (cervical trauma, thoracic herpes zoster, syringomyelia, multiple sclerosis, HIV infection, etc.) [82].

PSM typically arises at sleep onset, during relaxed wakefulness and drowsiness (with EEG characterized by diffuse alpha rhythm), and disappears as soon as the patient achieves sleep (with the appearance of the first sleep spindles in stage 2 NREM). Physiological sleep usually continues until the morning [83]. The jerks may recur quasi-periodically, every 10–20 s, for minutes or hours, hindering sleep

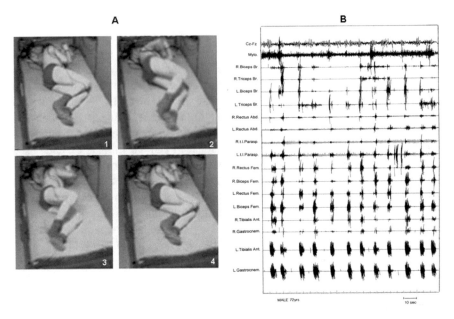

Fig. 13.2 Propriospinal myoclonus. (**a**) Videorecording of a jerk of propriospinal myoclonus in a 41-year-old man. (**b**) Excerpt from polysomnographic recordings in a 72-year-old man: myoclonic jerks recur at quasi-periodic intervals at sleep onset, and during relaxed wakefulness prior to falling asleep. The abnormal EMG activity originates in the right rectus abdominis muscle spreading thereafter to more rostral and caudal muscles (*mylo* mylohyoideus, *biceps br.* biceps brachii, *triceps br.* triceps brachii, *rectus abd.* rectus abdominis, *t.l. parasp.* thoracolumbar paraspinalis, *rectus fem.* rectus femoris, *biceps fem.* biceps femoris, *tibialis ant.* tibialis anterior, *gastrocnem.* gastrocnemius, *R.* right, *L.* left)

onset and eventually leading to a severe insomnia which can persist for years or even decades (Fig. 13.2). The jerks quickly disappear also whenever the patient is aroused (by somesthetic stimuli, or when asked to perform mental calculation, make a fist, or simply speak) and EEG then changes to desynchronized activity. Clonazepam (at a dose of 0.5–2 mg) can reduce muscular jerks making sleep more restful. Opiates may also be effective but carry the risk of dependence [83].

Nocturnal Frontal Lobe Epilepsy (NFLE)

NFLE is a peculiar form of partial epilepsy in which seizures are characterized by bizarre motor behavior or sustained dystonic posture. Seizures appear almost exclusively during sleep. The clinical spectrum of NFLE comprises distinct paroxysmal manifestations of variable duration and complexity arising during SWS and usually consisting of (1) *paroxysmal arousals* (PA), brief sudden awakenings associated with stereotyped and abnormal movements, recurring several times per night; (2) *nocturnal paroxysmal dystonia* (NPD), more complex motor episodes lasting for 1–2 min, characterized by violent motor behavior (choreo-athetosic, ballic and

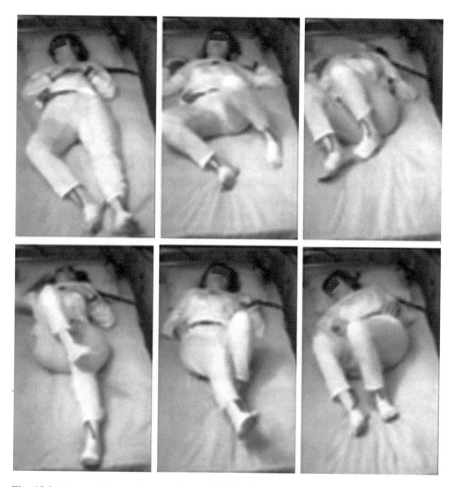

Fig. 13.3 Nocturnal frontal lobe epilepsy (NFLE). Videorecordings (excerpts taken at regular time intervals) of an NPD attack. During the attack, frantic wide-ranging movements display ballistic and dystonic patterns involving the trunk and limbs

nearly rhythmic leg or arm movements), vocalization, screaming, fearful and repetitive movements of the trunk and limbs, and dystonic-dyskinetic postures (Fig. 13.3); and (3) prolonged episodes, named *episodic nocturnal wandering* (ENW), or *agitated somnambulism* [84]. The three types of seizures often coexist in the same patient. If seizures recur frequently every night, patients may feel tired and weary on awakening in the morning and complain of daytime sleepiness. NFLE can be inherited as an autosomal dominant disorder and some mutations linked to familial cases of NFLE have been identified [85].

Distinguishing NFLE from paroxysmal non-epileptic sleep disorders is often difficult and sometimes impossible on clinical grounds alone, because a reliable description of motor events occurring during the night is often difficult to collect from a sleep partner. Therefore, video-polysomnography monitoring together with careful history taking may represent the only tool to distinguish NFLE from other non-epileptic paroxysmal motor disorders in sleep [86].

Effective treatment controlling or reducing the amount of nocturnal seizures improves insomnia and daytime somnolence.

REM Sleep Behavior Disorder (RBD)

REM Sleep Behavior Disorder (RBD) is a parasomnia characterized by abnormal and often violent motor agitation arising during REM sleep [87, 88]. Violent behavior can result in sleep disruption and severe injuries, including ecchymoses, lacerations, and fractures for the patient or bed partner, have been described [89]. Patients with RBD have a high proportion of aggressive content in their dreams associated with more or less purposeful gestures enacting attack or defense reactions, despite normal levels of daytime aggressiveness [87]. RBD usually occurs in the middle of the night or early hours of the morning and are caused by the loss of the physiological muscular atonia during REM sleep (REM sleep without atonia) (Fig. 13.4). RBD is more common in the older population and in male; the mean age at onset is 60 years. At the moment, two main types of RBD are recognized: acute-onset and chronic RBD. Acute-onset RBD is usually related to the effects of medications, such as the use of tricyclic antidepressant and SSRI, or to withdrawal of barbiturates, benzodiazepines, alcohol, or meprobamate. In this context, RBD is usually a transient manifestation, resolving spontaneously after a few days. Chronic RBD can present alone, without concomitant medical disorders, known as idiopathic or is

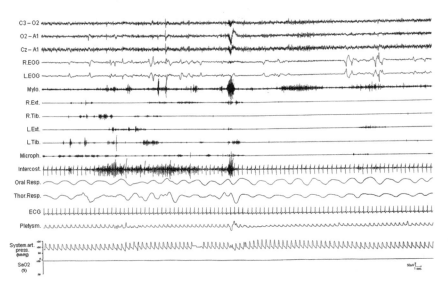

Fig. 13.4 Polysomnogram of a patient with REM sleep behavior disorder (RBD). The normal muscle atonia of REM sleep is disrupted (see sustained EMG activity of the mylohyoideus muscle)

more commonly reported in patients with neurodegenerative disorders, especially synucleinopathy [90, 91], sometimes as a heralding symptom [43, 90, 91]. Clonazepam (0.5–2 mg before bedtime) is highly effective and well tolerated in 80–90 % of cases [89].

Other less common sleep-related movement disorders which may disrupt sleep include the following:

Excessive Fragmentary Hypnic Myoclonus (EFHM)

Excessive fragmentary hypnic myoclonus (EFHM) is a pathological motor activity consisting of small myoclonic twitches and fasciculation potentials during NREM sleep [92]. It is an abnormal intensification of the physiologic hypnic myoclonia and is characterized by sudden arrhythmic asynchronous and asymmetric brief twitches involving different body areas. EFHM may be an isolated phenomenon or associated with other sleep disorders such as sleep apnea, RLS, RBD, and excessive daytime drowsiness. If severe, EFHM may disturb sleep onset and continuity, causing insomnia [93].

Facio-Mandibular Myoclonus

Facio-mandibular myoclonus is a rare sleep-related movement disorder and usually does not affect sleep. It consists of sudden forceful myoclonus of the masticatory muscles, evident only during sleep, often associated with biting of the tongue and lips and, in such cases, simulating epileptic seizures during sleep [94–96]. The myoclonus usually starts in adult life, and may be familial. Rhythmic or prolonged tonic contractions of the masticatory muscles may damage the tongue and oral mucosa resulting in a burning pain that disturbs sleep [94].

Generalized Overactivity Syndrome (Agrypnia Excitata)

There are at least three neurological conditions (fatal insomnia, Morvan syndrome and delirium tremens) in which the inability to sleep is typically associated with motor and sympathetic or noradrenergic overactivation. Agrypnia (from the Greek "to chase sleep") excitata (AE) are the terms aptly defining the clinical conditions in which organic insomnia is associated with a generalized activation syndrome [97–99].

Fatal Familial Insomnia

Fatal familial insomnia (FFI) is an autosomal dominant disease caused by a point mutation at codon 178 of the prion protein gene (PRPN). Nearly 50 FFI kindreds have been described to date in addition to nine sporadic (non-genetic) cases (SFI) around the world in every ethnic group.

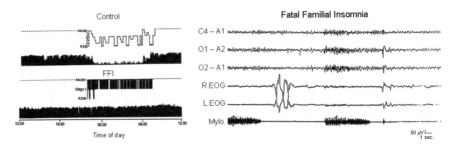

Fig. 13.5 Fatal familial insomnia (FFI). *Left*: Hypnograms and 24-h actigraphic recordings in a healthy control individual and in an FFI patient. *Right*: Excerpt of polysomnographic recording (PSG) in FFI. The hypnogram fluctuates from stage 1 NREM to REM sleep. Actigraphic recording shows continuous motor activity throughout the 24 h. The polysomnographic tracing is characterized by wake or subwake EEG patterns interspersed with short episodes of REM sleep

The disease begins, on average, at the age of 50 years with a variable duration from 8 months to 7 years. The early cardinal symptoms are apathy (attention deficit and indifference to surroundings), drowsiness and stupor, accompanied by enacted dreams (gestures mimicking daily-life activities with a dream content), autonomic hyperactivation (hyperhidrosis, sialorrhea, tachycardia, hypertension, mild fever, etc.), and motor signs (ataxia, dysarthria, evoked and spontaneous myoclonus) [100]. Signs and symptoms of sympathetic overactivity are associated with a marked and progressive increase in catecholamine secretion. In addition, 24-h serial studies document autonomic (blood pressure and body temperature) and hormonal (cortisol, norepinephrine) circadian oscillations that progressively subside until they disappear almost completely. On the contrary, melatonin secretion is reduced and lacks the nocturnal peak.

Longitudinal polysomnographic studies document that spindles and delta sleep, the typical EEG features of synchronized sleep, markedly reduced from disease onset, are completely absent in the most advanced stages (Fig. 13.5), whereas wake or subwakefulness EEG patterns (stage 1 NREM) interspersed by recurrent brief REM sleep episodes without atonia persist throughout day and night, and actigraphic recordings performed during several weeks or even months preceding death document persistent motor activity throughout the 24 h (Fig. 13.5). At this stage even intravenous administration of barbiturates or benzodiazepines fails to generate spindle-like activity and delta rhythms [101].

PET scan in short evolution FFI cases discloses a brain hypometabolism confined to the thalamus, while hypometabolism still predominates in the thalamus but is widespread to the cerebral cortex (namely frontotemporal cortex) and basal ganglia in long evolution cases.

FFI neuropathology is dominated by selective degeneration of the mediodorsal and anteroventral thalamic nuclei. Other thalamic nuclei and some limbic cortical regions (the caudal orbital cortex and anterior cingulate gyrus) are less consistently and less severely involved [101, 102].

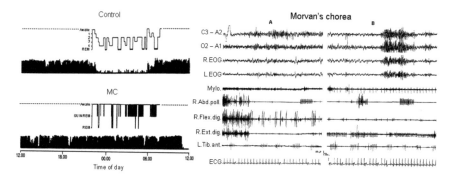

Fig. 13.6 Morvan syndrome (MS). *Left*: Hypnograms and 24-h actigraphic recordings in a healthy control individual and in an MS patient, (MC). *Right*: Excerpts of polysomnographic recordings (PSG) in an MS patient. The hypnogram fluctuates from wakefulness to REM sleep. Actigraphic recording shows continuous motor activity throughout the 24 h. PSG: (*A*) the patient is agitated and presents dream-enacting behavior. Characteristic continuous muscle fiber activity on the electromyogram is also present. ECG shows multiple arrhythmic abnormalities; (*B*) sleep-like behavior: the patient is quiet, but the EEG lacks any characteristic sleep pattern

Morvan Syndrome (MS)

First described by Morvan in 1890, MS is an autoimmune limbic encephalopathy, characterized by severe insomnia accompanied by autonomic overactivity (profuse perspiration, tachycardia, hypertension, and fever), fasciculations, cramps, and motor agitation [103]. Mental confusion with vivid hallucinations and enacted dreams (behaviorally similar to those observed in FFI patients) appear in the most severe cases [104]. MS arises at any age and has a spontaneous remission, in a few weeks or months, in 80–90% of the cases. The remainder have a malignant progression of the disease until death. In 1974 Fisher-Perroudon and co-workers demonstrated that sleep disappeared at least 4 months before death in a typical case of MS [105]. We described serial polysomnographic recordings in a malignant evolution case documenting the abolition of spindle and delta sleep in the full-blown stage of the disease [104]. Short episodes of REM sleep recurring in clusters emerged from a subwake EEG pattern (stage 1 NREM) during day and night in the months before death (Fig. 13.6). Enacted dreams mimicking daily life activities coincided with REM sleep episodes as in FFI. Motor agitation persisting day and night, central sympathetic overactivation accompanied by persistently high norepinephrine levels, and reduced melatonin secretion characterized the patients we observed [104, 106]. Serum IgG in our first case bound strongly to neurons in the hippocampus, thalamus, and striatum of rat brain, whereas direct immunochemistry on frozen sections of the patient's brain tissue showed areas of antibody leakage in the thalamus. Postmortem brain examination was unremarkable in our case as in the few other cases.

Silber et al., briefly reporting a case of MS with benign outcome, also emphasized the striking similarities between the polygraphic aspects in their cases and those observed in FFI [107].

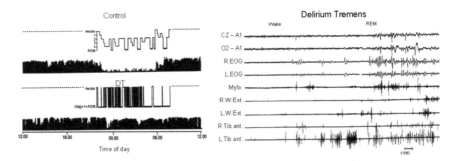

Fig. 13.7 Delirium tremens (DT). *Left*: Hypnograms and 24-h actigraphic recordings in a healthy control individual and in a DT patient. *Right*: Excerpt of polysomnographic recording (PSG) in a DT patient. The hypnogram and PSG are characterized by fluctuation from wakefulness to stage 1+REM sleep. Actigraphy shows a continuous motor overactivity with a loss of the 24-h circadian rest-activity cycle

Delirium Tremens (DT)

Delirium tremens (DT) is the well-known acute psychotic syndrome linked to sudden alcohol or benzodiazepine withdrawal after chronic abuse [108]. DT is clinically characterized by severe insomnia, anxiety, confusion associated with visual hallucinations, and dream enactment. Tremor and motor violent agitation associated with sleeplessness and sympathetic hyperactivity (perspiration, tachycardia, hypertension, mild fever) are other common signs. During the acute phase of the disease, polysomnographic recordings disclosed complete sleep-wake disruption with a drastic reduction of spindle and delta sleep. A state between subwakefulness (stage 1) and protracted REM sleep episodes (so-called stage 1+REM) becomes the predominant PSG pattern as Kotorii et al. reported [108] (Fig. 13.7). Enacted dreams mimicked daily life activities as in FFI and MS and coincided with REM sleep episodes [109]. Even though the pathogenetic mechanism of DT is not fully understood, we can assume that sudden alcohol or benzodiazepine (BDZ) withdrawal results in a transient homeostatic imbalance within the limbic system, due to the sudden dramatic changes in GABAergic synapses, downregulated by chronic alcohol abuse [109].

Agrypnia Excitata: A Generalized Activation Syndrome

The striking clinical and polygraphic similarities shared by FFI, MS, and DT suggest that they have a common pathogenetic mechanism, despite the widely different etiology and clinical course. Clinically, the picture is characterized by severe insomnia, hallucinations, dream-enacting behavior (oneiric stupor), motor agitation, and sympathergic activation. Hormonal functions are consistently involved (cortisol and catecholamine secretion is high, melatonin secretion, at least in FFI and MS, is markedly reduced). Polygraphically, FFI, MS, and DT are characterized by the disappearance of SWS (spindle and delta activity) and EEG signs of "subwakefulness" alternating or intermingling with REM sleep episodes. The intralimbic disconnection caused by degeneration of the visceral thalamus triggers the generalized activation associated with the inability to sleep characteristic of FFI [110]. Autoantibodies binding to the (voltage dependent) potassium channels of thalamo-limbic neurons, giving rise to a sort of autoimmune limbic encephalopathy, could explain the clinical picture of MS [104, 111]. Sudden alcohol (or BDZ) withdrawal generates the same clinical features because previous alcohol (or BDZ) abuse had strongly downregulated the inhibitory GABAergic synapses within the thalamo-limbic circuits [109].

Summing up, an anatomical or functional intralimbic disconnection resulting in the prevalence of activating over de-activating systems is the cause of the generalized activation syndrome—agrypnia excitata—shared by FFI, MS, and DT [112].

References

1. Schutte-Rodin S, Broch L, Buysse D, Dorsey C, Sateia M. Clinical guideline for the evaluation and management of chronic insomnia in adults. J Clin Sleep Med. 2008;4:487–504.
2. Passarella S, Duong MT. Diagnosis and treatment of insomnia. Am J Health Syst Pharm. 2008;65:927–34.
3. Lugaresi E, Cirignotta F, Zucconi M, Mondini S, Lenzi PL, Coccagna G. Good and poor sleepers: epidemiological survey of the San Marino Population. In: Guilleminault C, Lugaresi E, editors. Sleep/wake disorders: natural history, epidemiology, and long-term evolution. New York: Raven; 1983. p. 1–12.
4. Ohayon MM. Epidemiology of insomnia: what we know and what we still need to learn. Sleep Med Rev. 2002;6:97–111.
5. Avidan AY. Sleep changes and disorders in the elderly patient. Curr Neurol Neurosci Rep. 2002;2:178–85.
6. Smagula SF, Stone KL, Fabio A, Cauley JA. Risk factors for sleep disturbances in older adults: evidence from prospective studies. Sleep Med Rev. 2016;25:21–30.
7. Krystal AD. Insomnia in women. Clin Cornerstone. 2003;5:41–50.
8. Manber R, Chambers AS. Insomnia and depression: a multifaceted interplay. Curr Psychiatry Rep. 2009;11:437–42.
9. Roth T, Roehrs T, Pies R. Insomnia: pathophysiology and implications for treatment. Sleep Med Rev. 2007;11:71–9.
10. Winkelman JW. Insomnia disorder. N Engl J Med. 2015;373:1437–44.
11. Buysse DJ. Insomnia. JAMA. 2013;309:706–16.
12. Nofzinger EA, Buysse DJ, Germain A, Price JC, Miewald JM, Kupfer DJ. Functional neuroimaging evidence for hyperarousal in insomnia. Am J Psychiatry. 2004;161:2126–8.
13. Drake CL, Scofield H, Roth T. Vulnerability to insomnia: the role of familial aggregation. Sleep Med. 2008;9:297–302.
14. Happe S. Excessive daytime sleepiness and sleep disturbances in patients with neurological diseases: epidemiology and management. Drugs. 2003;63:2725–37.
15. Hoyt BD. Sleep in patients with neurologic and psychiatric disorders. Prim Care. 2005;32:535–48.
16. Rao V, Spiro J, Samus QM, et al. Insomnia and daytime sleepiness in people with dementia residing in assisted living: findings from the Maryland Assisted Living Study. Int J Geriatr Psychiatry. 2008;23:199–206.

17. Cipriani G, Lucetti C, Danti S, Nuti A. Sleep disturbances and dementia. Psychogeriatrics. 2015;15:65–74.
18. Potvin O, Lorrain D, Forget H, et al. Sleep quality and 1-year incident cognitive impairment in community-dwelling older adults. Sleep. 2012;35:491–9.
19. Guarnieri B, Adorni F, Musicco M, et al. Prevalence of sleep disturbances in mild cognitive impairment and dementing disorders: a multicenter Italian clinical cross-sectional study on 431 patients. Dement Geriatr Cogn Disord. 2012;33:50–8.
20. Lim AS, Kowgier M, Yu L, Buchman AS, Bennett DA. Sleep fragmentation and the risk of incident Alzheimer's disease and cognitive decline in older persons. Sleep. 2013;36:1027–32.
21. Bombois S, Derambure P, Pasquier F, Monaca C. Sleep disorders in aging and dementia. J Nutr Health Aging. 2010;14:212–7.
22. Motohashi Y, Maeda A, Wakamatsu H, Higuchi S, Yuasa T. Circadian rhythm abnormalities of wrist activity of institutionalized dependent elderly persons with dementia. J Gerontol A Biol Sci Med Sci. 2000;55A:M740–3.
23. McCurry SM, Logsdon RG, Teri L, et al. Characteristics of sleep disturbance in community-dwelling Alzheimer's disease patients. J Geriatr Psychiatry Neurol. 1999;12:53–9.
24. Sloane PD, Mitchell CM, Preisser JS, Phillips C, Commander C, Burker E. Environmental correlates of resident agitation in Alzheimer's disease special care units. J Am Geriatr Soc. 1998;46:862–9.
25. Mishima K, Okawa M, Satoh K, Shimizu T, Hozumi S, Hishikawa Y. Different manifestations of circadian rhythms in senile dementia of Alzheimer's type and multi-infarct dementia. Neurobiol Aging. 1997;18:105–9.
26. Ancoli-Israel S, Ayalon L. Diagnosis and treatment of sleep disorders in older adults. Am J Geriatr Psychiatry. 2006;14:95–103.
27. Deschenes CL, McCurry SM. Current treatments for sleep disturbances in individuals with dementia. Curr Psychiatry Rep. 2009;11:20–6.
28. Morin CM, Bootzin RR, Buysse DJ, et al. Psychological and behavioral treatment of insomnia: update of the recent evidence (1998–2004). Sleep. 2006;29:1398–414.
29. Gammack JK. Light therapy for insomnia in older adults. Clin Geriatr Med. 2008;24:139–49.
30. Morgenthaler TI, Lee-Chiong T, Alessi CA, et al. Practice parameters for the clinical evaluation and treatment of circadian rhythm sleep disorders. An American Academy of Sleep Medicine report. Sleep. 2007;30:1445–59.
31. Jennum P, Santamaria J, Members of the Task Force. Report of an EFNS task force on management of sleep disorders in neurologic disease (degenerative neurologic disorders and stroke). Eur J Neurol. 2007;14:1189–200.
32. Wirz-Justice A, Werth E, Savaskan E, et al. Haloperidol disrupts, clozapine reinstates the circadian rest-activity cycle in a patient with early—onset Alzheimer disease. Alzheimer Dis Assoc Disord. 2000;14:212–5.
33. Mahlberg R, Walther S. Actigraphy in agitated patients with dementia. Monitoring treatment outcomes. Z Gerontol Geriatr. 2007;40:178–84.
34. Cardinali DP, Furio AM, Brusco L. Clinical aspects of melatonin intervention in Alzheimer's disease progression. Curr Neuropharmacol. 2010;8:218–27.
35. Roth T, Seiden D, Sainati S, et al. Effects of ramelteon on patient—reported sleep latency in older adults with chronic insomnia. Sleep Med. 2006;7:312–8.
36. Ylikoski A, Martikainen K, Sieminski M, Partinen M. Parkinson's disease and insomnia. Neurol Sci. 2015;36:2003–10.
37. Christensen JA, Nikolic M, Warby SC, et al. Sleep spindle alterations in patients with Parkinson's disease. Front Hum Neurosci. 2015;9:233.
38. Turner R, D'Amato C, Chervin R, Blaivas M. The pathology of REM sleep behavior disorder with comorbid Lewy body dementia. Neurology. 2000;55:1730–2.
39. Ferman TJ, Boeve BF. Dementia with Lewy bodies. Neurol Clin. 2007;25:741–60.

40. McKeith IG, Dickson DW, Lowe J, et al; Consortium on DLB. Diagnosis and management of dementia with Lewy bodies: third report of the DLB Consortium. Neurology. 2005;65:1863–72.
41. Iranzo A. Sleep and breathing in multiple system atrophy. Curr Treat Options Neurol. 2007;9:347–53.
42. Stanzani-Maserati M, Gallassi R, Calandra-Buonaura G, et al. Cognitive and sleep features of multiple system atrophy: review and prospective study. Eur Neurol. 2014;72:349–59.
43. Plazzi G, Corsini R, Provini F, et al. REM sleep behavior disorders in multiple system atrophy. Neurology. 1997;48:1094–7.
44. Vetrugno R, Liguori R, Cortelli P, et al. Sleep-related stridor due to dystonic vocal cord motion and neurogenic tachypnea/tachycardia in multiple system atrophy. Mov Disord. 2007;22:673–8.
45. Chokroverty S. The assessment of sleep disturbance in autonomic failure. In: Bannister R, Mathias CJ, editors. Autonomic failure. A textbook of clinical disorders of the nervous system. 3rd ed. London: Oxford University Press; 1992. p. 442–61.
46. Vetrugno R, Provini F, Cortelli P, et al. Sleep disorders in multiple system atrophy: a correlative video-polysomnographic study. Sleep Med. 2004;5:21–30.
47. Pierangeli G, Provini F, Maltoni P, et al. Nocturnal body core temperature falls in Parkinson's disease but not in Multiple-System Atrophy. Mov Disord. 2001;16:226–32.
48. Auger RR, Boeve BF. Sleep disorders in neurodegenerative diseases other than Parkinson's disease. In: Montagna P, Chokroverty S, editors. Handbook of clinical neurology, Sleep disorders part 2, vol. 99 (3rd series). The Netherlands: Elsevier; 2011. p. 1011–50.
49. Bhidayasiri R, Jitkritsadakul O, Colosimo C. Nocturnal manifestations of atypical Parkinsonian disorders. J Parkinsons Dis. 2014;4:223–36.
50. Olson EJ, Boeve BF, Silber MH. Rapid eye movement sleep behaviour disorder: demographic, clinical and laboratory findings in 93 cases. Brain. 2000;123:331–9.
51. Cooper AD, Josephs KA. Photophobia, visual hallucinations, and REM sleep behavior disorder in progressive supranuclear palsy and corticobasal degeneration: a prospective study. Parkinsonism Relat Disord. 2009;15:59–61.
52. Boeve BF, Silber MH, Ferman TJ, et al. Clinicopathologic correlations in 172 cases of rapid eye movement sleep behavior disorder with or without a coexisting neurologic disorder. Sleep Med. 2013;14:754–62.
53. Piano C, Losurdo A, Della Marca G, et al. Polysomnographic findings and clinical correlates in Huntington Disease: a cross-sectional cohort study. Sleep. 2015;38:1489–95.
54. Hertenstein E, Tang NK, Bernstein CJ, Nissen C, Underwood MR, Sandhu HK. Sleep in patients with primary dystonia: a systematic review on the state of research and perspectives. Sleep Med Rev. 2016;26:95–107.
55. Ghosh D, Rajan PV, Das D, Datta P, Rothner AD, Erenberg G. Sleep disorders in children with Tourette syndrome. Pediatr Neurol. 2014;51:31–5.
56. Osorio I, Daroff RB, Richey ET, Simon JB. Absence of REM and altered NREM sleep in patients with spinocerebellar degeneration and slow saccades. Trans Am Neurol Assoc. 1978;103:225–9.
57. Boesch SM, Frauscher B, Brandauer E, Wenning GK, Högl B, Poewe W. Disturbance of rapid eye movement sleep in spinocerebellar Ataxia type 2. Mov Disord. 2006;21:1751–4.
58. Tuin I, Voss U, Kang JS, et al. Stages of sleep pathology in spinocerebellar ataxia type 2 (SCA2). Neurology. 2006;67:966–72.
59. Friedman JH, Fernandez HH, Surdarsky LR. REM behavior disorder and excessive daytime somnolence in Machado-Joseph Disease (SCA3). Mov Disord. 2003;18:1520–2.
60. Iranzo A, Muñoz E, Santamaria J, Vilaseca I, Milà M, Tolosa E. REM sleep behavior disorder and vocal cord paralysis in Machado-Joseph disease. Mov Disord. 2003;18:1179–83.
61. Schöls L, Haan J, Riess O, Amoiridis G, Przuntek H. Sleep disturbance in spinocerebellar ataxias: is the SCA3 mutation a cause of restless legs syndrome? Neurology. 1998;51:1603–7.

62. Fukutani Y, Katsukawa K, Matsubara R, Kobayashi K, Nakamura I, Yamaguchi Y. Delirium associated with Joseph disease. J Neurol Neurosurg Psychiatry. 1993;56:1207–12.
63. Silva GM, Pedroso JL, Dos Santos DF, et al. NREM-related parasomnias in Machado-Joseph disease: clinical and polysomnographic evaluation. J Sleep Res. 2015. doi:10.1111/jsr.12330.
64. Ekbom KA. Restless legs. Acta Med Scand. 1945;158:1–123.
65. Allen RP, Picchietti D, Hening WA, Trenkwalder C, Walters AS, Montplaisir J. Restless legs syndrome: diagnostic criteria, special considerations, and epidemiology. A report from the restless legs syndrome diagnosis and epidemiology workshop at the National Institutes of Health. Sleep Med. 2003;4:101–19.
66. Allen RP, Picchietti DL, Garcia-Borreguero D, et al; International Restless Legs Syndrome Study Group. Restless legs syndrome/Willis—Ekbom disease diagnostic criteria: updated International Restless Legs Syndrome Study Group (IRLSSG) consensus criteria—history, rationale, description, and significance. Sleep Med. 2014;15:860–73.
67. Lugaresi E, Cirignotta F, Coccagna G, Montagna P. Nocturnal myoclonus and restless legs syndrome. In: Fahn S et al., editors. Advances in neurology, Myoclonus, vol. 43. New York: Raven; 1986. p. 295–307.
68. Allen RP, Walters AS, Montplaisir J, et al. Restless legs syndrome prevalence and impact: REST general population study. Arch Intern Med. 2005;165:1286–92.
69. Winkelmann J, Shormair B, Lichtner P, et al. Genome-wide association study of restless legs syndrome identifies common variants in three genomic regions. Nat Genet. 2007;39: 1000–6.
70. Rye DB. The molecular genetics of Restless Legs Syndrome. Sleep Med Clin. 2015;10: 227–33.
71. Stiasny K, Oertel WH, Trenkwalder C. Clinical symptomatology and treatment of restless legs syndrome and periodic limb movement disorder. Sleep Med Rev. 2002;6:253–65.
72. Simakajornboon N, Dye TJ, Walters AS. Restless Legs Syndrome/Willis—Ekbom disease and growing pains in children and adolescents. Sleep Med Clin. 2015;10:311–22.
73. Picchietti DL, Bruni O, de Weerd A, et al; International Restless Legs Syndrome Study Group (IRLSSG). Pediatric restless legs syndrome diagnostic criteria: an update by the International Restless Legs Syndrome Study Group. Sleep Med. 2013;14:1253–9.
74. Hening W. The clinical neurophysiology of the restless legs syndrome and periodic limb movements. Part I: diagnosis, assessment, and characterization. Clin Neurophysiol. 2004;115:1965–74.
75. Vignatelli L, Billiard M, Clarenbach P, et al. EFNS guidelines on management of restless legs syndrome and periodic limb movement disorder in sleep. Eur J Neurol. 2006;13:1049–65.
76. Trenkwalder C, Paulus W. Restless legs syndrome: pathophysiology, clinical presentation and management. Nat Rev Neurol. 2010;6:337–46.
77. Lugaresi E, Coccagna G, Mantovani M, Lebrun R. Some periodic phenomena arising during drowsiness and sleep in man. Electroencephalogr Clin Neurophysiol. 1972;32:701–5.
78. Terzano MG, Mancia D, Salati MR, Costani G, Decembrino A, Parrino L. The cyclic alternating pattern as a physiological component of normal NREM sleep. Sleep. 1985;8:137–45.
79. Provini F, Vetrugno R, Meletti S, et al. Motor pattern of periodic limb movements during sleep. Neurology. 2001;57:300–4.
80. Brown P, Thompson PD, Rothwell JC, Day BL, Marsden CD. Axial myoclonus of propriospinal origin. Brain. 1991;114:197–214.
81. Vetrugno R, Provini F, Plazzi G, et al. Focal myoclonus and propriospinal propagation. Clin Neurophysiol. 2000;111:2175–9.
82. Antelmi E, Provini F. Propriospinal myoclonus: the spectrum of clinical and neurophysiological phenotypes. Sleep Med Rev. 2015;22:54–63.
83. Montagna P, Provini F, Plazzi G, Liguori R, Lugaresi E. Propriospinal myoclonus upon relaxation and drowsiness: a cause of severe insomnia. Mov Disord. 1997;12:66–72.
84. Provini F, Plazzi G, Tinuper P, Vandi S, Lugaresi E, Montagna P. Nocturnal frontal lobe epilepsy. A clinical and polygraphic overview of 100 consecutive cases. Brain. 1999;122:1017–31.

85. Steinlein OK. Genetic heterogeneity in familial nocturnal frontal lobe epilepsy. Prog Brain Res. 2014;213:1–15.
86. Tinuper P, Provini F, Bisulli F, et al. Movement disorders in sleep: guidelines for differentiating epileptic from non-epileptic motor phenomena arising from sleep. Sleep Med Rev. 2007;11:255–67.
87. American Academy of Sleep Medicine. International classification of sleep disorders. 3rd ed. Darien, IL: American Academy of Sleep Medicine; 2014.
88. Schenck CH, Bundlie SR, Ettinger MG, Mahowald MW. Chronic behavioral disorders of REM sleep: a new category of parasomnia. Sleep. 1986;9:293–308.
89. Schenck CH, Hurwitz TD, Mahowald MW. REM sleep behaviour disorder: an update on a series of 96 patients and a review of the world literature. J Sleep Res. 1993;2:224–31.
90. Boeve BF, Silber MH, Ferman TJ, Lucas JA, Parisi JE. Association of REM sleep behavior disorder and neurodegenerative disease may reflect an underlying synucleinopathy. Mov Disord. 2001;16:622–30.
91. Howell MJ, Schenck CH. Rapid eye movement sleep behavior disorder and neurodegenerative disease. JAMA Neurol. 2015;72:707–12.
92. Broughton R, Tolentino MA. Fragmentary pathological myoclonus in NREM sleep. Electroencephalogr Clin Neurophysiol. 1984;57:303–9.
93. Vetrugno R, Plazzi G, Provini F, Liguori R, Lugaresi E, Montagna P. Excessive fragmentary hypnic myoclonus: clinical and neurophysiologic findings. Sleep Med. 2002;3:73–6.
94. Vetrugno R, Provini F, Plazzi G, et al. Familial nocturnal facio-mandibular myoclonus mimicking sleep bruxism. Neurology. 2002;58:644–7.
95. Loi D, Provini F, Vetrugno R, D'Angelo R, Zaniboni A, Montagna P. Sleep-related faciomandibular myoclonus: a sleep-related movement disorder different from bruxism. Mov Disord. 2007;22:1819–22.
96. Aguglia U, Gambardella A, Quattrone A. Sleep-induced masticatory myoclonus: a rare parasomnia associated with insomnia. Sleep. 1991;14:80–2.
97. Lugaresi E, Provini F. Agypnia Excitata: clinical features and pathophysiological implications. Sleep Med Rev. 2001;5:313–22.
98. Montagna P, Lugaresi E. Agrypnia Excitata: a generalized overactivity syndrome and a useful concept in the neurophysiopathology of sleep. Clin Neurophysiol. 2002;113:552–60.
99. Provini F, Cortelli P, Montagna P, Gambetti P, Lugaresi E. Fatal insomnia and agrypnia excitata: sleep and the limbic system. Rev Neurol (Paris). 2008;164(8–9):692–700.
100. Montagna P, Gambetti P, Cortelli P, Lugaresi E. Familial and sporadic fatal insomnia. Lancet Neurol. 2003;2:167–76.
101. Lugaresi E, Medori R, Montagna P, et al. Fatal familial insomnia and dysautonomia with selective degeneration of thalamic nuclei. N Engl J Med. 1986;315:997–1003.
102. Parchi P, Petersen RB, Chen SG, et al. Molecular pathology of Fatal Familial Insomnia. Brain Pathol. 1998;8:539–48.
103. Morvan A. De la chorée fibrillaire. Gaz Heb Méd Chirurg. 1890;27:173–200.
104. Liguori R, Vincent A, Clover L, et al. Morvan's syndrome: peripheral and central nervous system and cardiac involvement with antibodies to voltage—gated potassium channels. Brain. 2001;124:2417–26.
105. Fischer-Perroudon C, Trillet M, Mouret J, et al. Investigations polygraphiques et métaboliques d'une insomnie durable avec hallucinations. Rev Neurol (Paris). 1974;130:111–25.
106. Baiardi S, Provini F, Avoni P, Pasquinelli M, Liguori R. Immunotherapy of oneiric stupor in Morvan syndrome: efficacy documented by actigraphy. Neurology. 2015;84:2457–9.
107. Silber MH, Nippoidt TB, Karnes PS, Goerss JB, Patel T, Kane L. Morvan's fibrillary chorea resembling fatal familial insomnia. Sleep Res. 1995;24:431.
108. Kotorii T, Nakazawa Y, Yokoyama T, et al. The sleep pattern of chronic alcoholics during the alcohol withdrawal period. Folia Psychiatr Neurol Jpn. 1980;34:89–95.
109. Plazzi G, Montagna P, Meletti S, Lugaresi E. Polysomnographic study of sleeplessness and oneiricisms in the alcohol withdrawal syndrome. Sleep Med. 2002;3:279–82.

110. Lugaresi E, Tobler I, Gambetti P, Montagna P. The pathophysiology of fatal familial insomnia. Brain Pathol. 1998;8:521–6.
111. Vincent A, Buckley C, Schott JM, et al. Potassium channel antibody-associated encephalopathy: a potentially immunotherapy-responsive form of limbic encephalitis. Brain. 2004;127:701–12.
112. Lugaresi E, Provini F, Montagna P. The neuroanatomy of sleep. Considerations on the role of the thalamus in sleep and a proposal for a caudorostral organization. Eur J Anat. 2004;8:85–93.

Chapter 14
Insomnia in Psychiatric Disorders

Zachary L. Cohen and Katherine M. Sharkey

Abstract Insomnia is a common feature of mental illness and data have emerged indicating that sleep disturbance can be a risk factor for developing a psychiatric disorder and for worsening of pre-existing mental illness. Management of insomnia without accounting for underlying psychiatric disorders can be expected to result in suboptimal outcomes. Although associations between insomnia and mental illness are likely bidirectional, evidence suggests that treating comorbid insomnia can improve sleep and psychiatric outcomes. This chapter reviews the prevalence and features of insomnia in patients with frequently encountered psychiatric disorders, including mood disorders, anxiety disorders, substance-use disorders, and psychotic disorders, as well as specific treatment strategies where applicable. Further study of the subtleties of sleep disturbance among patients with different mental disorders may elucidate the genetic, neurochemical, and neurophysiological mechanisms underlying overlapping syndromes of insomnia and psychiatric illness.

Keywords Major depressive disorder • Bipolar disorder • Generalized anxiety disorder • Panic disorder • Post-traumatic stress disorder • Substance-use disorders • Schizophrenia

Z.L. Cohen, B.A.
The Warren Alpert Medical School of Brown University, Providence, RI, USA

K.M. Sharkey, M.D., Ph.D. (✉)
Sleep for Science Research Laboratory, Division of Pulmonary, Critical Care, and Sleep Medicine, Rhode Island Hospital, Brown University,
300 Duncan Drive, Providence, RI 02906, USA
e-mail: Katherine_Sharkey@brown.edu

© Springer International Publishing Switzerland 2017
H.P. Attarian (ed.), *Clinical Handbook of Insomnia*, Current Clinical Neurology,
DOI 10.1007/978-3-319-41400-3_14

267

Introduction

Over 18 % of US adults experience mental illness annually, with an estimated 4.2 %, or ~10 million, diagnosed with serious mental illness that results in substantial functional impairment [1]. The costs of mental illness are staggering, not only in terms of human suffering, but also in societal burden, including costs of care, lost income, and economic impact of disability. Disturbed sleep can contribute to the onset, persistence, and severity of psychiatric disorders, including increased risk of suicide attempts and death by suicide [2]. In addition to insomnia, other common sleep disorders may contribute to sleep disturbance in patients with mental illness. For instance, many psychiatric medications increase weight gain and thus obstructive sleep apnea should be considered as a source of disturbed sleep in overweight patients taking psychoactive medications that cause weight gain. Similarly, several psychiatric medications (e.g., selective serotonin reuptake inhibitors [SSRIs], lithium, tricyclic antidepressants) have been implicated in restless leg syndrome and periodic limb movement disorder and thus iatrogenic causes of sleep disturbance should not be overlooked in patients taking these medications for psychiatric illness.

Depression

Major depressive disorder (MDD)—defined as a period of at least 2 weeks during which an individual experiences either sad mood or loss of interest or pleasure, and at least four other functional symptoms, i.e., difficulties with sleep, eating, concentration, suicidality, energy, and/or self-esteem—is one of the most prevalent mental disorders, affecting an estimated 6.7 % of the US population each year [1]. Sleep disturbance is a common feature of MDD, and insomnia can precede the onset of other depressive symptoms [3, 4] and persist after other signs of the depressive episode have diminished [5]. Subjective complaints of sleep disturbance occur in 65–75 % of patients with MDD with specific insomnia symptoms, depending on the depression phenotype [6]. For instance, in addition to difficulties with sleep onset and sleep maintenance, patients with MDD with melancholic features experience premature awakenings, i.e., "early-morning insomnia," whereas MDD with atypical features is characterized by excessive daytime sleepiness and hypersomnia. Polysomnographic studies show abnormalities in sleep architecture among individuals with MDD, including prolonged sleep latency, decreased sleep efficiency, shortened REM latency, increased percent REM sleep, increased rapid eye movement density during REM sleep, and decreased slow-wave sleep [6, 7].

Treatment strategies for comorbid insomnia and depression encompass both behavioral and pharmacologic techniques. Cognitive-behavioral therapy for insomnia (CBT-I) is favored by many sources as the most appropriate first-line treatment and has been shown to improve symptoms of insomnia and depression in patients with both disorders [8, 9]. Clinical guidelines recommend tailoring pharmacotherapy based on individual factors including specific insomnia symptom(s), side

Table 14.1 Effects of commonly used antidepressants on sleep

Medication	Sleep continuity	Slow Wave Sleep	REM sleep
SSRIs Example: sertraline	↓	↓/↔	↓
SNRIs Example: venlafaxine	↓	↓/↔	↓
Tricyclics Example: amitriptyline	↑	↑/↔	↓
Mirtazapine	↑	↑	↔
Bupropion	↔	↑/↔	↑
Trazodone	↑	↑	↓

SSRIs selective serotonin reuptake inhibitors, *SNRIs* serotonin and norepinephrine reuptake inhibitors
↑ = increased, ↓ = decreased, ↔ = negligible effect
References: [62–64]

effects, and medication interactions [10]. Thus, clinicians should exert caution when adding sedative-hypnotics to other medications that may be employed for treatment of depression. Table 14.1 shows the effects of commonly used antidepressants on sleep. As shown, some antidepressant medications facilitate sleep, for instance, mirtazapine, trazodone, and amitriptyline. Other pharmacotherapy for depression, however, can disrupt sleep, most notably SSRIs and serotonin and norepinephrine reuptake inhibitors (SNRIs). Little is known about acute versus chronic effects of antidepressants on sleep measures.

Regardless of what treatment is utilized, it is critical to address symptoms of insomnia in patients with concomitant MDD because of evidence that depressed patients with concomitant insomnia have more severe and persistent disease, increased suicidality, and higher rates of relapse. Furthermore, it is crucial to ensure that patients with MDD who report insomnia are not suffering from an occult sleep disorder, as sleep disorders such as obstructive sleep apnea have been observed to be more prevalent among patients with MDD and insomnia compared with the general population [11].

Bipolar Disorder

Bipolar disorder is a mood disorder with a lifetime prevalence of 0.5–1 % that is associated with significant morbidity and mortality and is characterized by episodes of mania lasting 1 week or more. During manic episodes, individuals with bipolar disorder experience an abnormally elevated, expansive, or irritable mood in conjunction with increased energy/activity levels and at least three other behavioral symptoms such as grandiosity, pressured speech, decreased attention span, increased goal-directed or risk-taking behavior, and/or decreased need for sleep. In addition to manic episodes, patients with bipolar illness also experience depressive episodes (similar in character to MDD episodes) and inter-episodic periods of relative euthymia. The decreased

Table 14.2 Effects of medications FDA approved for bipolar disorder on sleep

Medication	Sleep continuity	Slow Wave Sleep	REM sleep
Lithium [65, 66]	↔	↑	↓
Divalproex [67, 68]	↔	↔	↔
Lamotrigine [69]	↔	↓	↑
Olanzapine [70–72]	↑	↑*	↑*
Risperidone [72, 73]	↔/↑	↔	↓
Quetiapine [74, 75]	↑	↔/↓	↓
Lurasidone [76]	↑^	↑^	↓^
Ziprasidone [77, 78]	↑	↑	↓/↔
Aripiprazole	No data	No data	No data
Carbamazepine [79, 80]	↑/↔	↑/↔	↔
Asenapine	No data	No data	No data

* = a sex difference with women affected more than men has been reported
^ = in rats
↑ = increased, ↓ = decreased, ↔ = negligible effect

sleep need during the manic phase of bipolar illness is characterized by short sleep times, but few complaints of difficulty falling or staying asleep. Thus, despite short sleep duration, patients in a manic episode do not subjectively report insomnia, but rather report that their sleep needs are fulfilled with little or no sleep. The few studies that examined sleep during mania using polysomnography have shown longer sleep-onset latency, poorer sleep efficiency, and reduced sleep period time compared to normal controls [12], as well as increased percentage of stage 1 sleep, shortened REM latency, and increased REM density, similar to patients with MDD [13].

During inter-episodic periods, about 70 % of patients with bipolar disorder report insomnia [14]. In contrast, during the depressive phase, the most commonly reported sleep complaint is hypersomnia, estimated to occur in 40–80 % of patients [15]. Thus, sleep disturbance occurs across the entire spectrum of bipolar mood states and ranges from decreased need for sleep to difficulty initiating and maintaining sleep, to complaints of excessive sleepiness and sleeping too long. Indeed, one cohort study of more than 2000 patients with bipolar disorder demonstrated variability in sleep duration across 1 week of more than 2 h and 45 min [16]. Given these data, it is not surprising that behavioral therapies aimed at stabilizing sleep and circadian rhythms and improving sleep duration and regularity have been adopted [17]. Table 14.2 shows sleep effects of medications such as mood stabilizers and antipsychotics that are used to treat BPD.

Anxiety Disorders

Anxiety disorders are the most prevalent psychiatric illnesses with over 18 % of US adults affected by anxiety disorders on an annual basis [18]. Anxiety disorders affect women more than men and onset tends to occur in the teens and young adulthood. Sleep difficulties are common among those with anxiety disorders and insomnia is one criterion for diagnosing generalized anxiety disorder. Likewise, individuals with insomnia frequently report anxiety and psychological distress, including apprehension about going to sleep and rumination while attempting to fall asleep. Despite the high prevalence of anxiety disorders and the frequency with which sleep disturbance is encountered in patients with anxiety, polysomnographic (PSG) studies of anxiety disorders are scant. In general, however, patients with anxiety disorders have decreased sleep efficiency and shortened total sleep time when studied with PSG.

Generalized Anxiety Disorder

Patients with generalized anxiety disorder (GAD) experience chronic and persistent worrying that interferes with their day-to-day functioning. Insomnia is one of six functional symptoms of GAD [19], and at least half of the other defining symptoms (i.e., fatigue, irritability, trouble concentrating) may be related to shortened and disrupted sleep. The majority of patients with GAD report at least one symptom of insomnia. Sleep maintenance issues are the most common—reported by more than 60%—followed by early-morning awakenings, and difficulty with sleep initiation, both reported by about 50% of GAD patients.

Polysomnographic recordings of patients with GAD corroborate patients' subjective reports of insomnia. Compared to controls, PSG in patients with GAD show increased sleep latency, decreased sleep efficiency, increased stage N1 and N2 sleep, decreased slow-wave sleep, and decreased REM sleep [20]. Interestingly, the sleep-related clinical presentation of GAD is similar to that of psychophysiologic insomnia. Thus, when a patient's anxiety is focused almost exclusively on poor sleep and its effects on daytime functioning, psychophysiologic insomnia is the most appropriate diagnosis, whereas GAD is a more appropriate diagnosis when anxiety is global and permeates most aspects of functioning.

Cognitive/behavioral therapy is employed frequently to treat GAD, and modules specifically designed to address insomnia (i.e., CBT-I components such as sleep restriction, stimulus control) articulate well with the overall goals of CBT for GAD. Benzodiazepines such as alprazolam, lorazepam, and clonazepam are utilized for pharmacologic management of GAD. This drug class tends to increase sleep continuity and stage N2 sleep, and decrease REM sleep. SSRI, SNRI, and tricyclic antidepressants are also used to treat GAD.

Panic Disorder

Panic disorder is characterized by the abrupt, unexpected onset of attacks of intense fear/discomfort accompanied by at least four physical symptoms, such as dizziness, choking, palpitations, trembling, chest pain, sweating, or fear of dying. An estimated 2.7% of US adults have panic disorder and women are twice as likely as men to be affected. Social withdrawal and avoidance of usual activities—sometimes progressing to agoraphobia—are some of the most debilitating consequences of panic disorder, and a high percentage of patients with panic disorder also suffer from comorbid major depressive disorder.

Between 70 and 90% of patients with panic disorder are estimated to also experience insomnia. Polysomnographic studies in patients with panic disorder show prolonged sleep latency, reduced sleep efficiency, and decreased percentage of slow wave–sleep compared to healthy controls [21, 22]. About 30% of panic disorder patients report recurrent panic attacks associated with sudden awakening from sleep. Nocturnal panic attacks typically emerge from N2 or N3 sleep, with palpitations, dyspnea, and flushing reported as the most frequent symptoms. Since obstructive sleep apnea (OSA) is common in the general population and may be associated with symptoms that are similar to a panic attack, patients that awaken from sleep with panic may need evaluation for OSA, particularly if they also report snoring, daytime sleepiness, or other symptoms of sleep-disordered breathing. Nocturnal panic should be distinguished from night terrors, which are usually followed by no recollection of the nocturnal event and are not associated with daytime panic symptoms.

As with generalized anxiety disorder, the mainstays of treatment for panic disorder are psychotherapy and/or pharmacologic approaches that include benzodiazepines and antidepressants.

Posttraumatic Stress Disorder

Posttraumatic stress disorder (PTSD) follows an event where an individual is subject to or a witness of a terrifying experience involving physical harm or threat of physical harm. The lifetime prevalence of PTSD is estimated at 7–8% of the US population, with women more likely to develop PTSD than men. PTSD causes symptoms in three domains: re-experiencing of the trauma (e.g., flashbacks, frightening thoughts, and nightmares), hyperarousal (including insomnia, easy startle, and feeling irritable or "on edge"), and avoidance (emotional numbness, difficulty remembering the trauma, and loss of interest in previously pleasurable activities).

Two of the cardinal diagnostic criteria for PTSD—insomnia and nightmares—directly affect sleep quality and quantity. Indeed, in a Canadian survey of approximately 1800 community-dwelling adults, ~70% of those with PTSD reported sleep disturbances. The most commonly reported symptom was sleep maintenence insomnia (endorsed by 46.6%) followed by early-morning awakenings (reported by 42.9%) and difficulty initiating sleep (reported by 41.2%) [23]. Several studies suggest that individuals who experienced insomnia prior to their exposure to a traumatic event are more likely to develop PTSD [23–26].

Polysomnographic studies of patients with PTSD show inconsistent findings, including differences between PTSD patients and healthy controls in both REM and NREM sleep. A meta-analysis that examined 20 studies including nearly 800 patients with PTSD showed increased N1 percent, increased REM density, and decreased slow-wave sleep compared to control participants [27]. Research investigating the neurobiology of associations between PTSD and disturbed sleep implicates increased amygdala activity and impaired functioning of the medial prefrontal cortex in abnormal sleep regulation in PTSD patients [28].

Patients with PTSD and sleep complaints may benefit from behavioral and pharmacologic treatments. For instance, patients with PTSD and nightmares show decreased nightmares and improvements in other insomnia symptoms from the alpha-antagonist, prazosin, and image rehearsal therapy (IRT), a modality that employs cognitive and behavioral strategies to alter distressing dream content. Evidence also supports the use of CBT-I, as well as mirtazapine, tricyclic antidepressants, and nefazodone for treatment of insomnia in PTSD patients [29].

Obsessive Compulsive Disorder

Obsessive-compulsive disorder (OCD) is characterized by recurrent intrusive thoughts (obsessions) and/or repetitive behaviors (compulsions) that cause anxiety and impair daytime functioning. OCD affects approximately 1 % of the population and up to 50 % of patients are classified as severe or are refractory to treatment. Although sleep difficulties are not part of the diagnostic criteria for OCD, differences in sleep have been observed between patients with OCD and healthy comparison groups. Furthermore, cognitive domains that show impairment in OCD (i.e., response inhibition, cognitive processing) are affected by sleep disturbance, raising the possibility that improving sleep may also diminish OCD symptoms [30].

Compared to healthy controls, patients with OCD have prolonged sleep latency, decreased total sleep time, and increased wake after sleep onset [31, 32]. Polysomnographic studies also have shown decreased REM latency and increased REM density in OCD patients, similar to the sleep of patients with major depression. It has been suggested that the sleep disturbances observed among OCD patients are a result of comorbid depression, rather than OCD [33], but other studies have refuted this claim [34]. Furthermore, patients with OCD also exhibit delayed sleep–wake-phase disorder (DSPD) more commonly than healthy controls or patients with MDD [30, 35, 36]. Although there are no extensive trials of interventions for sleep disturbances in patients with OCD, at least one case report has shown improvement of OCD symptoms and DSPD with chronotherapy techniques [37].

Attention-Deficit Hyperactivity Disorder

Attention-deficit hyperactivity disorder (ADHD) affects an estimated 9 % of US adolescents and 4 % of US adults, and is diagnosed more commonly in males than females. ADHD is characterized by inattention, impulsivity, and increased motor activity, and the neurobiological correlates of these clinical features, e.g., the dorsolateral and ventrolateral prefrontal cortex and the dorsal anterior cingulate cortex, are also negatively affected by insufficient sleep [38]. Epidemiologic studies show that patients with ADHD have increased reports of insomnia and delayed sleep–wake-phase disorder [39], though it is not clear whether these associations reflect the underlying ADHD or represent side effects of stimulants commonly used to treat ADHD. Given the daytime impairment associated with ADHD and insufficient sleep, it is imperative that ADHD patients with comorbid insomnia be assessed for adequate sleep quality and quantity.

Schizophrenia and Psychotic Disorders

Schizophrenia is a severe psychotic illness that affects about 1 % of adults. Although sleep disturbance is reported commonly by patients with schizophrenia, the estimated prevalence of insomnia among schizophrenic patients is variable, with estimates ranging between 16 and 87 % [40]. In one study of outpatients diagnosed with schizophrenia or schizoaffective disorders, 44 % met the criteria for insomnia [41]. Common features of insomnia in medicated and medication-naïve schizophrenic patients include prolonged sleep latency, decreased sleep efficiency, poor subjective sleep quality, shorter total sleep time, and disrupted circadian rhythmicity [40]. Polysomnographic studies of patients with schizophrenia show decreased sleep spindle activity compared to healthy controls [42]. Sleep disturbances in schizophrenia are linked more closely with "positive" symptoms such as hallucinations, delusions, and disorganized thought processes, whereas negative symptoms like social withdrawal, anhedonia, and poor self-care are not as strongly correlated with insomnia [40]. Furthermore, several studies have found that poor sleep quality has a negative effect on quality of life in patients with schizophrenia.

Although antipsychotic medications are sedating, many patients treated chronically with antipsychotic medications continue to experience insomnia symptoms. For instance, one survey of 101 patients with schizophrenia showed that insomnia symptoms persisted even with treatment with benzodiazepine receptor agonists in about 40 % of patients [43], though other work suggests that the BDZ agonist zopiclone is more effective than benzodiazepines in this population [44]. Two studies tested melatonin at doses between 2 and 12 mg to treat insomnia in patients with schizophrenia: one study showed an increase in objective sleep efficiency [45] and the second showed improvements in self-reported sleep quality and sleep fragmentation [46]. Daytime sedation from use of hypnotics is a concern in this population given the sedation caused by antipsychotic medications and the prevalence of negative symptoms. Few studies have examined whether treating insomnia in patients with psychotic disorders improves the psychotic symptoms. An exception is an open trial of cognitive-behavioral treatment for insomnia in patients with delusions, which showed that CBT-I improved sleep and psychotic symptoms [47].

Substance-Use Disorders

An estimated 10% of US adults have some form of drug-use disorder during their lifetime. The prevalence of sleep disturbance in patients with substance abuse is high with 80–90% of opioid-dependent patients [48] and 50–60% of alcohol-dependent patients reporting sleep difficulties [49]. Links between substance-use disorders and insomnia vary depending on the substance, whether use is acute or chronic, and whether the individual is using the substance actively or is withdrawing from its use. In general, chronic use of substances is associated with more sleep disturbance, including increased sleep-onset latency and less total sleep time.

There is likely a mixed etiology of sleep difficulties among substance-dependent patients, including neurochemical effects of the specific substance, concomitant drug use, other comorbid psychiatric disorders, and behaviors adopted to sustain drug use. For example, the prolonged sleep latency associated with chronic drug use and/or withdrawal may lead to later bedtimes, which can result in more night-time light exposure that could delay endogenous circadian phase and further exacerbate sleep-onset insomnia [49]. Insomnia and substance-use disorders are frequently intertwined, such that sleep difficulties may lead to the initiation of substance use, substance use may disturb sleep directly, and substance withdrawal may result in insomnia, which, in turn, may promote escalation of substance abuse or relapse [50].

Alcohol

Between 50 and 60% of patients with alcohol-use disorders (AUDs) report difficulty falling and/or staying asleep [49]. Although the etiology of insomnia in AUD patients is likely multifactorial and variable, proposed mechanisms include concomitant mood disorders, genetic risk, and underlying dysfunction in sleep and circadian regulatory mechanisms [49]. A large body of research suggests that insomnia can precipitate and perpetuate alcohol-use disorders, as well as increase the risk of relapse, with prolonged latency to sleep onset emerging as the strongest predictor of resuming alcohol use [49].

Polysomnographic (PSG) studies reveal that acute alcohol ingestion reduces the amount of wakefulness during the first 3–4 h of sleep, but increases wakefulness during the second half of the night. Alcohol withdrawal results in disrupted sleep, including increased N1 sleep, decreased slow-wave sleep, shortened REM latency, and increased REM sleep percent [49]. Sleep architecture abnormalities have been shown to persist for over 2 years in patients with AUDs, despite cessation of alcohol use [51].

Treatment for insomnia in patients with AUDs consists of addressing the underlying AUD and utilization of behavioral and pharmacologic treatments. Many patients with AUDs will require adjunct therapy because of persistence of symptoms despite abstinence. CBT-I and progressive relaxation have both been shown to improve insomnia in patients with AUDs, but have not shown parallel decreases in drinking. Evidence supports the use of topiramate [52] and gabapentin [53, 54] both to improve sleep disturbance and decrease alcohol use in patients with AUDs and insomnia. Trazodone, on the other hand, has been shown to improve insomnia but increase alcohol use [55].

Marijuana

Acute effects of marijuana span a wide range from euphoria and behavioral activation to drowsiness and relaxation. Subjective experience of marijuana's effects on sleep reflects this breadth, with marked individual differences reported, though in general a reduction in sleep latency is described most frequently. PSG studies of the effects of marijuana on sleep also have conflicting results; overall the most consistent finding is a decrease in REM sleep and REM density in individuals who have used marijuana before sleep [56]. Heavy marijuana users often report sleep difficulties when they are trying to quit marijuana, and there are clinical trials under way to determine whether adjunctive pharmacologic or behavioral treatments for insomnia can help marijuana users stop more easily.

Opiates

Subjective sleep disturbance is reported by 75–84% of opiate-dependent patients in methadone maintenance treatment [48, 57]. Symptoms of depression and anxiety, greater nicotine dependence, benzodiazepine use, bodily pain, and unemployment are associated with increased subjective sleep complaints. Opioids alter cholinergic, adenosinergic, and GABAergic neurotransmission and can therefore cause sleep disturbance through several different mechanisms. Polysomnographic studies show decreased REM and slow-wave sleep with opioid use [58]. In addition, central sleep apnea is observed in about 30% of chronic opioid users [58]. Although several studies have investigated whether concurrent insomnia treatment can decrease opioid use, no definitive treatment has been shown to address sleep disturbance in this population.

Nicotine

Nicotine is a stimulant that acts at acetylcholine receptors and is typically used by smoking tobacco. An estimated 21% of US adults smoke cigarettes. Acute use of nicotine results in decreased subjective sleep quality, prolonged sleep latency, and reduced sleep efficiency [59]. In chronic smokers withdrawing from nicotine, poly-somnographic studies show an increase in arousal index and wake time [60]. Relapse of tobacco use is associated with more subjective sleep complaints during withdrawal, less REM sleep, and longer REM latency [60].

Caffeine

Caffeine is an adenosine antagonist stimulant that is typically consumed in coffee and tea. Use of caffeine produces subjective reports of sleep disturbance the night following ingestion. PSG changes with caffeine include prolonged sleep latency, decreased total sleep time, decreased REM sleep, and decreased slow-wave sleep [61]. Excessive caffeine use is a frequent contributor to clinical complaints of insomnia.

Stimulants

An estimated 1.7 million Americans abuse or are dependent on cocaine. Serious medical and psychiatric complications result from cocaine and stimulant abuse, including disturbed sleep and insomnia. Acute effects of cocaine include prolonged sleep latency, decreased total sleep time, and REM suppression [56]. In cocaine withdrawal, polysomnography has documented increased sleep latency, decreased total sleep time, and REM rebound with shorter REM latency and increased percent REM sleep [56]. Stimulants (e.g., amphetamines and methylphenidate) are used therapeutically in the treatment of narcolepsy, attention-deficit hyperactivity disorder, and depression. Patients using prescribed stimulants require careful clinical monitoring to ensure that they are not experiencing insomnia as a side effect and to decrease the risk of stimulant abuse.

Conclusion

Insomnia is frequently comorbid with psychiatric illness and data indicate that in many disorders, treating insomnia can not only improve patients' disturbed sleep but can also lead to amelioration of the underlying mental illness. Treatment of insomnia with behavioral treatments and pharmacologic therapies should be tailored to the specific disorder. Other sleep disorders that may be contributing to disturbed sleep in patients with psychiatric disease should not be overlooked. Research that utilizes careful phenotyping of the types of sleep disturbance encountered across psychiatric diagnoses may further our understanding of underlying mechanisms of mental illness and its links to insomnia.

References

1. Substance Abuse and Mental Health Services Administration. Results from the 2013 National Survey on Drug Use and Health: Mental Health Findings. Rockville, MD: Substance Abuse and Mental Health Services Administration; 2014. Contract No.: HHS Publication No. (SMA) 14–4887.
2. Bernert RA, Nadorff MR. Sleep disturbances and suicide risk. Sleep Med Clin. 2015;10(1):35–9. Epub 2015/06/10.
3. Ford DE, Kamerow DB. Epidemiologic study of sleep disturbances and psychiatric disorders. An opportunity for prevention? JAMA. 1989;262(11):1479–84. Epub 1989/09/15.
4. Breslau N, Roth T, Rosenthal L, Andreski P. Sleep disturbance and psychiatric disorders: a longitudinal epidemiological study of young adults. Biol Psychiatry. 1996;39(6):411–8. Epub 1996/03/15.
5. Perlis ML, Giles DE, Buysse DJ, Tu X, Kupfer DJ. Self-reported sleep disturbance as a prodromal symptom in recurrent depression. J Affect Disord. 1997;42(2–3):209–12. Epub 1997/02/01.
6. Peterson MJ, Benca RM. Sleep in mood disorders. Sleep Med Clin. 2008;3(2):231–49.
7. Benca RM, Obermeyer WH, Thisted RA, Gillin JC. Sleep and psychiatric disorders. A meta-analysis. Arch Gen Psychiatry. 1992;49(8):651–68. discussion 69–70. Epub 1992/08/01.
8. Manber R, Edinger JD, Gress JL, San Pedro-Salcedo MG, Kuo TF, Kalista T. Cognitive behavioral therapy for insomnia enhances depression outcome in patients with comorbid major depressive disorder and insomnia. Sleep. 2008;31(4):489–95. Epub 2008/05/07.
9. Ashworth DK, Sletten TL, Junge M, Simpson K, Clarke D, Cunnington D, et al. A randomized controlled trial of cognitive behavioral therapy for insomnia: an effective treatment for comorbid insomnia and depression. J Couns Psychol. 2015;62(2):115–23. Epub 2015/04/14.
10. Schutte-Rodin S, Broch L, Buysse D, Dorsey C, Sateia M. Clinical guideline for the evaluation and management of chronic insomnia in adults. J Clin Sleep Med. 2008;4(5):487–504. Epub 2008/10/16.
11. Ong JC, Gress JL, San Pedro-Salcedo MG, Manber R. Frequency and predictors of obstructive sleep apnea among individuals with major depressive disorder and insomnia. J Psychosom Res. 2009;67(2):135–41. Epub 2009/07/21.
12. Linkowski P, Kerkhofs M, Rielaert C, Mendlewicz J. Sleep during mania in manic-depressive males. Eur Arch Psychiatry Neurol Sci. 1986;235(6):339–41. Epub 1986/01/01.
13. Hudson JI, Lipinski JF, Keck Jr PE, Aizley HG, Lukas SE, Rothschild AJ, et al. Polysomnographic characteristics of young manic patients. Comparison with unipolar depressed patients and normal control subjects. Arch Gen Psychiatry. 1992;49(5):378–83. Epub 1992/05/11.
14. Harvey AG, Schmidt DA, Scarna A, Semler CN, Goodwin GM. Sleep-related functioning in euthymic patients with bipolar disorder, patients with insomnia, and subjects without sleep problems. Am J Psychiatry. 2005;162(1):50–7. Epub 2004/12/31.
15. Kaplan KA, Gruber J, Eidelman P, Talbot LS, Harvey AG. Hypersomnia in inter-episode bipolar disorder: does it have prognostic significance? J Affect Disord. 2011;132(3):438–44. Epub 2011/04/15.
16. Gruber J, Harvey AG, Wang PW, Brooks 3rd JO, Thase ME, Sachs GS, et al. Sleep functioning in relation to mood, function, and quality of life at entry to the Systematic Treatment Enhancement Program for Bipolar Disorder (STEP-BD). J Affect Disord. 2009;114(1–3):41–9. Epub 2008/08/19.
17. Kaplan KA, Harvey AG. Behavioral treatment of insomnia in bipolar disorder. Am J Psychiatry. 2013;170(7):716–20. Epub 2013/07/04.
18. Kessler RC, Chiu WT, Demler O, Merikangas KR, Walters EE. Prevalence, severity, and comorbidity of 12-month DSM-IV disorders in the National Comorbidity Survey Replication. Arch Gen Psychiatry. 2005;62(6):617–27. Epub 2005/06/09.
19. American Psychiatric Association. Diagnostic and statistical manual of mental disorders. 5th ed. Arlington, VA: American Psychiatric Publishing; 2013.

20. Monti JM, Monti D. Sleep disturbance in generalized anxiety disorder and its treatment. Sleep Med Rev. 2000;4(3):263–76. Epub 2003/01/18.
21. Lepola U, Koponen H, Leinonen E. Sleep in panic disorders. J Psychosom Res. 1994;38 Suppl 1:105–11. Epub 1994/01/01.
22. Arriaga F, Paiva T, Matos-Pires A, Cavaglia F, Lara E, Bastos L. The sleep of non-depressed patients with panic disorder: a comparison with normal controls. Acta Psychiatr Scand. 1996;93(3):191–4. Epub 1996/03/01.
23. Ohayon MM, Shapiro CM. Sleep disturbances and psychiatric disorders associated with post-traumatic stress disorder in the general population. Compr Psychiatry. 2000;41(6):469–78. Epub 2000/11/22.
24. Harvey AG, Bryant RA. The relationship between acute stress disorder and posttraumatic stress disorder: a prospective evaluation of motor vehicle accident survivors. J Consult Clin Psychol. 1998;66(3):507–12. Epub 1998/06/27.
25. Koren D, Arnon I, Lavie P, Klein E. Sleep complaints as early predictors of posttraumatic stress disorder: a 1-year prospective study of injured survivors of motor vehicle accidents. Am J Psychiatry. 2002;159(5):855–7. Epub 2002/05/03.
26. Mellman TA, Pigeon WR, Nowell PD, Nolan B. Relationships between REM sleep findings and PTSD symptoms during the early aftermath of trauma. J Trauma Stress. 2007;20(5):893–901. Epub 2007/10/24.
27. Kobayashi I, Boarts JM, Delahanty DL. Polysomnographically measured sleep abnormalities in PTSD: a meta-analytic review. Psychophysiology. 2007;44(4):660–9. Epub 2007/05/25.
28. Germain A, Buysse DJ, Nofzinger E. Sleep-specific mechanisms underlying posttraumatic stress disorder: integrative review and neurobiological hypotheses. Sleep Med Rev. 2008;12(3):185–95. Epub 2007/11/13.
29. Pigeon WR, Gallegos AM. Posttraumatic stress disorder and sleep. Sleep Med Clin. 2015;10(1):41–8. Epub 2015/06/10.
30. Nota JA, Sharkey KM, Coles ME. Sleep, arousal, and circadian rhythms in adults with obsessive-compulsive disorder: a meta-analysis. Neurosci Biobehav Rev. 2015;51:100–7. Epub 2015/01/21.
31. Insel TR, Gillin JC, Moore A, Mendelson WB, Loewenstein RJ, Murphy DL. The sleep of patients with obsessive-compulsive disorder. Arch Gen Psychiatry. 1982;39(12):1372–7. Epub 1982/12/01.
32. Kluge M, Schussler P, Dresler M, Yassouridis A, Steiger A. Sleep onset REM periods in obsessive compulsive disorder. Psychiatry Res. 2007;152(1):29–35. Epub 2007/02/24.
33. Bobdey M, Fineberg N, Gale TM, Patel A, Davies HA. Reported sleep patterns in obsessive compulsive disorder (OCD). Int J Psychiatry Clin Pract. 2002;6(1):15–21. Epub 2002/01/01.
34. Voderholzer U, Riemann D, Huwig-Poppe C, Kuelz AK, Kordon A, Bruestle K, et al. Sleep in obsessive compulsive disorder: polysomnographic studies under baseline conditions and after experimentally induced serotonin deficiency. Eur Arch Psychiatry Clin Neurosci. 2007;257(3):173–82. Epub 2006/12/07.
35. Mukhopadhyay S, Fineberg NA, Drummond LM, Turner J, White S, Wulff K, et al. Delayed sleep phase in severe obsessive-compulsive disorder: a systematic case-report survey. CNS Spectr. 2008;13(5):406–13. Epub 2008/05/23.
36. Turner J, Drummond LM, Mukhopadhyay S, Ghodse H, White S, Pillay A, et al. A prospective study of delayed sleep phase syndrome in patients with severe resistant obsessive-compulsive disorder. World Psychiatry. 2007;6(2):108–11. Epub 2008/02/01.
37. Coles ME, Sharkey KM. Compulsion or chronobiology? A case of severe obsessive-compulsive disorder treated with cognitive-behavioral therapy augmented with chronotherapy. J Clin Sleep Med. 2011;7(3):307–9. Epub 2011/06/17.
38. Cortese S, Brown TE, Corkum P, Gruber R, O'Brien LM, Stein M, et al. Assessment and management of sleep problems in youths with attention-deficit/hyperactivity disorder. J Am Acad Child Adolesc Psychiatry. 2013;52(8):784–96. Epub 2013/07/25.
39. Hysing M, Lundervold AJ, Posserud MB, Sivertsen B. Association between sleep problems and symptoms of attention deficit hyperactivity disorder in adolescence: results from a large population-based study. Behav Sleep Med. 2015:1–15. Epub 2015/10/28.

40. Soehner AM, Kaplan KA, Harvey AG. Insomnia comorbid to severe psychiatric illness. Sleep Med Clin. 2013;8(3):361–71. Epub 2014/10/11.
41. Palmese LB, DeGeorge PC, Ratliff JC, Srihari VH, Wexler BE, Krystal AD, et al. Insomnia is frequent in schizophrenia and associated with night eating and obesity. Schizophr Res. 2011;133(1–3):238–43. Epub 2011/08/23.
42. Ferrarelli F, Huber R, Peterson MJ, Massimini M, Murphy M, Riedner BA, et al. Reduced sleep spindle activity in schizophrenia patients. Am J Psychiatry. 2007;164(3):483–92. Epub 2007/03/03.
43. Haffmans PM, Hoencamp E, Knegtering HJ, van Heycop ten Ham BF. Sleep disturbance in schizophrenia. Br J Psychiatry. 1994;165(5):697–8. Epub 1994/11/01.
44. Kajimura N, Kato M, Okuma T, Sekimoto M, Watanabe T, Takahashi K. A quantitative sleep-EEG study on the effects of benzodiazepine and zopiclone in schizophrenic patients. Schizophr Res. 1995;15(3):303–12. Epub 1995/05/01.
45. Shamir E, Laudon M, Barak Y, Anis Y, Rotenberg V, Elizur A, et al. Melatonin improves sleep quality of patients with chronic schizophrenia. J Clin Psychiatry. 2000;61(5):373–7. Epub 2000/06/10.
46. Suresh Kumar PN, Andrade C, Bhakta SG, Singh NM. Melatonin in schizophrenic outpatients with insomnia: a double-blind, placebo-controlled study. J Clin Psychiatry. 2007;68(2):237–41. Epub 2007/03/06.
47. Freeman D, Startup H, Myers E, Harvey A, Geddes J, Yu LM, et al. The effects of using cognitive behavioural therapy to improve sleep for patients with delusions and hallucinations (the BEST study): study protocol for a randomized controlled trial. Trials. 2013;14:214. Epub 2013/07/13.
48. Stein MD, Herman DS, Bishop S, Lassor JA, Weinstock M, Anthony J, et al. Sleep disturbances among methadone maintained patients. J Subst Abus Treat. 2004;26(3):175–80. Epub 2004/04/06.
49. Brower KJ. Assessment and treatment of insomnia in adult patients with alcohol use disorders. Alcohol. 2015;49(4):417–27. Epub 2015/05/11.
50. Roth T. Does effective management of sleep disorders reduce substance dependence? Drugs. 2009;69 Suppl 2:65–75. Epub 2010/02/06.
51. Drummond SP, Gillin JC, Smith TL, DeModena A. The sleep of abstinent pure primary alcoholic patients: natural course and relationship to relapse. Alcohol Clin Exp Res. 1998;22(8):1796–802. Epub 1998/12/03.
52. Johnson BA, Rosenthal N, Capece JA, Wiegand F, Mao L, Beyers K, et al. Improvement of physical health and quality of life of alcohol-dependent individuals with topiramate treatment: US multisite randomized controlled trial. Arch Intern Med. 2008;168(11):1188–99. Epub 2008/06/11.
53. Anton RF, Myrick H, Wright TM, Latham PK, Baros AM, Waid LR, et al. Gabapentin combined with naltrexone for the treatment of alcohol dependence. Am J Psychiatry. 2011;168(7):709–17. Epub 2011/04/02.
54. Mason BJ, Quello S, Goodell V, Shadan F, Kyle M, Begovic A. Gabapentin treatment for alcohol dependence: a randomized clinical trial. JAMA Intern Med. 2014;174(1):70–7. Epub 2013/11/06.
55. Friedmann PD, Rose JS, Swift R, Stout RL, Millman RP, Stein MD. Trazodone for sleep disturbance after alcohol detoxification: a double-blind, placebo-controlled trial. Alcohol Clin Exp Res. 2008;32(9):1652–60. Epub 2008/07/12.
56. Schierenbeck T, Riemann D, Berger M, Hornyak M. Effect of illicit recreational drugs upon sleep: cocaine, ecstasy and marijuana. Sleep Med Rev. 2008;12(5):381–9. Epub 2008/03/04.
57. Peles E, Schreiber S, Adelson M. Variables associated with perceived sleep disorders in methadone maintenance treatment (MMT) patients. Drug Alcohol Depend. 2006;82(2):103–10. Epub 2005/09/13.
58. Wang D, Teichtahl H. Opioids, sleep architecture and sleep-disordered breathing. Sleep Med Rev. 2007;11(1):35–46. Epub 2006/12/05.
59. Jaehne A, Unbehaun T, Feige B, Herr S, Appel A, Riemann D. The influence of 8 and 16 mg nicotine patches on sleep in healthy non-smokers. Pharmacopsychiatry. 2015;48(7):291. Epub 2015/10/09.

60. Jaehne A, Unbehaun T, Feige B, Cohrs S, Rodenbeck A, Riemann D. Sleep changes in smokers before, during and 3 months after nicotine withdrawal. Addict Biol. 2015;20(4):747–55. Epub 2014/05/07.
61. Roehrs T, Roth T. Caffeine: sleep and daytime sleepiness. Sleep Med Rev. 2008;12(2):153–62. Epub 2007/10/24.
62. Winokur A, Gary KA, Rodner S, Rae-Red C, Fernando AT, Szuba MP. Depression, sleep physiology, and antidepressant drugs. Depress Anxiety. 2001;14(1):19–28. Epub 2001/09/25.
63. Mayers AG, Baldwin DS. Antidepressants and their effect on sleep. Hum Psychopharmacol. 2005;20(8):533–59. Epub 2005/10/18.
64. Krystal AD. Psychiatric disorders and sleep. Neurol Clin. 2012;30(4):1389–413. Epub 2012/10/27.
65. Kupfer DJ, Reynolds 3rd CF, Weiss BL, Foster FG. Lithium carbonate and sleep in affective disorders. Further considerations. Arch Gen Psychiatry. 1974;30(1):79–84. Epub 1974/01/01.
66. Hudson JI, Lipinski JF, Frankenburg FR, Tohen M, Kupfer DJ. Effects of lithium on sleep in mania. Biol Psychiatry. 1989;25(5):665–8. Epub 1989/03/01.
67. Placidi F, Scalise A, Marciani MG, Romigi A, Diomedi M, Gigli GL. Effect of antiepileptic drugs on sleep. Clin Neurophysiol. 2000;111 Suppl 2:S115–9. Epub 2000/09/21.
68. Bazil CW. Effects of antiepileptic drugs on sleep structure: are all drugs equal? CNS Drugs. 2003;17(10):719–28. Epub 2003/07/23.
69. Placidi F, Marciani MG, Diomedi M, Scalise A, Pauri F, Giacomini P, et al. Effects of lamotrigine on nocturnal sleep, daytime somnolence and cognitive functions in focal epilepsy. Acta Neurol Scand. 2000;102(2):81–6. Epub 2000/08/19.
70. Lindberg N, Virkkunen M, Tani P, Appelberg B, Virkkala J, Rimon R, et al. Effect of a single-dose of olanzapine on sleep in healthy females and males. Int Clin Psychopharmacol. 2002;17(4):177–84. Epub 2002/07/20.
71. Gimenez S, Romero S, Gich I, Clos S, Grasa E, Antonijoan RM, et al. Sex differences in sleep after a single oral morning dose of olanzapine in healthy volunteers. Hum Psychopharmacol. 2011;26(7):498–507. Epub 2011/09/29.
72. Gimenez S, Clos S, Romero S, Grasa E, Morte A, Barbanoj MJ. Effects of olanzapine, risperidone and haloperidol on sleep after a single oral morning dose in healthy volunteers. Psychopharmacology. 2007;190(4):507–16. Epub 2007/01/06.
73. Sharpley AL, Bhagwagar Z, Hafizi S, Whale WR, Gijsman HJ, Cowen PJ. Risperidone augmentation decreases rapid eye movement sleep and decreases wake in treatment-resistant depressed patients. J Clin Psychiatry. 2003;64(2):192–6. Epub 2003/03/14.
74. Cohrs S, Rodenbeck A, Guan Z, Pohlmann K, Jordan W, Meier A, et al. Sleep-promoting properties of quetiapine in healthy subjects. Psychopharmacology. 2004;174(3):421–9. Epub 2004/03/19.
75. Keshavan MS, Prasad KM, Montrose DM, Miewald JM, Kupfer DJ. Sleep quality and architecture in quetiapine, risperidone, or never-treated schizophrenia patients. J Clin Psychopharmacol. 2007;27(6):703–5. Epub 2007/11/16.
76. Murai T, Nakamichi K, Shimizu I, Ikeda K. Lurasidone suppresses rapid eye movement sleep and improves sleep quality in rats. J Pharmacol Sci. 2014;126(2):164–7. Epub 2014/09/19.
77. Baskaran A, Summers D, Willing SL, Jokic R, Milev R. Sleep architecture in ziprasidone-treated bipolar depression: a pilot study. Ther Adv Psychopharmacol. 2013;3(3):139–49. Epub 2013/10/30.
78. Cohrs S, Meier A, Neumann AC, Jordan W, Ruther E, Rodenbeck A. Improved sleep continuity and increased slow wave sleep and REM latency during ziprasidone treatment: a randomized, controlled, crossover trial of 12 healthy male subjects. J Clin Psychiatry. 2005;66(8):989–96. Epub 2005/08/10.
79. Legros B, Bazil CW. Effects of antiepileptic drugs on sleep architecture: a pilot study. Sleep Med. 2003;4(1):51–5. Epub 2003/11/01.
80. Gann H, Riemann D, Hohagen F, Muller WE, Berger M. The influence of carbamazepine on sleep-EEG and the clonidine test in healthy subjects: results of a preliminary study. Biol Psychiatry. 1994;35(11):893–6. Epub 1994/06/01.

Index

A

Absenteeism, 65
Acromegaly, 207
Actigraphy, 80, 143
Active self-management, 88
Acupuncture, 187, 193
Acute insomnia, 244
Adolescent insomnia, 144
Agrypnia excitata (AE)
    delirium tremens, 260, 261
    FFI, 257–258, 260
    Morvan syndrome, 259, 261
Alcohol-use disorders (AUDs),
        275–276
American Academy of Sleep Medicine
        (AASM), 6, 144, 153
American Gastroenterological
        Association, 204
American Psychiatric Association (APA), 5
American Psychological Association, 153
Antihistamines, 209
Anxiety disorders
    GAD, 271
    panic disorder, 271–272
    PTSD, 272–273
Attention-deficit hyperactivity disorder
        (ADHD), 273–274

B

Behavioral insomnias of childhood (BIC)
    ICSD, 136, 137
    limit-setting type, 136
    mixed type, 136
    pathophysiology

bedtime routines, 137
environmental and circadian factors,
        142–144
feeding behavior, 139
origins, 138
parental guilt, 140
parental reinforcement, 138–139
psychopathology and temperament,
        140–142
sentinel event, 140
sleep disorders, 144
sleep-onset association type, 136
treatment
    behavioral interventions,
        152–153
    extinction techniques, 149–151
    feeding schedules, 149
    positive routines, 151
    schedule modification, 151–152
    sleep hygiene training, 152
Behavioral sleep medicine, 79
Benign prostatic hyperplasia (BPH), 206
Benzodiazepine receptor agonists (BzRAs)
    discontinuation effects, 109
    efficacy of, 105–106
    mechanism of action, 103–104
    pharmacokinetics, 104–105
    residual effects
        amnestic effect, 107
        complex behaviors during sleep, 108
        driving performance, 106–107
        fall risk, 107
        mortality risk, 108–109
        sedation, 106
    tolerance, dependence, abuse potential, 109

© Springer International Publishing Switzerland 2017
H.P. Attarian (ed.), *Clinical Handbook of Insomnia*, Current Clinical Neurology,
DOI 10.1007/978-3-319-41400-3

Benzodiazepines, 203
Bipolar disorder, 269–270
Braxton-Hicks contractions, 163

C
Caffeine, 277
Cambridge-Hopkins Restless Legs
        Syndrome, 164
Cardiovascular disease (CVD), 60, 63–65,
        200–202
Central sleep apnea (CSA), 201
Cheyne-Stokes respirations, 201
Child Behavior Checklist (CBCL), 148
Child Depression Inventory (CDI), 148
Childhood sleep problems
    assessment
        CBCL, 148
        CDI, 148
        CRS-R, 148
        daytime impairment, 146
        parent–child interactions, 146
        SCARED, 148
        sleep logs/diaries, 146, 147
        sleep questionnaires, 146, 147
        wrist actigraphy, 147
    BIC (*see* Behavioral insomnias of
        childhood (BIC))
Children's Sleep Habits Questionnaire
        (CSHQ), 147
Chronic insomnia disorders (CID)
    clinical assessment
        history, 32
        patient-compliant therapy, 35
        polysomnography, 35
        sleep applications, 34
        sleep complaints, 33
        sleep logs, 34
        symptoms, 32
        testing environment, 35
        tools, 33
    clinical features, 28–30
    diabetes, 62
    differential diagnosis, 35–36
    ICSD, 144, 145
    neurological diseases, 244
    prognosis, 59
    subtypes
        drug/substance, 31
        idiopathic insomnia, 31
        inadequate sleep hygiene, 31
        medical disorder, 31
        mental disorder, 31

        paradoxical insomnia, 31
        psychophysiological insomnia, 30
Chronic kidney disease (CKD), 203–204
Chronic obstructive pulmonary disease
        (COPD), 202–203
Circadian rhythm disorders, 36
Citalopram, 187
Clonazepam, 112
Cognitive behavioral therapy (CBT)
    abbreviated versions, 91
    complicating factors
        mental and medical disorders
            comorbidity, 89
        poor treatment compliance, 88–89
        sedative hypnotics, 89–90
    efficacy, 90–91
    first-line interventions
        cognitive restructuring approach, 85–86
        phototherapy, 87
        relaxation training, 86–87
        SCT, 81
        sleep hygiene education, 83–84
        SRT, 81–82
    postmenopause, 187, 191
    relaxation training, 80
    technology-based interventions, 91–92
    therapeutic regimen, 80–81
Cognitive behavioral therapy for insomnia
        (CBT-I)
    breast cancer, 210
    MDD, 268
    postmenopause, 191
    school-age children, 153–154
"Cognitive Behavioral Therapy for Insomnia:
        A Session by Session Guide", 80
Connors Rating Scale-Revised (CRS-R), 148
Continuous positive airway pressure (CPAP),
        171, 172
Corticobasal degeneration (CBD),
        248, 250
Co-sleeping, 142
Cushing's syndrome, 207

D
Danger zone, 151
Delirium tremens (DT), 249, 260, 261
Dexlansoprazole, 205
Diagnostic and Statistical Manual on
        Mental Disorders-5th edition
        (DSM-V), 5, 183
Doxepin, 111
Dual-orexin receptor antagonist (DORA), 110

E
Edmonton Symptom Assessment Scale (ESAS), 230
Epidemiology
    adolescent groups, 15
    age, 17
    categories, 15
    country, 14–16
    economic impact, 22
    ethnocultural variables, 18
    factors, 18–19
    gender, 16, 17
    hypnotic use, 21
    morbidity and mortality, 20–21
    pediatric populatio, 15
    psychiatric disorders, 19–20
    shift work, 18
Episodic nocturnal wandering (ENW), 255
Epworth Sleepiness Scale (ESS), 186
Escitalopram, 187, 189
Esomeprazole, 205
Eszopiclone, 106, 187, 189
Excessive fragmentary hypnic myoclonus (EFHM), 249, 257

F
Facio-mandibular myoclonus, 249, 257
Fatal familial insomnia (FFI), 249, 257–258, 260
Fetal movements, 163
Folate deficiency, 165
Follicle-stimulating hormone (FSH), 182
Food and Drug Administration (FDA), 168
Free-running circadian disorder, 208

G
Gabapentin, 115, 187, 190
Gastric acid secretion, 205
Gastroesophageal reflux, 163
Gastrointestinal disorders, 204–205
General anxiety disorder (GAD), 35
Generalized anxiety disorder (GAD), 271
Good sleepers (GS), 66
Graduated extinction (GE) techniques, 150–151

H
Heartburn, 163
High-frequency power (HFP) ratios, 43
Hmg-CoA reductase inhibitors, 201

Homeostatic model assessment (HOMA), 63
Huntington's disease (HD), 248, 250
Hypercapnic states, 202
Hypertension (HTN), 63
Hyperthyroidism, 206

I
Idiopathic insomnia, 31
Inadequate sleep hygiene, 31
Insomnia
    AASM, 6
    agrypnia excitata (see Agrypnia excitata (AE))
    APA-DSM-V, 5
    behavioral perspective, 76–77
    behavioral sleep medicine assessment, 79
    burden of illness, 60, 65–67
    CBT-I, school-age children, 153–154
    cognitive perspective, 77–78
    comorbidity, 9
    CVD, 60, 63–65
    daytime complaints, 9
    definitions, 4–5, 8
    duration of illness, 7
    historical perspectives, 4
    medical conditions
        cancer, 209–210
        cardiovascular disease, 200–202
        CKD, 203–204
        COPD, 202–203
        endocrine disorders, 206–207
        genitourinary conditions, 206
        GERD, 204–205
        ocular disorder, 208
    menopause (see Menopause)
    metabolic disorders, 60, 62–63
    neurocognitive function, 60–62
    neurocognitive perspective, 78
    neurological diseases
        CBD, 248, 250
        dementia, 245–246
        Huntington's disease, 248, 250
        Lewy body disease, 247, 248
        MSA, 247, 248
        Parkinson's disease, 247, 248
        progressive dystonia, 248, 250
        PSP, 248
        SCA, 248, 250
        Tourette's syndrome, 248, 250
    pathophysiology
        brain metabolism, 43
        daytime fatigue/dysphoria, 44

Insomnia (*cont.*)
  depression, 51
  development of, 48–50
  EEG criteria, 42
  elevated blood pressure/hypertension,
    50–51
  glycemic control/diabetes, 51
  immune function, 52
  LFP and HFP, 43
  MMPI, 45
  mortality, 52
  MSLT, 43–45
  NREM sleep, 43
  POMS, 44
  poor sleep (*see* Poor sleep)
  positron emission tomography, 43
  whole-body metabolic rate, 43
  in pregnancy (*see* Pregnancy)
  PSG assessment, 79–80
  psychiatric disorders (*see* Psychiatric
    disorders)
  secondary, 9
  severity of illness, 8
  sleep-related movement (*see* Sleep-related
    movement disorders)
  subjective complaint, 9
  WHO-ICD, 6
"Insomnia: Psychological Assessment and
    Management", 80
Insomnia Severity Index (ISI), 91, 186, 210
Insomnia symptoms (SYMPT), 66
Insomnia syndrome (SYND), 66
International Agency for Research
    on Cancer, 228
International Classification of Diseases
    (ICD-10), 5
International Classification of Sleep Disorders
    (ICSD), 136, 137
International Classification of Sleep Disorders-
    3rd edition (ICSD-3), 6, 7
International Menopause Society and the
    World Health Organization, 182
International Restless Legs Syndrome
    Study Group (IRLSSG),
    164, 168
Isoflavones, 187, 190

K
Kampo, 187, 191

L
Lewy body disease (LBD), 247, 248
Low-frequency power (LFP), 43

Lung cancer, 223
Luteinizing hormone (LH), 182

M
Major depressive disorder (MDD), 268–269
Marijuana, 276
Master circadian pacemaker, 208
Melatonin, 203
Melatonin receptor agonists, 110
Menopause
  climacteric
    clinical evaluation, 184–186
    definition, 182
    hypoestrogenism, 184
    prevalence, 184
    sleep impairment, 184
  definition, 182
  menopausal transition, 182–183
  postmenopause (*see* Postmenopause)
Metabolic disorders, 60, 62–63
Metastatic cancer, 226
Mirtazapine, 113–114, 187, 190
Morvan syndrome (MS), 249, 259, 261
Mother-infant sleep problems, 141
Multiple sleep latency tests (MSLT), 43–45
Multiple system atrophy (MSA), 247–249

N
National Comprehensive Cancer Network
    (NCCN), 230
Nicotine, 276
NIH State-of-the-Science Conference, 4
Nocturia, 162
Nocturnal angina, 200
Nocturnal frontal lobe epilepsy (NFLE), 249,
    254–256
Nocturnal paroxysmal dystonia (NPD), 254
Non-benzodiazepine receptor, 203
Nord-Trondelag Health Studies, 201

O
Obsessive-compulsive disorder (OCD), 273
Obstructive sleep apnea (OSA). *See* Sleep-
    disordered breathing (SDB)
Opiate, 276
Oral corticosteroids, 209
Overlap syndrome, 203

P
Pan-Canadian practice guidelines, 230
Panic disorder, 271–272

Paradoxical insomnia, 31
Parasomnias, 144
Parental guilt, 140
Parental reinforcement, 138–139
Parkinson's disease (PD), 248
Paroxysmal arousals (PA), 254
Paroxysmal nocturnal dyspnea (PND), 201
PDQ® Sleep Disorders, 230
Pediatric Sleep Questionnaire (PSQ), 147
Perimenopausal symptoms, 17
Periodic limb movement disorder (PLMD), 36
Periodic limb movements in sleep (PLMS), 253
Pharmacological treatment of insomnia
    alpha$_1$-adrenergic antagonists, 116
    anticonvulsant drugs, 115
    antidepressants
        mirtazapine, 113–114
        trazodone, 113
        tricyclic antidepressants, 114
    antipsychotic drug, 114
    BzRAs (see Benzodiazepine receptor
        agonists (BzRAs))
    comorbid conditions, 120–121
    contraindication, 117–118
    histamine (H1) antagonists
        diphenhydramine/doxylamine, 112
        doxepin, 111
    indications, 117
    medications, 98–100
    melatonin, 116
    melatonin receptor agonists
    orexin antagonists, 110–111
    sleep maintenance, 119
    sleep onset only, 119
    sleep-wake behavior, 98–103
    starting treatment, 118
    stopping treatment, 118
Phototherapy, 87
Phyto-female complex, 191
Pittsburgh Sleep Quality Index (PSQI), 186, 191
Poly-pharmacy, 200
Polysomnographic (PSG) assessment, 79–80
Poor sleep
    effect of, 46–47
    insomnia patients, 47–48
Postmenopause
    acupuncture, 187, 193
    antidepressants
        citalopram, 187
        citalopram and fluoxetine, 189
        desvenlafaxine, 189
        escitalopram, 187, 189
        gabapentin, 187, 190
        mirtazapine, 187, 190
        paroxetine, 189

quetiapine, 187, 189
        venlafaxine, 189
    CBT, 187, 191
    clinical manifestations, 183
    definition, 182
    early, 182
    herbal and nutritional supplements
        isoflavones, 187, 190
        Kampo, 187, 191
        phyto-female complex, 191
        pycnogenol, 187, 191
        valerian root, 190
    high-intensity exercise, 187, 192
    hormone therapy, 187, 188
    hypnosis, 187, 192
    late, 182
    massage therapy, 187, 192
    pathophysiology, 182–183
    sedatives/hypnotics
        eszopiclone, 187, 189
        ramelteon, 187, 189
        zolpidem, 187, 188
    yoga, 187, 192
Postpartum depression, 141
Posttraumatic stress disorder (PTSD), 272–273
Pramipexole, 168
Prazosin, 116
Pregnancy
    hormonal changes, sleep, 160–161
    implications, 173
    nocturnal arousals change, 162–164
    RLS (see Restless legs syndrome (RLS))
    SDB (see Sleep-disordered breathing
        (SDB))
    sleep disruption, 160
    sleep duration, 161–162
    sleep patterns, 161
    treatment, 173–174
Prevalence of. See Epidemiology
Primary care-friendly, CBT, 91
Profile of Mood States (POMS), 44
Progressive dystonia, 248
Progressive supranuclear palsy (PSP), 248, 250
Prolactin, 166
Propriospinal myoclonus (PSM), 249, 253–254
Psychiatric disorders
    ADHD, 273–274
    alcohol and substance abuse, 61
    anxiety (see Anxiety disorders)
    bipolar disorder, 269–270
    depression, 60
    eszopiclone/fluoxetine cotherapy, 61
    MDD, 268–269
    OCD, 273
    persistent symptoms, 61

Psychiatric disorders (*cont.*)
   risk factor, 60
   schizophrenia, 274
   substance-use disorders
      AUDs, 275–276
      caffeine, 277
      marijuana, 276
      nicotine, 276
      opiate, 276
      sleep disturbance, 275
      stimulants, 277
Psychophysiological insomnia, 30
Pycnogenol, 187, 191

Q
Quetiapine, 187

R
Ramelteon, 110, 187, 189
Relaxation training, 80, 86–87
REM sleep behavior disorder (RBD), 249,
      256–257
Restless legs syndrome (RLS)
   pregnancy
      alcohol, 167
      carbidopa/levodopa, 168
      cesarean delivery, 166
      coffee consumption, 165
      estradiol levels, 165
      estrogen levels, 165
      ferritin level, 166
      folate deficiency, 165
      folate supplementation, 167
      impact of, 166
      iron deficiency, 165
      medications, 167
      non-pharmacologic therapy, 167
      non-pharmacologic treatment, 167
      obstructive sleep apnea, 167
      opioids, 168
      oral iron supplementation, 166
      pharmacologic agents, 167
      pharmacologic treatment, 168
      pramipexole, 168
      preeclampsia risk, 166
      prevalence, 164
      prolactin, 166
      ropinirole, 168
      rotigotine, 168
      sleep duration, 165
      tobacco use, 165, 167

PLMD, 36
   sleep disorders, 144
   sleep-related movement disorders, 248,
      251–252
Ropinirole, 168
Rotigotine, 168

S
Schizophrenia, 274
Screen for Child Anxiety-Related Emotional
      Disorders (SCARED), 148
Secondary insomnia, 9, 205
Short-term insomnia, 144, 145
Simple/unmodified extinction, 149
Sleep-disordered breathing (SDB)
   conservative treatment measures, 172
   CPAP, 171, 172
   diagnosis, 171
   gestational diabetes, 170
   impaired fetal growth, 170
   maternal and fetal health outcomes, 170
   maternal health risks, 171
   mild sleep apnea, 170
   nocturnal awakenings, 169
   obesity, 171
   physiologic changes, 168
   preeclampsia, 170
   pregnancy
   frequency and severity, 169
   pregnancy-induced hypertension, 170, 171
   preterm birth, 171
   prevalence, 169
   sleep fragmentation, 169
Sleep disturbance
   advanced stage, 226
   chemotherapy, 222, 224
   circadian rhythms, 228
   contributing factors, 233–236
   health-related quality of life, 223
   negative consequences, 223
   post treatment and long-term
      survivorship, 225
   pretreatment, 223
   prevalence and impact, 223
   radiation therapy, 224
   risk factors, 226–228
   screening and assessing sleep, 230–233
   symptom cluster, 222, 228–230
Sleep Habits Questionnaire, 147
Sleep hygiene education, 83–84
Sleep hygiene training, 152
Sleep logs, 146

Sleep-related movement disorders
   delirium tremens, 249
   EFHM, 257
   excessive fragmentary hypnic
       myoclonus, 249
   facio-mandibular myoclonus, 249, 257
   FFI, 249
   Morvan syndrome, 249
   NFLE, 254–256
   nocturnal frontal lobe epilepsy, 249
   PLMS, 253
   propriospinal myoclonus, 249
   PSM, 253–254
   RBD, 256–257
   REM, 249
   RLS, 248, 251–252
Sleep restriction therapy (SRT), 81–82
Sleep-state misperception, 31
Snoring, 169
Spielman model, 78
Speilman's three-factor model, 226
Spinocerebellar ataxia (SCA), 248, 250–251
Stimulus control therapy (SCT), 81
STOP Questionnaire, 234
Sundowning, 245
Suprachiasmatic nuclei (SCN), 208
Suvorexant, 110
Symptom cluster, 228–230
Systolic blood pressure (SBP), 64

T
Theophylline, 202
Tiotropium, 202
Total wake time (TWT), 64
Tourette's syndrome (TS), 248, 250
Trazodone, 113
Tricyclic antidepressants (TCAs),
     114, 202

V
Valerian root, 190
Veterans Health Administration
     system (VA), 90

W
Wake after sleep onset (WASO), 64, 161
Wake-to-sleep transition, 141
Work productivity and activity impairment
     (WPAI), 65
Work-related accidents, 66
World Health Organization (WHO), 5
Wrist actigraphy, 147

Z
Zolpidem, 105, 187, 188
Zopiclone, 108